OPHTHALMOLOGY MONOGRAPHS

Surgery of the Eyelid, Orbit, and Lacrimal System

VOLUME 3

American Academy of Ophthalmology

655 Beach Street

P.O. Box 7424

San Francisco, CA 94120-7424

This continuing medical education activity was planned and produced in accordance with the Essentials of the Accreditation Council for Continuing Medical Education.

Surgery of the Eyelid, Orbit, and Lacrimal System

VOLUME 3

Edited by

William B. Stewart, MD

California Pacific Medical Center

AMERICAN ACADEMY OF OPHTHALMOLOGY

LEO

LIFELONG
EDUCATION FOR THE
OPHTHALMOLOGIST

LEO

LIFELONG
EDUCATION FOR THE
OPHTHALMOLOGIST

Ophthalmology Monograph 8, *Surgery of the Eyelid, Orbit, and Lacrimal System*, is one component of the Lifelong Education for the Ophthalmologist (LEO) framework, which assists members in planning their continuing medical education. LEO includes an array of clinical education products and programs that members may select to form individualized, self-directed learning plans for updating their clinical knowledge. Active members or fellows who use LEO components may accumulate sufficient CME credits to earn the LEO Award. Contact the Academy's Clinical Education Division for further information on LEO.

Library of Congress Cataloging-in-Publication Data
(Revised for vol. 3)

Surgery of the eyelid, orbit, and lacrimal system.

    (Ophthalmology monographs ; 8)
    Includes bibliographical references and index.
    1. Eyelids—Surgery.   2. Eye-sockets—Surgery.
3. Lacrimal apparatus—Surgery. I. Stewart,
William B. (William Bennett), 1943–   . II. Series.
[DNLM: 1. Eye Diseases—surgery. 2. Orbit—surgery.
3. Eyelids—surgery. 4. Lacrimal Apparatus—surgery.
5. Surgery, Plastic. W1 OP372L v.8 1993
WW 205 S961 1993]
RE121.S87 1993   617.7′1   93-19768
ISBN 1-56055-069-4 (v. 1)
ISBN 1-56055-070-8 (v. 2)
ISBN 1-56055-071-6 (v. 3)

99 98 97 96 95 5 4 3 2 1

Contributors

Richard L. Anderson, MD
Salt Lake City, Utah

Jurij R. Bilyk, MD
Huntington Valley, Pennsylvania

Roger A. Dailey, MD
Portland, Oregon

William A. Danz, BCO
San Francisco, California

Richard K. Dortzbach, MD
Madison, Wisconsin

Jonathan J. Dutton, MD, PhD
Durham, North Carolina

Steven Fagien, MD
Boca Raton, Florida

Patrick M. Flaharty, MD
Fort Myers, Florida

Robert Alan Goldberg, MD
Los Angeles, California

Don O. Kikkawa, MD
La Jolla, California

Peter S. Levin, MD
Mountain View, California

Mark R. Levine, MD
Beachwood, Ohio

John V. Linberg, MD
Morgantown, West Virginia

John G. McHenry, MD, MPH
Detroit, Michigan

Loan K. Nguyen, MD
Fresno, California

Bhupendra C. Patel, MD
Salt Lake City, Utah

James R. Patrinely, MD
Houston, Texas

Janet L. Roen, MD
New York, New York

John W. Shore, MD
Boston, Massachusetts

David B. Soll, MD
Philadelphia, Pennsylvania

Stephen M. Soll, MD
Philadelphia, Pennsylvania

Thomas C. Spoor, MD, MS
Detroit, Michigan

Samuel Stal, MD
Houston, Texas

Orkan George Stasior, MD
Albany, New York

Mary A. Stefanyszyn, MD
Wynnewood, Pennsylvania

Randal S. Weber, MD
Houston, Texas

John L. Wobig, MD
Portland, Oregon

John E. Wright, FRCS
London, England

Steven R. Young, BCO
Oakland, California

Contents

Chapter 29   PERIORBITAL AND CRANIOFACIAL SURGERY **60**

James R. Patrinely, MD
Samuel Stal, MD
Randal S. Weber, MD

PART VIII   THE ANOPHTHALMIC SOCKET **83**

Chapter 30   ENUCLEATION AND EVISCERATION **84**

Mark R. Levine, MD
Steven Fagien, MD

Chapter 33 **OVERVIEW OF OCULAR PROSTHETICS** **133**

Steven R. Young, BCO

Chapter 36 **BLOWOUT FRACTURES OF THE ORBITAL FLOOR** **204**

Richard K. Dortzbach, MD
Don O. Kikkawa, MD

Chapter 37 **LATE REPAIR OF POSTTRAUMATIC DEFORMITIES** **224**

Jurij R. Bilyk, MD
John W. Shore, MD

PART X   THE LACRIMAL SYSTEM   **253**

Chapter 38   EVALUATION OF THE LACRIMAL SYSTEM   **254**

Loan K. Nguyen, MD
John V. Linberg, MD

Chapter 39   **SURGERY OF THE LACRIMAL SYSTEM**   **270**

John L. Wobig, MD
Roger A. Dailey, MD

Foreword

I consider it an honor to have been asked to share my thoughts as a foreword to this teaching text for the specialty of ophthalmic plastic and reconstructive surgery.

My counsel can be summed up in one word: read. Read this book carefully; it has been written by experienced surgeons who wish to pass on their skills to you. Read the literature; many of the same problems faced today have been dealt with in the past, and the techniques forgotten. Or these same techniques can be used to better correct other problems. The greater your base knowledge, the more likely you are to improve your results and to evaluate new techniques.

I have never viewed other ophthalmic plastic surgeons as competitors, rather as colleagues. The most important learning experiences for me at meetings are not the lectures, but the conversations with other ophthalmic surgeons, who have unselfishly helped me solve difficult problems. If you can observe other surgeons operate, I would encourage you to do so.

Probably the most important pearl I learned in my practice was to listen carefully to my patients. Concentrating on what they say is the only way you can truly understand what is bothering them and why they are seeking your expertise. If you listen carefully, you can often identify those patients you have no hope of pleasing.

Develop a routine for questioning and examining patients. If you do so, you will not forget to ask an important question or omit a crucial part of the examination. When examining the patient, first get a general overall view of the person, then study the face, especially noting any facial asymmetry. Feel the skin and muscle tone of the face, as well as the underlying bony structure. This detailed examination should be done even if the patient is presenting with a small lid lesion. Many lesions tend to be multiple, so assume this to be the case until you have proved otherwise. Be certain to record your findings, because you never know who will be reading the chart next. We have all been guilty of this omission at some time in a busy practice.

Even though a patient is pleased with the result of your efforts, be critical (of yourself) and think about how you can improve the results on the next patient who presents with the same or a similar problem. Do not be satisfied with only acceptable results; be your own severest critic.

If two different techniques give the same result, use the one that is easier and faster. But if a more difficult and longer operation yields a superior result, use it. Some exceptions to this advice exist, particularly if the patient's age and medical condition are considered.

Patients should be fully informed of at least the most serious complications. Do not be afraid of scaring patients away. If learning what might happen is enough to deter patients from having a cosmetic operation, they are not good candidates for the procedure. Be honest with your patients and yourself; both will benefit.

Ophthalmic plastic surgery is a stimulating specialty, with new techniques and materials being developed all the time. If you sincerely try to do your best—the only guarantee I ever give a patient—you will never be bored and your patients will be the beneficiaries of your best effort and engagement.

Richard R. Tenzel, MD

Preface

As the preface to this monograph on ophthalmic plastic and reconstructive surgery is written, contemporary medicine is in a period of significant transformation. Issues of vital importance are being debated—issues related to the practice, organization, application, accessibility, financing, and ethics of our profession and its expansive frame of reference. The power and universality of the health and healing arena touch all individuals, institutions, and their local as well as extended communities. The need for a more accessible and affordable health care system challenges not only our individual knowledge and skills but also our sense of service, compassion, and responsibility. Our work needs to nourish our communities and ourselves. More than ever, our knowledge base needs to be comprehensive and our surgical expertise up to date and appropriately applied.

The knowledge and skills necessary to practice our specialty continue to expand, increasing the challenge to keep current. Attempting to serve that need is the objective of this monograph, which is not intended to be just a surgical atlas, but a resource for diagnosis and management as well. The manual from which this monograph derives, *Ophthalmic Plastic and Reconstructive Surgery*, was published in 1984. In one sense, that was a short time ago; in medical terms, however, it was an eon because so much in the specialty has changed over the past decade. The magnitude of these changes is reflected in the expansion of the original work from one book to three volumes. Although some material from the manual could be retained, it had to be updated, edited, reorganized, and reworked. Many chapters were rewritten, and an all-new art program was created to complement the updated text.

The breadth and detail of the field require a large number of experts to create a timely and valuable publication. The strength and timeliness of the work are due to the efforts of the many individuals who participated in this ongoing educational venture. I am extremely grateful for the generous gift that each of the contributors to this monograph has made to all who read this book and to those they care for. I hope this spirit continues to pervade our specialty and that this book will serve as a model of what can be accomplished when our work is done with generosity and caring as well as skill and intellect.

William B. Stewart, MD

Editor's Note to Volume 3

The Academy's Ophthalmology Monograph 8, *Surgery of the Eyelid, Orbit, and Lacrimal System*, comprises three volumes:

VOLUME 1 (1993) addresses general concepts, principles, and techniques.

VOLUME 2 (1994) engages the challenging field of eyelid surgery.

VOLUME 3 (1995) covers orbital and lacrimal system surgery.

This book, Volume 3, exemplifies the expansion in both knowledge base and applicable procedures of the field of ophthalmic plastic and reconstructive surgery. The realm of orbital and lacrimal system surgery, in particular, has been altered in major ways by technologic advances. Incorporating revised material from previous editions of the manual *Ophthalmic Plastic and Reconstructive Surgery* as well as new material, this volume is a blend of refinement of classic understanding, approaches, and procedures with emerging and controversial topics.

The practice of medicine and surgery evolves as new information and techniques become available and as data and procedures that fail the test of time are discarded. This growth cycle keeps the profession vibrant and fertile. Always, our scientific system and data base need to be combined with the art and intuition that together create the truly wise and skilled ophthalmic surgeon.

The preparation of this three-volume monograph demanded a great generosity from a great number of contributing authors—71 in all. Their task required a constant balancing act between accessible brevity and appropriate inclusiveness. The editor and the Academy are extremely grateful to the contributors and hope that the collaborative result is of meaningful service to the readers and their patients.

William B. Stewart, MD

PART VII

Orbital Surgery

CHAPTER 25

Evaluation and Spectrum of Orbital Diseases[*]

Robert Alan Goldberg, MD

Orbital disorders are rare: the comprehensive ophthalmologist only occasionally has the opportunity to diagnose (or, if not alert, to overlook) a patient with orbital disease. This rarity breeds some unfamiliarity that may lead to discomfort or lack of confidence. This chapter endeavors to bolster confidence by providing a thoughtful, stepwise, and logical approach to the evaluation of orbital disease. The discussion begins with differential diagnosis, adds an intelligent history-taking and physical examination, and then focuses on efficient use of diagnostic tests to finally arrive at the correct diagnosis. The staging and management of two common orbital disorders, orbital inflammation and thyroid-related orbitopathy, will be discussed.

25-1

DIFFERENTIAL DIAGNOSIS

The differential diagnosis of orbital disease is extensive, and most listings of orbital disease divide the causes between histopathologic and mechanistic categories.[1-3] This type of grouping is intellectually sound and scientifically useful, but does not provide a framework that the clinical practitioner can easily grasp and directly use in sorting through the differential diagnosis of any given patient. In broad terms, orbital disease can be considered in terms of location, extent, and biologic activity.[4] The classification used in this chapter is broken down along clinical lines, and takes advantage of the fact that the orbit has a somewhat limited repertoire of ways that it can respond to pathologic conditions.

Orbital disease can be categorized into five basic clinical patterns: inflammatory, mass effect, structural, vascular, and functional. Although many cases cross over

[*]David A. Weinberg, MD, provided valuable assistance in the preparation of this chapter.

into several categories, the vast majority of clinical presentations fit predominantly into one of these patterns. As the clinician walks through each step of the evaluation process—history, physical examination, laboratory testing, orbital imaging—a conscious effort should be made to categorize the presentation within this framework.

If the practitioner approaches orbital disease with this framework of discrete patterns of clinical presentation, then at every step of the diagnostic pathway (history, physical examination, orbital imaging studies, and special tests), the clinician can draw from a defined set of differential diagnoses that characterize each pattern of orbital disease and use that information to efficiently and confidently orchestrate diagnosis and management. Often, as the practitioner moves along this diagnostic pathway, a difficult decision encountered is whether or not to perform an orbital biopsy. This framework can help guide the clinician in distinguishing those cases requiring tissue for histopathologic evaluation from those cases that can be safely managed, at least initially, without the security of a tissue diagnosis.

25-1-1 Inflammatory Clinical Pattern

A large percentage of orbital diseases have orbital inflammation as their primary pattern of clinical presentation (Table 25-1). These cases can be further broken down into acute inflammation (onset over hours to days), subacute inflammation (onset over days to weeks), and chronic inflammation (onset over weeks to months). The classical signs of inflammation are present: pain, redness, edema and chemosis, heat, and eventually dysfunction.

TABLE 25-1

Inflammatory Pattern of Presentation

Acute (Days)

Infection: preseptal cellulitis, orbital cellulitis, abscess

Acute idiopathic inflammation: scleritis, myositis, diffuse anterior, apical

Fulminant thyroid-related orbitopathy

Fulminant neoplasia

Hemorrhage into existing lesion: lymphangioma, hematic cyst, bone cyst

Subacute (Days to Weeks)

Infection: fungal, opportunistic

Specific: thyroid-related orbitopathy, Wegener's syndrome, sarcoidosis, vasculitis, etc

Nonspecific idiopathic ("pseudotumor")
    Diffuse
    Localized: scleritis, myositis, dacryoadenitis, perioptic neuritis

Chronic (Weeks to Months)

Idiopathic sclerosing inflammation of orbit

Specific: thyroid-related orbitopathy, Wegener's syndrome, sarcoidosis, vasculitis, etc

Masquerade: neoplasm (primary or metastatic)

Retained foreign body

TABLE 25-2

Mass Effect Pattern of Presentation

Soft Tissue

Localized

Cavernous hemangioma
Peripheral nerve tumor (schwannoma, meningioma)
Lymphoma
Lacrimal gland neoplasms
Optic nerve meningioma
Optic nerve glioma
Other soft-tissue neoplasms
Idiopathic sclerosing inflammation of orbit
    ("pseudotumor")
Metastatic neoplasm
Secondary tumor from paranasal sinuses
In infants and children: rhabdomyosarcoma,
    metastatic neuroblastoma, capillary
    hemangioma, lymphangioma

Cystic

Dermoid cyst
Epithelial and lacrimal duct cyst
Mucocele
Lacrimal sac mucocele (dacryocele)
Parasitic cyst (echinococcal, cysticercosis)
Hematocele
Lymphangioma or other hemorrhagic tumor

Bone

Sphenoid wing meningioma
Metastatic neoplasm
Osteoma, osteosarcoma, ossifying fibroma
Xanthomatous bone lesion
Plasmacytoma, myeloma, and other marrow
    neoplasms
Histiocytosis-X, eosinophilic granuloma
Fibrous dysplasia and other idiopathic ossifying
    syndromes

25-1-2 Mass Effect Clinical Pattern

Tumors presenting primarily with mass effect are characterized by displacement of the globe (axial or nonaxial proptosis) and in some cases a palpable eyelid mass (Table 25-2).

25-1-3 Structural Clinical Pattern

Orbital diseases that present a structural orbital pattern are characterized by enophthalmos, bony asymmetry produced by major structural shifts in the bony orbital framework, or pulsatile proptosis when the bony barrier between the orbit and the intracranial cavity is missing (Table 25-3). The presence of a structural lesion can often be strongly suspected on these clinical grounds, but orbital imaging studies confirm the diagnosis and characterize the precise anatomic nature of the structural defect.

25-1-4 Vascular Clinical Pattern

The grouping of vascular orbital lesions is somewhat problematic, in that vascular lesions span the spectrum from true active vascular lesions, such as arteriovenous malformation and orbital varix, to neoplasms of cells of vascular origin, such as hemangiopericytomas. Even though their biologic origin is from vascular tissue, vascular neoplasms behave clinically like soft-tissue tumors, do not have the characteristics of active vascular lesions, and, for the purposes of this clinically based classification, are not included in the vascular pattern of presentation. The true active vascular lesions in the orbit are characterized by a clinical pattern of dynamic change, either slow dynamic change related to pos-

tural changes in venous pressure in the case of varices and related lesions connected to the venous system, or pulsation, thrill, bruit, and generalized vascular congestion seen in arterial lesions such as arteriovenous malformation or cavernous sinus fistulas (Table 25-4).

25-1-5 Functional Clinical Pattern

The functional pattern of presentation is characterized by functional deficit out of proportion to mass or inflammation (Table 25-5). Though primarily optic nerve dysfunction, occasionally involvement of other neurovascular structures at the orbital apex, with ophthalmoplegia or sensory deficit, is seen. The clinical presentation is characterized by decreased vision with an afferent pupillary defect, or ophthalmoplegia.

25-2

HISTORY-TAKING

In both the history-taking and the physical examination, the clinician (armed with the differential diagnosis discussed above) needs to "think biologically." What is the pattern of disease in the framework above, and is there evidence for destruction of tissue? Destructive biology, which characterizes neoplasia and sometimes severe inflammation, manifests clinically as loss of function: sensorimotor deficits such as optic neuropathy, limitation of movement, or decreased sensation.

Historical information that should be obtained includes the time course of onset; old photographs can be very useful to verify the presence or absence of orbital

---

TABLE 25-3

Structural Pattern of Presentation

Acquired Structural Alterations

Trauma (including postoperative)
Destructive lesions of bone (dermoid cyst, bone cyst, neoplasm)

Congenital Structural Alterations

Encephalocele, meningocele
Sphenoid wing hypoplasia (neurofibromatosis 1)

TABLE 25-4

Vascular Pattern of Presentation

Dynamic* Lesions

Orbital arteriovenous malformation
Cavernous sinus fistula
Dural arteriovenous malformation (fistula)
Varix

**That is, pulsating or responding to changing venous pressure.*

TABLE 25-5

Functional Pattern of Presentation

Optic Nerve Tumors

Glioma
Meningioma

Orbital Apical Neoplasms

Lymphoma
Idiopathic sclerosing inflammation of orbit
Tolosa-Hunt syndrome

Compression

Fibrous dysplasia or other bony overgrowths
Sphenoid wing meningioma
Indirect optic nerve trauma

changes. Historical evidence of infiltration or compression (pain, decreased vision, double vision, numbness) should be carefully sought. Systemic disease affects the orbit, and symptoms of thyroid dysfunction, systemic vasculitis, inflammation, or neoplasia may help refine the differential diagnosis as well as detect generalized disease requiring therapy. Previous trauma or surgery, including nasal, sinus, intracranial, or facial, must not be overlooked.

25-3

PHYSICAL EXAMINATION

A careful examination of the globe and ocular adnexa may offer important clues to the underlying diagnosis. A complete, dilated eye examination should be performed in conjunction with a comprehensive orbital examination, which includes assessment for proptosis, resistance to retropulsion of the globe, palpable orbital masses, associated eyelid abnormalities, ocular pulsations, and orbital bruits. Proptosis is quantified by exophthalmometry. A difference of greater than 2 mm between the two eyes on exophthalmometry is likely pathologic. It should be noted whether the proptosis is axial (indicative of a mass behind the globe, usually intraconal) or if the globe is displaced horizontally or vertically (with the direction of proptosis generally opposite the location of the orbital mass lesion). Location of orbital lesions is often helpful in guiding the differential diagnosis. For example, mucoceles are usually superonasal, while lacrimal gland lesions tend to be centered superotemporally.

General physical examination may include inspection of skin, oropharynx, and nasopharynx; palpation of the lymph nodes; auscultation of the lungs; and neurologic testing when indicated. A more thorough systemic examination could reveal evidence of an occult malignancy (breast or prostate mass) or a systemic inflammatory disorder (rheumatoid arthritis, Wegener's granulomatosis, sarcoidosis).

Evaluation of afferent (visual physiology and sensation) and efferent (extraocular motility) function of the eye is an essential part of the examination. This will assist in localization of the lesion, assessment of disease progression on serial examinations, and decision-making regarding the need for prompt intervention, such as surgery or systemic corticosteroids. Eye examination must include testing of visual acuity, pupillary function and assessment for a relative afferent pupillary defect (Marcus Gunn pupil), confrontation visual fields (with formal perimetry when indicated), extraocular motility, and ocular alignment (alternate cover test), in addition to slit-lamp examination, tonometry, and dilated fundus examination. Refraction is important, to confirm that decreased vision is truly refractive in nature. If the vision is not correctable to 20/20, then an explanation must be found (corneal epitheliopathy, cataract, maculopathy, choroidal striae, or optic neuropathy). Dyschromatopsia in the affected eye lends further support for optic nerve involvement in a patient with decreased vision and a relative afferent pupillary defect. Corneal sensation should be evaluated, and any evidence of dysfunction of cranial nerve II, III, IV, V, VI, or VII noted. A lesion between the orbital apex and the cavernous sinus may affect multiple cranial nerves with minimal or no proptosis. Forced-duction testing may differentiate restrictive from paretic muscle dysfunction and may be useful in some cases.

Table 25-6 summarizes ocular, periocular, and systemic signs that are clinically significant to orbital disease.

TABLE 25-6

Clinical Significance of Ocular, Periocular, and Systemic Signs

Signs	Diagnoses to Consider
Ocular	
Subconjunctival salmon-colored lesion	Lymphoma
Granulomatous uveitis/retinal periphlebitis	Sarcoidosis
Dilated and tortuous episcleral vessels/elevated IOP/dilated retinal veins	Carotid–cavernous sinus fistula, dural or orbital arteriovenous malformation
Increased IOP on upgaze	Thyroid-related orbitopathy
Optociliary shunt vessels	Optic nerve meningioma
Orbital/Periocular	
S-shaped lid deformity	Plexiform neurofibroma/lacrimal gland fossa mass
Lid retraction/lid lag	Thyroid-related orbitopathy
Prominent lid veins/proptosis worse on bending over or Valsalva maneuver	Orbital varix
Ocular pulsations	Neurofibromatosis, meningoencephalocele
Orbital bruit	Carotid–cavernous sinus fistula, dural or orbital arteriovenous malformation
Lid ecchymosis	Neuroblastoma, leukemia, lymphangioma; trauma
Unilateral vesicular skin lesions	Herpes zoster ophthalmicus
Enophthalmos	Trauma, chronic sinusitis, metastatic breast cancer (scirrhous carcinoma)
Systemic	
Scalp tenderness	Giant-cell arteritis
Prominent temple	Sphenoid wing meningioma
Black eschar in nose or mouth	Mucormycosis, phycomycosis
Café-au-lait spots	Neurofibromatosis
Generalized lymphadenopathy	Lymphoma
Weight loss	Malignant neoplasm
Multiple system infection	Immune system compromise

25-4

LABORATORY EVALUATION

Particularly in the case of inflammatory disease, orbital disorders are often manifestations of systemic abnormalities. Laboratory testing not only helps to narrow the differential diagnosis by pinpointing systemic disease that may account for orbital findings, but also may be important in identifying systemic disorders that require treatment independent of the orbital pathology. Systemic disorders that commonly affect the orbit and can be evaluated with laboratory testing include Graves' thyroid disease (T_3, T_4, sensitive TSH), sarcoidosis (angiotensin-converting enzyme, chest x-ray), Wegener's granulomatosis (antinuclear cytoplasmic antibody), myasthenia gravis (acetylcholine receptor antibodies), and specific autoimmune disorders such as lupus or Sjogren's.

25-5

ORBITAL IMAGING

Orbital imaging is the cornerstone of diagnosis. Imaging technology is continually improving, allowing the practitioner to increasingly refine the differential diagnosis and make an accurate presumed diagnosis based on the imaging findings.

The comprehensive ophthalmologist should have a basic understanding of the relative advantages and disadvantages of each imaging modality, should know which study should be ordered in different clinical situations, and should be able to order the test (eg, orientation of view, slice thickness, intravenous contrast) to obtain the most information in an efficient and cost-effective manner. Guidelines for ordering orbital imaging studies are summarized in Table 25-7.

25-5-1 Ultrasonography

Orbital ultrasonography has generally been replaced by computed tomography (CT) and magnetic resonance imaging (MRI) in orbital diagnosis, but it still plays an important role in selected instances. In thyroid-related orbitopathy, ultrasound often demonstrates enlarged extraocular muscles,[5] but this finding is nonspecific and does not typically refine the differential diagnosis. However, ultrasound may be useful to stage the disease.[6] Ultrasonography has high resolution in the area of the sclera and optic nerve insertion and is particularly useful to evaluate scleritis and other anterior inflammations that produce sub-Tenon's fluid. Ultrasonography lacks the resolution of CT and MRI in the deep orbit, but has one very significant advantage: it is performed in real time, so that dynamic changes can be readily observed. For example, with eye movements, the optic nerve can be observed to move around a tumor that is separate from the nerve, differentiating it from a tumor attached to the nerve. Also, vascular tumors can be identified by active

TABLE 25-7

Guidelines for Ordering Orbital Imaging Studies

Study	Most Useful	Less Useful	Contraindications	How to Order
Ultrasonography	Vascular tumors (color-flow doppler) Anterior inflammations Dynamic imaging	Deep orbital tumors Bony tumors		Clarify differential diagnosis Skilled operator required
Computed tomography (CT)	Trauma Orbital mass Bone tumors	Orbital apex and cavernous sinus	Pregnancy (relative) Intravenous dye with renal dysfunction Dye allergy	Fine orbital cuts 1.5-mm width at 1.0-mm intervals Direct coronal scans
Magnetic resonance imaging (MRI)	Orbital apex, optic nerve, cavernous sinus, skull base tumors Vascular lesions Inflammatory lesions Staging Graves' disease	Bony trauma	Claustrophobia Metal in patient: pacemaker, ocular foreign body	Clarify differential diagnosis Orbital surface coil
Magnetic resonance angiography (MRA)	High-flow vascular lesions: arteriovenous fistula, cavernous dural fistula	Smaller or low-flow lesions	Claustrophobia Metal in patient: pacemaker, ocular foreign body Paramagnetic dye allergy (rare)	Clarify differential diagnosis
Arteriography	High-flow vascular lesions: arteriovenous fistula, cavernous dural fistula Small lesions Neuro-interventional therapy		Dye allergy	Clarify differential diagnosis

pulsation or, in the case of venous lesions, by compressibility and demonstrable change in size with Valsalva maneuver. Color-flow doppler ultrasonography is particularly sensitive for demonstrating vascular flow and can demonstrate arterialized, retrograde flow in the orbital veins in cases of cavernous dural fistula or arteriovenous malformation.

25-5-2 Computed Tomography

Especially at centers where it is less expensive and more easily obtained, computed tomography is the single most useful orbital imaging modality. Compared to MRI, CT scanning is faster, less expensive, and less sensitive to movement artifact. The resolution and soft-tissue contrast are adequate to visualize almost any pathologic orbital process, and the bony resolution is superior to all other modalities, making CT ideal for evaluation of orbital trauma or bony tumors. To obtain optimal images, the entire orbit should be scanned in fine resolution; fine 1.5-mm cuts at 1.0-mm intervals provide the best possible detail, although thicker slices suffice for many types of disease conditions. Direct coronal scans are obtained by tilting the patient's neck back, and although coronal scans are sometimes limited by

neck mobility or by artifacts from dental fillings, they allow excellent views of the extraocular muscles and optic nerve and provide the best view of the orbit to evaluate the roof or floor (for example, blowout fractures) or the extraocular muscles. Contrast CT studies provide more information; however, the iodinated intravenous dye may be contraindicated in patients with renal dysfunction, eg, diabetic patients.

25-5-3 Magnetic Resonance Imaging

In the orbit, magnetic resonance imaging provides similar information to that obtained with computed tomography without exposure to ionizing radiation. Technologic advances are gradually making MRI cost-competitive to CT, and "open" scanners are reducing the claustrophobia induced by confinement in a tight closed gantry. Nevertheless, at present in most centers, MRI is still more expensive and more difficult for the patient. MRI provides soft-tissue and bone-marrow resolution superior to CT and is particularly useful to evaluate tumors of the cavernous sinus and skull base, including optic nerve tumors that enter the cranial cavity. MRI scans can be taken in any plane without repositioning the patient—an especially useful feature for patients with limited neck mobility. T2-weighted images may be useful for staging Graves' orbitopathy by assessing muscle edema, an indicator of active inflammation.[7] Because bone is not differentiated from air, MRI is not useful for evaluating orbital fractures or differentiating bone and calcium.

MRI and CT can be synergistic in their contribution to diagnosis and, particularly in difficult cases, both studies may be better than either alone. The radiologist has a number of tools to improve orbital images, including surface coils for increased resolution, various fat-suppression protocols, and intravenous contrast agents (gadolinium). The best results are obtained when the radiologist knows the differential diagnosis so that the appropriate studies can be obtained. Therefore, it is essential to provide the radiologist with as much clinical information as possible and to review the films with the radiologist.

25-5-4 Angiography and Arteriography

In the case of orbital vascular lesions characterized by flowing blood and vascular lesions of the cavernous sinus, standard orbital imaging studies often need to be supplemented by specific techniques to evaluate vascular flow patterns. Newer, noninvasive modalities such as magnetic resonance angiography and color-flow doppler ultrasonography can occasionally provide adequate diagnostic information to guide diagnosis and management. Standard arteriography is the gold standard to detect and characterize the most subtle lesions, and in modern centers often allows direct treatment by a transarterial or transvenous route. Arteriography carries a small but real risk of serious complications such as stroke. Working closely with the radiologist is imperative to achieve good diagnostic results with minimal risk when dealing with suspected orbital vascular tumors.

25-6

ORBITAL BIOPSY

Orbital biopsy must be approached with respect. To maximally benefit a patient whose tissue is required for diagnosis, a number of factors must be taken into account. The decision to perform biopsy should be weighed against the relative risks and benefits. In general, the threshold for biopsy should be low, although in the setting of lesions that are benign clinically and radiographically, observation may be appropriate. Also, certain inflammations may be appropriately treated medically, under close observation. Fine-needle aspiration biopsy, in a center with a skilled cytopathologist, is a very useful tool that can obviate the need for a trip to the operating room in cases such as lymphoma or metastatic carcinoma that would not otherwise need surgery.[8,9] Open biopsy must be performed with care and skill to produce a diagnostic tissue sample with as little damage as possible to normal structures.[10] The removed tissue must be handled gently and fixed immediately; preoperative consultation with a pathologist will identify any special handling of the tissue or special fixatives that might be necessary.*

---

*See also Chapter 26, "Surgical Exploration of the Orbit," in this volume.—ED.

25-7

MANAGEMENT OF ORBITAL DISORDERS

25-7-1 Orbital Inflammation

An inflamed orbit with redness and compromised ophthalmic function is a dramatic presentation that, particularly in the fulminant form, can be frightening for both patient and diagnostician. As with all orbital disease, a careful, methodical, and studied approach to formulating and working through a differential diagnosis is required. The history helps to sort through possible antecedent factors such as trauma, foreign body, sinus disease, and pre-existing (local or systemic) disease, including thyroid dysfunction. The history also allows the clinician to characterize the inflammatory disease with regard to timing of onset: Is the presentation acute (evolving over days), subacute (days to weeks), or chronic (weeks to months)? These major categories of onset have significance with regard to constructing a differential diagnosis (see Table 25-1).

It is particularly important to identify treatable inflammations. Obvious in this group is infection, which requires specific and sometimes emergent treatment with antibiotics or surgery. Other inflammations that might respond to treatment include surgical diseases, such as retained foreign body, abscess, or neoplasia, or systemic diseases, such as Wegener's granulomatosis or sarcoidosis, which require systemic treatment that may be life-saving as well as vision-saving.

Because of its overwhelming statistical prominence in orbital disease, thyroid-related orbitopathy should be in the differential diagnosis of virtually every case of orbital inflammation. Atypical presentations of Graves' orbitopathy, such as strikingly asymmetric or acute onsets, occur and must be considered.

Unfortunately, the current state of medical knowledge does not allow for a specific diagnosis in many cases of orbital inflammation, hence the "generic" diagnosis idiopathic orbital inflammatory disease. This condition can take an acute, subacute, or chronic form and can involve a specific orbital structure (scleritis, myositis, dacryoadenitis, or perioptic neuritis, for example) or multiple orbital structures. The outdated term *pseudotumor* lumps together a rich variety of specific and nonspecific, diffuse and localized inflammatory syndromes. It should be abandoned for terminology that is as precise as possible with regard to both the localization and the cause of the inflammation.

A prime example of a specific type of inflammation that should not be called a pseudotumor is idiopathic sclerosing orbital inflammatory tumor.[11] This is a type of nonspecific inflammation that has a characteristic pathologic picture with desmoplasia and considerable fibrosis. These tumors form a slow-growing orbital mass that can be associated with significant infiltration and loss of function (Figure

25-1). Rather than being a "burned-out" acute nonspecific inflammation, these tumors probably represent an entirely different disease and should be treated early and aggressively. The optimal treatment has not been identified, but corticosteroids, surgical debulking, radiotherapy, and immunosuppression with cytotoxic drugs may play a role in selected cases.

25-7-2 Thyroid-Related Orbitopathy

Thyroid-related orbitopathy is by far the most common disease entity producing orbital signs and symptoms, and should always be considered in the differential diagnosis of a patient with proptosis or orbital inflammation. Although the classic presentation—with bilateral proptosis, inflammation, extraocular motility restriction, and eyelid retraction—is easily recognized, atypical presentations such as asymmetric or purely unilateral disease, acute severe inflammation, myositis, or subtle noninflamed disease are not infrequent and may be difficult to diagnose, particularly if the diagnostician fails to consider the diagnosis of Graves' disease.

Thyroid-related orbitopathy is primarily a clinical diagnosis. Unless atypical features such as marked asymmetry, euthyroid status, pain, unusual neurologic symptoms, unusual systemic disease, trauma, or paranasal sinus disease make the diagnosis suspect or raise the specter of a second coexisting orbital process, orbital imaging studies would not change the management of the patient and may be avoided. If imaging studies are desired to clarify the diagnosis, either CT or MRI

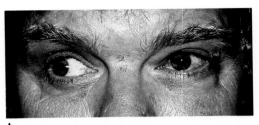

A

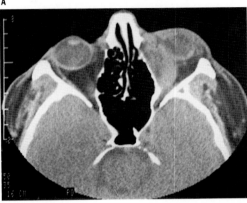

B

Figure 25-1 *Idiopathic sclerosing orbital inflammatory tumor. (A) 40-year-old man with slowly progressive painful proptosis and extraocular motility limitation. (B) Axial CT demonstrates homogeneous medial orbital mass involving medial rectus muscle and apex. Biopsy demonstrated mixed inflammatory response with marked fibrosis, consistent with idiopathic sclerosing inflammatory tumor of orbit. Tumor failed to respond to corticosteroids, radiation, and cytotoxic drugs, and patient eventually required exenteration for pain control.*

provides adequate information to rule out other considerations in the differential diagnosis. Aside from ruling out a tumor, vascular process, or other disorders in the differential diagnosis, imaging studies typically show fusiform expansion of one or more of the extraocular muscles, most often with thin tendons.[12] Large muscles (greater then 9 mm in width) or a "crowded" orbital apex indicates patients at risk for compressive optic neuropathy[13] as does restrictive myopathy.[14] Ultrasonography often shows enlarged extraocular muscles but lacks specificity and does not rule out other disorders; it is therefore not very useful in making treatment or diagnostic decisions, although some evidence suggests that it may be useful in staging the disease.[6] A reasonable guideline is to use orbital imaging as an aid with the differential diagnosis in atypical cases, to evaluate the optic nerve in cases of compressive optic neuropathy, as a method to document progression in association with clinical signs and symptoms, or as a planning tool for possible orbital decompression surgery.

No laboratory test definitively establishes the diagnosis of thyroid-related orbitopathy. Thyroid function associated with Graves' orbitopathy can be high, low, or normal, and an occasional patient with non–Graves' proptosis has thyroid dysfunction coincidentally. Nevertheless, the demonstration of autonomous thyroid functioning with an abnormally low sensitive TSH test makes the diagnosis of Graves' thyroid disease and therefore Graves' orbitopathy extremely likely. Perhaps the most important aspect of assessing thyroid function is to identify patients with hypothyroidism or hyperthyroidism, who should be evaluated by an internist or endocrinologist for long-term management of the thyroid component of the disease. The course of the orbitopathy is generally independent of thyroid function. For example, a hyperthyroid patient is not managed differently ophthalmologically from one who is hypothyroid. However, treatment of the thyroid gland may affect the orbitopathy: recent evidence suggests that radioactive iodine therapy may cause worsening of the eye disease,[15] and in many centers the movement is toward medical management of the thyroid disease with agents such as propothiouracil (PTU), combined with thyroxine replacement.

Graves' disease is a complex, multisymptom disorder with a chronic, unpredictable course, and patients with this disease benefit from a staged, orchestrated, and compassionate approach that includes educational and emotional support. When a patient with thyroid-related orbitopathy is evaluated, it is critically important to stage the disease: inflammatory phase and postinflammatory phase. Thyroid-related orbitopathy in most patients follows a fairly predictable course with an early inflammatory stage lasting 6 months to 2 years. This phase is characterized clini-

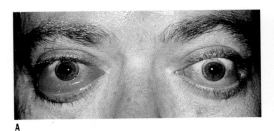

A

cally by inflammatory signs including eyelid erythema, chemosis, injection, and
edema and also by fluctuations that can
occur daily or weekly. During the inflammatory phase, treatment may include anti-
inflammatory medication such as corticosteroids or radiotherapy (Figure 25-2).[16]
One strategy is to offer a 2-month taper-
ing course of corticosteroids, and if there
is a rebound when the corticosteroids are
tapered, then radiotherapy (20 Gy given
in ten fractions) is offered along with another course of corticosteroids. Surgery is
less predictable and less successful when
performed during the inflammatory phase
and, except for unusual or emergent circumstances (such as marked exposure keratopathy or severe compressive optic neuropathy unresponsive to anti-inflammatory
therapy), is better deferred until the disease stabilizes into the postinflammatory
or chronic phase.

Although there can still be waxing and
waning smoldering inflammation, the postinflammatory phase is generally characterized by stability and lack of active inflammation, and staged reconstructive surgery
is often performed at this time (Figure
25-3).[17] The postinflammatory phase is often characterized by considerable orbital
congestion related to venous stasis in a
compressed orbit and manifested clinically

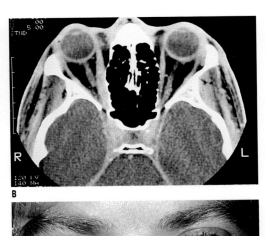

B

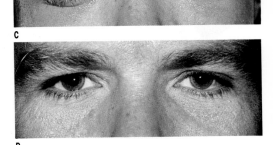

C

D

Figure 25-2 *Thyroid-related orbitopathy.*
(A) 35-year-old male developed bilateral acute
orbital cellulitis as initial onset of thyroid-related
orbitopathy. Lateral cantholysis and pulsed in-
travenous corticosteroids comprised initial ther-
apy. (B) Axial CT demonstrates proptosis and
moderate enlargement of medial rectus muscle
belly. (C) After 1 week of corticosteroid therapy,
inflammation decreased significantly. Cortico-
steroids were tapered over a 3-month period.
(D) 1 year later, well after corticosteroids were
discontinued, patient demonstrates minimal in-
flammation; no surgery was required.

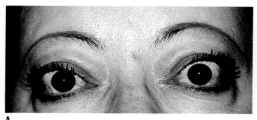

A

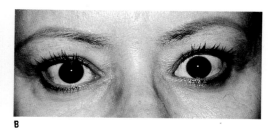

B

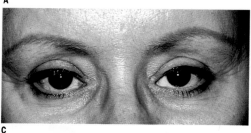

C

Figure 25-3 *Postinflammatory phase of thyroid-related orbitopathy. (A) Patient with stable congestive thyroid-related orbitopathy, 2 years into course. No compressive optic neuropathy is present, but patient has swelling and periocular pressure sensation related to orbital congestion, as well as exposure keratopathy from proptosis. (B) Same patient after orbital decompression: edema and chemosis, as well as orbital pressure sensation, improved following release of orbital apical crowding and venous congestion. When proptosis was reduced, exposure keratopathy was slightly improved. (C) Same patient following eyelid repositioning surgery; exposure keratopathy substantially improved.*

by edema, chemosis, and commonly a painful pressure sensation. These congestive symptoms must be differentiated from frank inflammation, because congestive disease in the postinflammatory stage responds poorly to anti-inflammatory medications but often responds well to orbital apical decompression surgery, which restores venous outflow.

Compressive optic neuropathy is a vision-threatening complication of Graves' orbitopathy that requires careful management.[18] It can occur in inflamed orbits early in the course of the disease or late, in the postinflammatory stage, and in proptotic or nonproptotic orbits. It is often but not always associated with orbital apical crowding on imaging studies and with increased intraocular pressure on upgaze. In the inflammatory stage, anti-inflammatory therapy is often effective. Because radiotherapy takes one or more months for maximal effect, corticosteroid therapy is generally preferred for all but the mildest cases, and pulsed corticosteroids can be used in more severe cases. Surgical decompression of the orbital apex is effective immediate treatment of compressive neuropathy and is utilized for cases that do not respond quickly (days to weeks) to medical treatment. For the most severe cases—for example, with counting-fingers vision or dense afferent pupillary defect—surgery and anti-inflammatory therapy are provided simultaneously. In the postinflammatory stage, medical therapy is less effective and surgery is the first line of treatment. The optic nerve has considerable reserve when it is compressed slowly, and even cases with severe loss of vision can respond to therapy.*

25-7-3 Benign Tumors

Benign tumors are characterized biologically by lack of infiltration into surrounding tissues. Therefore, they are often easily dissected from the orbit and surgery is indicated when the mass produces symptoms or signs. Orbital imaging studies occasionally pick up small benign orbital tumors. If these are asymptomatic, the best management is generally observation; many benign tumors such as schwannoma and cavernous hemangioma grow very slowly if at all. Benign masses should be excised completely if possible, to prevent recurrence. Benign mixed tumor of the lacrimal gland is an example of a tumor that can recur in malignant fashion if not completely excised; lacrimal gland tumors should be approached with care.[19] Recurrences can be much more difficult to manage than the initial tumor because of scar-tissue formation.

Some tumors—for example, dermoid cysts—are somewhat difficult to dissect because of chronic low-grade inflammation and possible erosion into surrounding bone; careful dissection and sometimes removal of significant amounts of bone are

required.[20] Other benign tumors—for example, lymphangioma and neurofibroma—tend to grow diffusely and intertwine extensively with normal structures, making complete removal difficult or impossible without endangering function. In these cases, subtotal resection is preferable. Optic nerve meningiomas cannot be surgically removed without causing functional damage to the nerve, so surgery is reserved for nonfunctioning nerves or for tumors that have been documented by gadolinium MRI to be growing into the cavernous sinus.

25-7-4 Vascular Tumors

From a treatment standpoint, orbital vascular tumors can be categorized by the degree of flow through the lesion. Low-flow vascular lesions such as orbital varices do not always require treatment. If treatment becomes necessary because of growth, compression of vital structures, or disfigurement, these lesions can be removed surgically with wide exposure and careful identification of the feeding veins. The lesions are fragile and surgery is difficult.

High-flow lesions represent abnormal connections between the arterial and venous circulations. These lesions often cause significant functional problems because of the profound alterations in blood flow. High-flow lesions are best treated with a multidisciplinary approach that includes neurovascular embolization combined with surgery.[21]

---

*See also Chapter 27, "Surgical Decompression of the Orbit," in this volume.—ED.

Capillary hemangiomas and lymphangiomas are examples of tumors that originate from vascular tissue but do not have abnormal connections to the vascular system. They can be removed surgically.[22-24] Capillary hemangiomas, particularly in the growing phase over the first year or two of life, often respond to oral or injected corticosteroids.[25]

25-7-5 Malignant Tumors

Malignant neoplasms have the biologic potential to spread aggressively in a localized area and to metastasize to distant sites. Decision-making must take this tendency into account. In general, if careful evaluation suggests that the tumor has not metastasized, cure is possible with complete local resection. In the orbit, resection often, but not always, involves removal of the globe. If a previous biopsy has been performed, the tract of the biopsy is included in the resection. Incisions for biopsies should be planned with this eventuality in mind. If the tumor has metastasized, there is usually not much role for surgery beyond obtaining an accurate biopsy or palliation. Tumors metastatic to the orbit from elsewhere in the body often respond to radiotherapy.[26]

Management decisions are made from permanent histopathologic material and in association with oncologists, radiotherapists, and related surgical specialists. Appropriate surgical treatment of malignant lesions can only be effected when coordinated with chemotherapy, immunotherapy, and radiation therapy. The needs and desires of the patient and family are of paramount importance in the application of all treatment protocols.

REFERENCES

1. Rootman J: *Diseases of the Orbit: A Multidisciplinary Approach.* Philadelphia: JB Lippincott Co; 1988.

2. Henderson JW: *Orbital Tumors.* New York: Raven Press; 1994.

3. Kennedy RE: An evaluation of 820 orbital cases. *Trans Am Ophthalmol Soc* 1984;82: 134–157.

4. Krohel GB, Stewart WB, Chavis RM: *Orbital Disease: A Practical Approach.* New York: Grune & Stratton; 1981.

5. Demer JL, Kerman BM: Comparison of standardized echography with magnetic resonance imaging to measure extraocular muscle size. *Am J Ophthalmol* 1994;118:351–361.

6. Prummel MF, Suttorp-Schulten MS, Wiersinga WM, et al: A new ultrasonographic method to detect disease activity and predict response to immunosuppressive treatment in Graves' ophthalmopathy. *Ophthalmology* 1993;100:556–561.

7. Hiromatsu Y, Kojima K, Ishisaka N, et al: Role of magnetic resonance imaging in thyroid-associated ophthalmopathy: its predictive value for therapeutic outcome of immunosuppressive therapy. *Thyroid* 1992;2:299–305.

8. Kennerdell JS, Slamovits TL, Dekker A, Johnson BL: Orbital fine-needle aspiration biopsy. *Am J Ophthalmol* 1985;99:547–551.

9. Glasgow BJ, Layfield LJ: Fine-needle aspiration biopsy of orbital and periorbital masses. *Diagn Cytopathol* 1991;7:132–141.

10. Rootman J, Stewart B, Goldberg RA: *Atlas of Orbital Surgery.* New York: Raven Press; 1995.

11. Rootman J, McCarthy M, White V, et al: Idiopathic sclerosing inflammation of the orbit: a distinct clinicopathologic entity. *Ophthalmology* 1994;101:570–584.

12. Patrinely JR, Osborn AG, Anderson RL, Whiting AS: Computed tomographic features of nonthyroid extraocular muscle enlargement. *Ophthalmology* 1989;96:1038–1047.

13. Feldon SE, Muramatsu S, Weiner JM: Clinical classification of Graves' ophthalmopathy: identification of risk factors for optic neuropathy. *Arch Ophthalmol* 1984;102:1469–1472.

14. Tanenbaum M, McCord CD Jr, Nunery WR: Graves' ophthalmopathy. In: McCord CD, Tanenbaum M, eds: *Oculoplastic Surgery.* New York: Raven Press; 1995:379–416.

15. Tallstedt L, Lundell G, Torring O, et al: Occurrence of ophthalmopathy after treatment for Graves' hyperthyroidism: The Thyroid Study Group. *N Engl J Med* 1992;326:1733–1738.

16. Kao SC, Kendler DL, Nugent RA, et al: Radiotherapy in the management of thyroid orbitopathy: computed tomography and clinical outcomes. *Arch Ophthalmol* 1993;111:819–823.

17. Shorr N, Seiff SR: The four stages of surgical rehabilitation of the patient with dysthyroid ophthalmopathy. *Ophthalmology* 1986;93:476–483.

18. Neigel JM, Rootman J, Belkin RI, et al: Dysthyroid optic neuropathy: the crowded orbital apex syndrome. *Ophthalmology* 1988;95:1515–1521.

19. Stewart WB, Krohel GB, Wright JE: Lacrimal gland and fossa lesions: an approach to diagnosis and management. *Ophthalmology* 1979;86:886–895.

20. Sherman RP, Rootman J, Lapointe JS: Orbital dermoids: clinical presentation and management. *Br J Ophthalmol* 1984;68:642–652.

21. Rootman J, Kao SC, Graeb DA: Multidisciplinary approaches to complicated vascular lesions of the orbit. *Ophthalmology* 1992;99:1440–1446.

22. Deans RM, Harris GJ, Kivlin JD: Surgical dissection of capillary hemangiomas: an alternative to intralesional corticosteroids. *Arch Ophthalmol* 1992;110:1743–1747.

23. Harris GJ, Sakol PJ, Bonavolontà G, De Conciliis C: An analysis of thirty cases of orbital lymphangioma: pathophysiologic considerations and management recommendations. *Ophthalmology* 1990;97:1583–1592.

24. Walker RS, Custer PL, Nerad JA: Surgical excision of periorbital capillary hemangiomas. *Ophthalmology* 1994;101:1333–1340.

25. Haik BG, Karcioglu ZA, Gordon RA, Pechous BP: Capillary hemangioma (infantile periocular hemangioma). *Surv Ophthalmol* 1994;38:399–426.

26. Goldberg RA, Rootman J, Cline RA: Tumors metastatic to the orbit: a changing picture. *Surv Ophthalmol* 1990;35:1–24.

CHAPTER 26

Surgical Exploration of the Orbit

John E. Wright, FRCS
Mary A. Stefanyszyn, MD

Access to the retrobulbar space is impeded by the bony walls of the orbit. Surgical exploration of the orbit is further complicated by the high concentration of delicate structures, especially in the orbital apex. Selection of the appropriate approach to biopsy and excision avoids damage to the complex oculomotor, neurosensory, and secretory structures responsible for normal ocular function. Current imaging techniques such as computed tomography (CT) and magnetic resonance imaging (MRI) greatly aid the clinician in delineating the position and extent of orbital lesions. Adequate exposure and visualization, good hemostasis, and atraumatic dissection are crucial to successful orbital surgery. Operative microscopy and fiberoptic illumination improve the accuracy of dissection. Hypotensive anesthesia, patient positioning, and local hemostasis using bipolar cautery help in maintaining a bloodless field.

Anterior orbital lesions can often be excised or biopsied without removal of bone; however, posterior lesions usually need removal of the lateral orbital wall for adequate exposure. If there is intracranial or paranasal sinus involvement, a combined approach with an otolaryngologist or a neurosurgeon is indicated. Well-demarcated and easily defined tumors, such as cavernous hemangiomas or dermoids, are dissected free and totally removed. More diffuse or infiltrating lesions, suggestive of inflammatory or malignant disease, undergo incisional biopsy. The decision to biopsy or to totally excise a lesion depends on the patient's clinical history, preoperative examination, and radiographic findings. Additionally, consultation should be obtained when needed from the radiologist, pathologist, or internist.

As the field of pathology becomes more sophisticated, the orbital surgeon needs to cooperate with the pathologist to ensure the proper handling of tissues for accurate diagnosis. The orbital surgeon should discuss with the pathologist the preoperative differential diagnosis and ask for guidance in the disposition of tissue. Accurate pathologic diagnosis may require special studies, including cytology, histochemistry, immunohistochemistry, and electron microscopy. Tissue for routine histologic examination is placed in paraformaldehyde. Electron microscopy requires appropriate

fixation in glutaraldehyde. Fresh-frozen tissue is best suited for immunohisto-chemistry. The pathologist needs to be available for frozen-section evaluation or to do cell impressions for cytology if necessary.

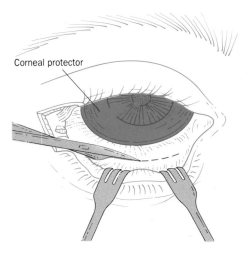

Corneal protector

Figure 26-1 *Conjunctival incision is made in inferior fornix. Lateral canthotomy with severance of lower crux of lateral canthal tendon has been performed, allowing good retraction of lower lid.*

26-1

ANTERIOR ORBITOTOMY

Excision of anterior lesions and biopsy of some posterior lesions can be performed with an anterior orbitotomy through either an eyelid skin approach or a conjunctival approach. The eyelid skin incision allows entry into the orbit by the extraperiosteal or transseptal route.

26-1-1 Transconjunctival Orbitotomy

Anterior periocular and orbital lesions can be explored through a conjunctival incision. Occasionally, it is necessary to detach one of the rectus muscles and introduce retractors between the muscle and the globe to gain entry and adequate visualization of the intraconal space. Lesions in the inferior orbit and fractures of the orbital floor can be approached through the inferior conjunctival fornix approach, often obviating the need for bone excision or deep extraperiosteal dissection. Lidocaine 2% with 1:100,000 epinephrine is injected in the inferior fornix and lateral canthal area to induce vasoconstriction. A lateral canthotomy with severance of the lower crus of the lateral canthal tendon is performed, and the lower eyelid is retracted downward, exposing the inferior fornix (Figure 26-1). A conjunctival incision is then performed, usually at the

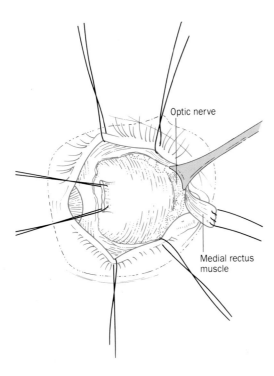

Optic nerve

Medial rectus
muscle

Figure 26-2 *Medial conjunctival orbitotomy with medial rectus muscle reflected away from globe, allowing entry into intraconal space. Note optic nerve and surrounding fatty tissue.*

junction of the bulbar and palpebral conjunctiva. The subconjunctival tissue, including the capsulopalpebral fascia, is incised with scissors directly to the periosteum of the inferior orbital rim. Rakes, vein retractors, or marginal sutures can be used to retract the lower eyelid and thus prevent buttonholing of the skin. A malleable retractor is used to retract the globe and any prolapsing orbital fat. If the mass is palpable and easily accessible within the orbital fat, bone excision or periosteal dissection can be avoided, especially if only a biopsy is necessary. If the lesion is large or posterior, a lateral orbitotomy can provide additional exposure.

The medial conjunctival approach is commonly used in the anterior medial orbit for obtaining biopsy material from the optic nerve or adjacent structures or when decompressing the nerve for chronic intracranial hypertension.* Surgically, the medial rectus is reflected from the globe as in a routine medial rectus strabismus procedure (Figure 26-2). A traction suture is passed through the insertion of the muscle, and the globe is rotated laterally. A retractor is placed on the inner aspect of the medial rectus muscle and is then retracted toward the midline. The intraconal surgical space can be explored and the structures on the medial side of the optic nerve examined with the operating microscope. Following biopsy or excision of the lesion, the rectus muscle is reattached with 5-0 or 6-0 polyglycolic sutures, and the conjunctiva is closed with 6-0 or 7-0

*See also Chapter 28, "Optic Nerve Sheath Decompression," in this volume. —ED.

collagen or polyglycolic absorbable sutures, sufficient gaps being left between sutures to allow seepage of any blood or serum that accumulates. An antibiotic ointment is instilled in the eye, and an eye pad is positioned over the closed eyelids with no pressure applied. Alternatively, the optic nerve can be approached laterally. A lateral canthotomy improves exposure, often making the removal of lateral orbital rim and disinsertion of the lateral rectus muscle unnecessary.

The intricate relationship between ocular and upper eyelid structures hinders the conjunctival approach to the anterior superior orbit. Damage to the levator muscle and the lacrimal ducts can be avoided by using a skin transseptal or extraperiosteal approach. Posterior superior lesions are best approached through a lateral orbitotomy or through an intracranial approach.

26-1-2 Transseptal Orbitotomy

Biopsy or excision of anterior tumors is often performed with a transseptal approach through a skin incision along natural wrinkle lines or eyelid folds. The orbicularis can be split and subcutaneous traction sutures placed to improve exposure and hemostasis. The orbital septum is incised with fine scissors, and the orbital fat retracted to improve exposure of the lesion. Attention must be paid to the levator and Müller's muscle in the upper eyelid, lower eyelid retractors, and other structures to assure good postoperative eyelid function. The orbicularis can be closed with absorbable sutures, and a drain placed if indicated. The skin is closed with 6-0 nylon suture or 6-0 mild chromic, and a light dressing applied. Depending on the extent or type of procedure, the patient is discharged the same day or the next. Mild chromic sutures dissolve, and nylon skin sutures are removed 5 to 7 days postoperatively.

26-1-3 Extraperiosteal Orbitotomy

The extraperiosteal approach is useful for lesions adjacent to the periosteum or involving bone. Osteomas and mucoceles of the ethmoid and frontal sinus, fractures of the orbital walls, and extensive dermoids can be explored this way. By staying in the extraperiosteal space as much as possible before entering the orbit, the surgeon limits the degree of damage to intraorbital structures. This operation should not be used to biopsy intraorbital lesions thought to be malignant, as the periosteum is a valuable barrier limiting spread and an important margin for surgical excision.

The extraperiosteal space can be reached through a skin incision overlying or outside the orbital rim. An inferior subciliary or upper eyelid skin crease incision can also be used; however, thorough knowledge of eyelid structures and careful dissection are necessary to prevent loss of normal eyelid function. An inferior fornix conjunctival approach provides an alternative in exploring the inferior extraperios-

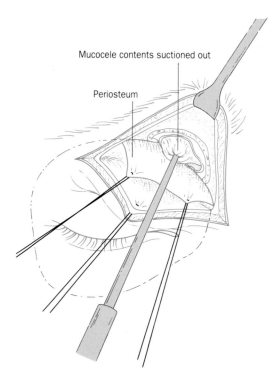

Mucocele contents suctioned out

Periosteum

Figure 26-3 *Superior nasal orbitotomy with extraperiosteal dissection is used for drainage of frontal sinus mucocele.*

teal space without a skin incision and extensive eyelid dissection. When exploring the superior extraperiosteal space, the surgeon must pay special attention to the nasal area to keep the periosteum near the trochlea intact. The periosteum should be reflected and replaced with minimal trauma. The supraorbital nerve should not be transected if it can be retracted out of the way. Regardless of approach, once the orbital margin is reached, the periosteum is incised and elevated from the rim using a periosteal elevator. Past the orbital rim, elevation is easy and malleable retractors or sutures placed at the edge of the orbital periosteum can be used to retract orbital contents out of the way. Over the area of interest, the periosteum is incised and the lesion exposed. Once the lesion is biopsied or excised, a drain is inserted in the extraperiosteal space and the conjunctival incision is closed with 6-0 absorbable collagen or polyglycolic sutures and the skin incision with 6-0 nylon or 6-0 mild chromic. Antibiotic ointment is instilled in the eye and along the incision, and a light patch is applied. The drain is removed the next day, and the following week nylon or residual sutures are removed.

A superior nasal orbitotomy with an extraperiosteal dissection is most commonly performed for a frontoethmoidal mucocele (Figure 26-3). Once the periosteum is incised and reflected out of the way, the mucocele is easily entered and the mucoid material suctioned out. The wall of the mucocele is excised or curetted and sinus drainage is re-established into the nasal cavity. For recurrent mucoceles, the sinus needs to be obliterated with adipose tissue. Intranasal drains are left in position for 2 to 3 weeks.

26-2

LATERAL ORBITOTOMY

The lateral orbitotomy is recognized as the best approach to the intraconal space and lateral orbit. Historically, the lateral approach to the orbit was first described by Krönlein in 1888.[1] His innovative approach employed a large, lateral, crescentic incision that was fashioned into a skin–fascia–muscle–bone flap hinged in the temporal area. The unsightly scar that sometimes resulted and lack of adequate working space led to further modifications. The Berke-Reese incision eliminated the curved flap with a straight horizontal cut extending from the lateral canthus for 30 to 40 mm.[2] Berke included a lateral canthotomy to permit wider retraction of the skin flaps, allowing better exposure; however, this necessitated careful lateral canthal reconstruction at the end of the operation. Stallard proposed the superior lateral orbitotomy with a curvilinear incision beginning in the eyebrow area, slanting downward, and extending laterally in a horizontal plane.[3] This approach as modified by Wright provides a wider operative field, avoids the lateral canthal angle, and provides excellent exposure to the lacrimal fossa.[4] The use of the coronal flap in performing a lateral orbitotomy has been advocated by Bonavolontà,[5] Kennerdell,[6] and Stewart[7] for selected patients, especially those with extensive lesions involving the apex and superior orbit. The discussion of lateral orbitotomy techniques that follows is limited to the modified Berke-Reese orbitotomy, the Stallard-Wright orbitotomy, and the coronal scalp flap orbitotomy.

26-2-1 Berke-Reese Lateral Orbitotomy

With the patient under general anesthesia, the lateral canthal area is injected with 2 to 3 cc of lidocaine 2% with 1:100,000 epinephrine. Intravenous antibiotics (Ancef 1 gram) and corticosteroids (dexamethasone 8 mg) are given intraoperatively and followed with a postoperative course of antibiotics and corticosteroids. Dosage protocols with respect to intraoperative and postoperative antibiotics and corticosteroids vary greatly among orbital surgeons. Postoperative corticosteroids most commonly include prednisone 40 mg tapered over 1 week or a Medrol 21 dose-pack. Oral cephalexin (Keflex) 500 mg qid is commonly used as a postoperative antibiotic.

The head of the operating table is elevated in a reverse Trendelenburg position to decrease orbital venous congestion. A moist Gelfoam disk, a protective corneal lens, or ointment can be used to protect the cornea. A lateral canthotomy is performed, with the upper and lower crura of the lateral canthal tendons being cut and detached from the lateral orbital rim. The canthotomy is extended laterally in a skin incision, and the skin–orbicularis flap is undermined from the temporalis fascia along its natural cleavage plane (Figure 26-4). Optionally, the canthus can be left intact, with the skin incision beginning near the lateral canthus. The skin–muscle

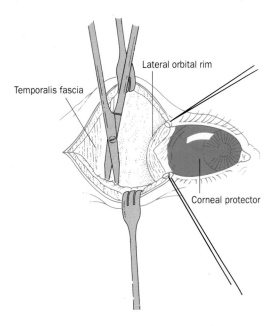

Figure labels: Temporalis fascia, Lateral orbital rim, Corneal protector

Figure 26-4 *Berke-Reese lateral orbitotomy. Lateral canthotomy has been performed, crura of lateral canthal tendon cut, and incision extended laterally. Scissors are used to separate skin–orbicularis flap from underlying temporalis fascia.*

flap is then retracted with rakes or 4-0 silk sutures. The periosteum overlying the frontal process of the zygoma and the zygomatic process of the frontal bone is then incised outside the orbital margin, and superior and inferior horizontal relaxing incisions are made so that the periosteum can be reflected from the orbital rim posteriorly to the anterior edge of the temporal fossa (Figure 26-5). Alternatively, the periosteum can be incised 2 mm behind and parallel to the orbital rim with a relaxing horizontal incision centrally.

After the dissection of the periosteum from the bone, the temporalis muscle is visualized and freed by an incision along the superior temporal crest. With care being taken not to damage its integrity, the orbital periosteum or periorbita is then dissected from the inner orbital wall using a periosteal elevator. Once the periosteum is loosened away from the orbital wall, a malleable retractor is used to reflect the orbital contents medially. Drill holes are placed on either side of the intended bone incision so that the bone can be wired or sutured into place on closing. With an oscillating saw, cuts are made in the lateral rim: one just above the body of the zygoma and one just superior to the frontozygomatic suture (Figure 26-6). During drilling and sawing, irrigating fluid is used to prevent heat necrosis of the bone, and suction is employed to prevent widespread scattering of bone fragments. The bone flap, measuring 2 to 3 cm in length, is removed in one piece by fracturing the thin lateral wall as the lateral orbital rim is removed using an end-cutting rongeur. A cutting Bovie is used to dissect the temporalis muscle. The bony fragment is

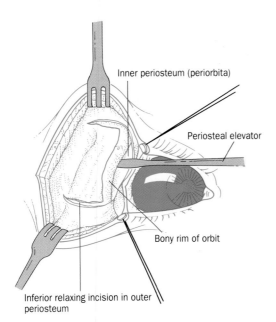

Inner periosteum (periorbita)

Periosteal elevator

Bony rim of orbit

Inferior relaxing incision in outer periosteum

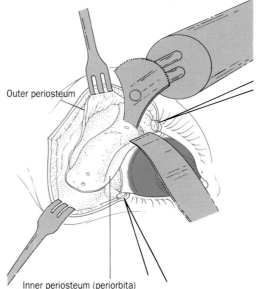

Outer periosteum

Inner periosteum (periorbita)

placed in warm Ringer's or antibiotic solution. The remaining lateral wall can be removed piecemeal using rongeurs. The periorbita is incised longitudinally and retracted with 4-0 silk sutures. The lateral rectus muscle is identified, and when necessary hooked and looped with silicone tubing, and rotated out of the way (Figure 26-7). A lesion in the muscle cone can be palpated or visualized and a decision made as to biopsy or total excision.

The key to successful exploration, biopsy, or excision is adequate exposure, sufficient magnification, and good illumination using operating loupes with a fiberoptic headlight or an operating microscope. Bipolar cautery, cottonoid sponges, cotton-tipped applicators, gentle irrigation, and suction help to maintain a bloodless field, thus allowing recognition of different

Figure 26-5 *(Left) Periosteum overlying lateral orbital rim is incised along rim margin with relaxing incisions superiorly and inferiorly. Inner orbital periosteum or periorbita is dissected from inner orbital wall using periosteal elevator.*

Figure 26-6 *(Right) Oscillating saw is used to cut lateral rim just above body of zygoma and superior to frontozygomatic suture. Drill holes have been placed on either side of incisions to be used in resuturing bony flap.*

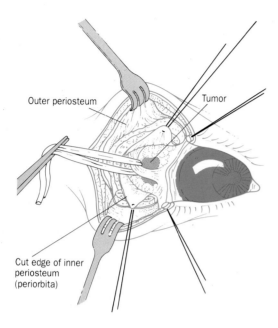

Outer periosteum

Tumor

Cut edge of inner
periosteum
(periorbita)

Figure 26-7 *Once bony flap is removed, periorbita is incised longitudinally and retracted out of the way. Medial rectus muscle is looped with silicone tubing and retracted, improving exposure of tumor.*

tissues. The margin between normal and abnormal structures is visualized and if the lesion is encapsulated and not adherent to surrounding structures, it is removed in toto. Delivery of the mass can be helped by gentle traction using forceps, a cryoprobe, or a suture passed through the lesion. Blunt dissection with cotton-tipped applicator sticks is useful, especially in removing well-encapsulated and not adherent lesions. Infiltrative lesions are biopsied and the diagnosis and extent of spread can sometimes be determined by frozen-section analysis. Excision may need to be delayed until permanent section and special pathologic studies have been done.

Closure begins with careful approximation of the anterior aspect of the periorbita using 5-0 or 4-0 absorbable chromic or polyglycolic sutures. The posterior limb of the incision can be left open to allow drainage from the orbit into the temporal area. The bone is replaced and wired into position using 30-gauge stainless-steel wire or 0 monofilament nylon. Occasionally, the bone is not replaced, especially when invasion by malignancy is suspected or if additional decompressive effect is desired. The upper and lower crura of the lateral canthal tendon and the lateral edges of the eyelid margin are sutured to the orbital periosteum with 4-0 Prolene or nylon sutures so as to reconstruct the canthal angle (Figure 26-8). The temporalis muscle is reattached to the superior temporal crest with 4-0 polyglycolic sutures. A drain is placed in the temporalis fossa and connected to suction, and negative pressure is maintained for 12 to 24 hours. Alternatively, a Penrose drain can be used for gravity drainage. Subcutaneous 5-0 or 6-0 absorbable collagen or polyglycolic sutures appose the deeper skin and muscle layer, and 5-0 or 6-0 subcuticular nylon completes the superficial skin closure. Antibiotic ointment is instilled in the eye. No pressure bandage is used, the head of the bed is elevated, and ice compresses are applied frequently.

26-2-2 Stallard-Wright Lateral Orbitotomy

The superolateral approach to the orbit as modified by Wright allows excellent exposure to lesions of the lacrimal gland, especially when it is necessary to resect the entire lateral wall and part of the orbital roof. An advantage of this approach is that the incision avoids the lateral canthal angle, thus simplifying closure.

The patient is prepped in the usual manner, and a large transparent plastic sheet is applied to the side of the face. This keeps the incision free from contamination and the eyelids closed over the cornea. The incision starts in the eyebrow near the supraorbital notch. It has a lazy-S shape, runs through the lateral half of the eyebrow, curving down some 3 to 4 mm outside the orbital margin, and passes toward the tragus across the zygomatic arch (Figure 26-9). The superior skin–muscle flap is undermined and the plane of dissection carried over the temporalis fascia. Three 4-0 silk traction sutures are placed in each flap and clipped to the head towels. The outer periosteum is incised 2 mm outside and parallel to the orbital rim. Once the level of the zygomatic arch is reached, the incision passes backward along the middle of the zygomatic arch. A

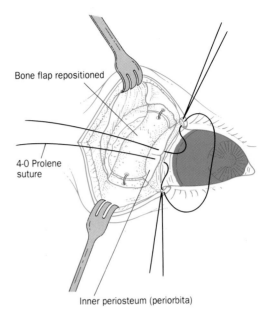

Bone flap repositioned

4-0 Prolene suture

Inner periosteum (periorbita)

Figure 26-8 *Bone is replaced and wired or sutured into position. Lateral canthal angle is reconstructed by suturing upper and lower crura of lateral canthal tendon to inner periosteum.*

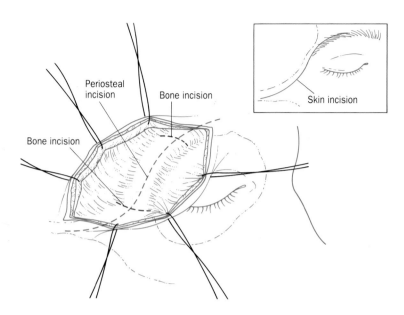

Figure 26-9 *Stallard-Wright lateral orbitotomy. Incision starts in eyebrow, runs laterally, curves downward along orbital rim, and continues laterally along zygomatic arch. Outer periosteum is incised parallel to orbital rim, curving inferiorly along zygomatic arch.*

Periosteal incision

Bone incision

Skin incision

Bone incision

relaxing periosteal incision can be made superiorly and the periosteum is reflected from the lateral wall. The orbitotomy is then performed as described previously for the Berke-Reese lateral orbitotomy.

In the case of an epithelial lacrimal gland tumor, once the lateral rim is removed, resection includes the periosteum overlying the lacrimal gland, the lesion, and, if necessary, the residual lacrimal gland tissue, including the palpebral lobe and ductules in the lateral fornix. If malignancy is present, this resection is enlarged to include the roof of the orbit, a portion of the temporal eyelid, and any involved tissues. The lower pole of the lacrimal gland is identified, together with the lateral rectus muscle. The lateral rectus muscle is freed and a traction stitch or silicone tubing is placed around the muscle belly so it can be retracted, thus giving access to the intraconal surgical space. The position and extent of the orbital tumor are confirmed by palpating the orbital contents. Dissection, biopsy, and removal are then performed as described previously, with emphasis on a blood-free field with good illumination and magnification. Hemostasis must be meticulous and intraorbital structures should be identified by careful dissection and division only under direct visualization, with application of bipolar cautery when necessary. Gentle irrigation and suction, combined with the generous use of cotton-tipped applicator sticks for blunt dissection, improves visualization and dissection.

Once the tumor has been removed from the orbit, all traction sutures are re-

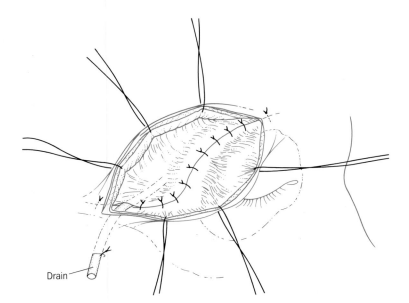

Drain

Figure 26-10 *Outer periosteum is sutured over replaced bony flap. Drain is placed underneath temporalis muscle and passed out through stab incision inferior to skin incision.*

moved and the incision is closed in layers similarly to the Berke-Reese orbitotomy. A 4-0 chromic catgut or polyglycolic suture is used to close the anterior limb of the periorbita, with the posterior limb left open for drainage. The bone, which has been in Ringer's solution, is sutured using stainless-steel wire or 0 monofilament nylon. The temporalis muscle is reattached to the superior temporal crest, and the periosteum is sutured over the lateral wall with 3-0 chromic catgut or 4-0 polyglycolic suture. A drain is placed underneath the temporalis muscle and passed to the exterior through a small stab incision just above the zygomatic arch (Figure 26-10). Interrupted buried subcutaneous 6-0 collagen or polyglycolic sutures are placed, and the skin edge is approximated with continuous 4-0 or 5-0 subcuticular nylon suture. Intravenous antibiotics and corticosteroids are given intraoperatively prior to the re-

placement of bone. Vaseline gauze is used to cover the incision, and a dressing applied to the incision. It is not necessary to patch the eye, and ice compresses can be applied. The drain is connected to suction until the next day. The subcuticular suture is removed in 10 to 14 days.

26-2-3 Coronal Scalp Flap Lateral Orbitotomy

The coronal scalp flap has been widely used for cosmetic surgery, sinus surgery, neurosurgery, and craniofacial reconstruction. Stewart and associates described the coronal scalp flap approach to the lateral orbitotomy in selected patients to improve exposure, especially for extensive lesions involving the apex and the superior orbit. Cosmesis is improved, as the scar is hidden in the hair of the scalp. A strip of hair posterior to the hairline is trimmed and shaved. Alternatively, the incision can be made at the hairline. The area of the incision is injected with lidocaine with epinephrine to aid in hemostasis. The incision extends from ear to ear and is deep to the galea aponeurotica, but above the temporalis fascia, thus avoiding bleeding from the temporalis muscle. The flap is then reflected inferiorly with dissection in the avascular subgaleal plane. Special attention is paid laterally in the temporal fossa because the facial nerve runs superficial to the temporal fascia and damage to it can result in paralysis of the eyebrow. The scalp is mobilized anteriorly, exposing the temporalis muscle, superior orbital rim, and lateral orbital rim to the level of the zygomatic arch. The supraorbital vessels and nerves are preserved. The temporalis muscle is disinserted from its attachment and is retracted posteroinferiorly. A lateral orbitotomy can then be performed in the usual manner. More extensive osteotomies and soft-tissue flaps can be fashioned if necessary. The temporalis muscle is reattached using 4-0 absorbable polyglycolic suture. The scalp is closed with 4-0 absorbable polyglycolic sutures, and the skin with running 5-0 nylon or Prolene sutures. A suction drain is placed and a Vaseline or nonadherent absorbent gauze is applied to the incision.

Intravenous antibiotics and corticosteroids are given intraoperatively and continued orally in the postoperative period.

Apical and extensive orbital lesions that need transcranial resection can also be approached through a coronal flap as described by Kennerdell and associates.[6] Superior orbital lesions such as frontal sinus mucoceles can also be readily approached this way.*

26-3

COMBINED ORBITOTOMIES

The lateral orbitotomy can be combined with medial and inferior approaches to get better exposure (Figure 26-11). Lesions in the medial posterior orbit are best visualized if a lateral orbitotomy is performed; the globe can then be displaced laterally and the medial space entered through a conjunctival incision. The medial rectus can be detached for better exposure of the optic nerve and the medial orbital apex. An operating microscope allows detailed evaluation of the optic nerve or any lesions near it. The muscle is reattached using 6-0 polyglycolic sutures, and the lateral orbitotomy is closed in the usual manner.

Lesions lying in the inferior or inferonasal orbit can be approached through the inferior fornix with a lateral cantholysis followed by a lateral bony orbitotomy if needed. If the lesion is easily palpable and resectable within the orbital fat, it is not necessary to elevate the periosteum or remove the lateral rim.

---

*See also Chapter 29, "Periorbital and Craniofacial Surgery," in this volume.—ED.

26-4

COMPLICATIONS OF ORBITAL SURGERY

Loss of vision, the most feared complication of orbital surgery, can be the result of traumatic manipulation of the optic nerve and its blood supply or secondary to optic nerve compression by blood or swelling. This complication occurs most commonly with optic nerve lesions or those surrounding the nerve. Ptosis and diplopia are common postoperative complications; however, they are usually transient and resolve within a few weeks. Neuroparalytic keratopathy, pupillary changes, hypesthesia of the forehead, temporalis muscle atrophy, seventh nerve weakness, keratitis sicca, cerebrospinal fluid leak, and infection are less common complications.

26-5

KEY POINTS IN ORBITAL SURGERY

Orbital surgery entails a number of areas that are of current interest:

1. *Imaging* Computed tomography (CT) and magnetic resonance imaging (MRI) have greatly aided the orbital surgeon in the diagnosis and localization of orbital tumors. The location of the tumor, its proximity to the optic nerve and other orbital structures, must be taken into consideration preoperatively and the most direct route of entry with the least risk and best exposure planned.

2. *Positioning* The patient is placed in a reverse Trendelenburg position to reduce arterial flow and venous back pressure. When a lateral orbitotomy is planned, the

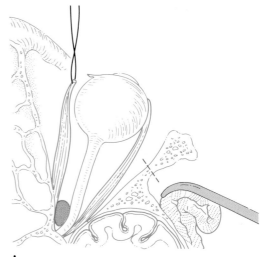

A

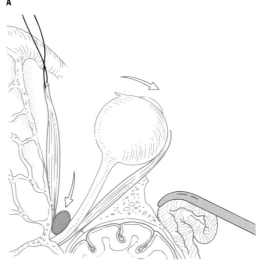

B

Figure 26-11 *Tumor in medial posterior orbit is best visualized by performing lateral orbitotomy, displacing globe laterally, and entering medial space through conjunctival incision. (A) Lateral bony rim in place. (B) Lateral bony rim removed.*

head is turned so as to expose the lateral aspect of the face. Adhesive plastic drapes help maintain a sterile field. Additionally, they provide a point of anchor for retracting sutures.

3. *Anesthesia and hemostasis* Hypotensive anesthesia helps in maintaining a bloodless field. Preoperative injection of lidocaine with epinephrine along the incision site contributes to vasoconstriction. The patient should be told not to use aspirin, anti-inflammatory drugs, and other medications that impair platelet aggregation and increase peripheral blood flow for 2 weeks preoperatively.

4. *Instruments* A variety of microsurgical, neurosurgical, and otolaryngologic instruments can be used for orbital surgery. Straight and curved malleable retractors, muscle hooks, and skin and vein retractors are used to achieve good exposure. Cottonoids and cotton-tipped applicators help in maintaining a bloodless field. Additionally, cotton-tipped applicators can be used for blunt dissection. Periosteal elevators, rongeurs, and bone-cutting instruments need to be available. Air-driven microsurgical bone-cutting instruments, including sagittal saws, oscillating saws, and drills, are light and easily manipulated. Microsurgical forceps, scissors, and microdissectors cause minimal trauma to tissues. Loupes ranging from 2 to 5 power, when combined with fiberoptic illumination, provide adequate visualization for most orbital procedures. The operative microscope is necessary, especially when operating on the optic nerve or at the orbital apex through an intracranial approach. Lasers are being introduced in the field of orbital surgery. The carbon dioxide laser is valuable in extirpating orbital lymphangiomas by maintaining hemostasis while debulking the tumor.

26-5-1 Surgical Pearls

Several surgical "pearls" may be helpful, especially to the less experienced surgeon:

1. Patience is key to a meticulous and bloodless dissection; rushing can result in disaster.

2. Clinicopathologic knowledge of orbital tumors is very important in choosing the best surgical approach and treatment. Cavernous hemangiomas can be punctured by a suture and partly drained, making removal easier. Similarly, hematic cysts and dermoid cysts can sometimes be drained anteriorly, allowing better exposure and making posterior dissection easier. If there is a suspicion of a benign mixed tumor of the lacrimal gland, care needs to be taken to remove the tumor in toto to prevent recurrence or malignant change. If malignancy or inflammation is suspected, a biopsy with the least manipulation is the first step. If metastatic disease is suspected, a fine-needle aspiration biopsy can be a viable option to open biopsy.

3. Imaging studies must be available in the operating room: the tumor may be hard to localize and a fresh look at the scans can be very helpful.

4. The ophthalmologist must know when to consult and enlist the help of the otolaryngologist, the craniofacial surgeon, and the neurosurgeon.

5. When obtaining a biopsy, the surgeon should make sure the specimen is adequate and placed in the appropriate solution, consulting with the pathologist when in doubt. Frozen sections can help to ensure that the right tissue was biopsied.

6. The size of the pupil should be monitored during the procedure. Dilation of the pupil indicates excess manipulation or retraction of the optic nerve and should be avoided.

7. The bipolar cautery is preferred for hemostasis in the intraconal space. Thrombin-soaked Gelfoam can help control oozing. Careful closure following tumor removal with appropriate drainage results in a good functional and cosmetic result.

REFERENCES

1. Krönlein RU: Zur Pathologie und operativen Behandlung der Dermoidcysten. *Beitr Klin Chir* 1888;4:149.

2. Berke RN: A modified Krönlein operation. *Arch Ophthalmol* 1954;51:609–632.

3. Stallard HB: A plea for lateral orbitotomy with certain modifications. *Br J Ophthalmol* 1960;44:718.

4. Wright JE: Surgery on the orbit. In: Symon L, ed: *Neurosurgery*. 3rd ed. London: Butterworth; 1979:430–437.

5. Bonavolontà G: Evolution of the lateral orbitotomy (coronal approach to the orbit). *Acta: XXIV International Congress of Ophthalmology*. Philadelphia: JB Lippincott Co; 1983;2:1036–1038.

6. Kennerdell JS, Maroon JC, Malton ML: Surgical approaches to orbital tumors. *Clin Plast Surg* 1988;15:273–282.

7. Stewart WB, Levin PS, Toth BA: Orbital surgery: the technique of coronal scalp flap approach to the lateral orbitotomy. *Arch Ophthalmol* 1988;106:1724–1726.

SUGGESTED READINGS

Goldberg RA, Lessner AM, Shorr N, Baylis HI: The transconjunctival approach to the orbital floor and orbital fat: a prospective study. *Ophthalmic Plast Reconstr Surg* 1990;6:241–246.

Henderson JW: *Orbital Tumors*. New York: Decker; 1980:580–601.

Kennerdell JS, Dekker A, Johnson BL, Dubois PJ: Fine-needle aspiration biopsy: its use in orbital tumors. *Arch Ophthalmol* 1979;97:1315–1317.

Krohel GB, Stewart WB, Chavis RM: *Orbital Disease: A Practical Approach*. New York: Grune & Stratton; 1981:95–116.

Leone CR Jr: Surgical approaches to the orbit. *Ophthalmology* 1979;86:930–941.

McCord CD Jr: Surgical approaches to orbital disease. In: McCord CD, Tanenbaum M, eds: *Oculoplastic Surgery*. New York: Raven Press; 1987:257–278.

Nowinski T, Anderson RL: Advances in orbital surgery. *Ophthalmic Plast Reconstr Surg* 1985;1:211–217.

Rootman J: *Diseases of the Orbit: A Multidisciplinary Approach*. Philadelphia: JB Lippincott Co; 1988:579–612.

Stallard HB: The evolution of lateral orbitotomy. *Trans Ophthalmol Soc UK* 1974;93:3–17.

CHAPTER 27

Surgical Decompression of the Orbit

Patrick M. Flaharty, MD
Bhupendra C. Patel, MD
Richard L. Anderson, MD

In 1835 Graves first described the characteristic exophthalmos of thyroid eye disease, and his name has since become synonymous with thyrotoxic ophthalmopathy. Graves' disease is relatively common, with a prevalence and incidence of 1% and 0.1%, respectively.[1] Although subtle signs of ophthalmopathy are present in most patients with Graves' disease, only 30% have obvious eye findings and only 5% develop ophthalmopathy severe enough to warrant specific treatment with radiotherapy, immunosuppression, or orbital decompression surgery.

OVERVIEW OF GRAVES' DISEASE

While the onset of Graves' disease usually occurs when people are in their forties, thyroid optic neuropathy tends to occur in the fifties and sixties, underscoring the importance of careful long-term followup of these patients.[2,3] The ophthalmopathy of Graves' disease is usually associated with hyperthyroidism, but occurs in euthyroid and hypothyroid patients as well. The clinical course of the ophthalmopathy does not directly correlate with the thyroid status, although more than 80% of thyroid patients who develop severe ophthalmopathy do so within 18 months of the detection of the thyroid disease.[4] The early findings of thyroid ophthalmopathy include conjunctival injection, lacrimation, ocular surface irritation, orbital and periorbital swelling, and mild eyelid retraction. Progression of the disease can result in severe orbital congestion, massive enlargement of the extraocular muscles with secondary diplopia, proptosis, compressive optic neuropathy, prominent eyelid retraction, spontaneous subluxation of the globe anterior to the eyelids, and exposure keratopathy. Treatment options for these serious complications of Graves' disease include systemic corticosteroids, radiation therapy, and orbital decompression surgery.*

Radiation therapy has shown promise in the treatment of the acute congestive phase of Graves' ophthalmopathy.[5-7] The role of radiation therapy in the management of thyroid optic neuropathy is controversial. Some orbital specialists have found radiation therapy useful in the management of compressive optic neuropathy and reserve orbital decompression surgery for patients who fail radiation therapy. Others feel that compressive optic neuropathy from Graves' disease is best managed with orbital decompression surgery and reserve orbital radiation for patients who fail to respond favorably to decompression surgery. These surgeons contend that orbital radiation causes a short-term increase in orbital congestion and may not have its maximal effect for several months after treatment, while orbital decompression surgery gives immediate relief of the optic nerve compression.[5] Radiation therapy is generally less effective than orbital decompression surgery in reducing severe proptosis. The long-term effects of orbital radiation in the treatment of thyroid eye disease have yet to be adequately studied.

Systemic corticosteroids are an effective temporizing measure in the acute management of thyroid optic neuropathy, but side effects make this an unattractive alternative for the long-term management of these patients.[5] Corticosteroids are very effective for the short-term relief of orbital congestion and are often used perioperatively with orbital decompression surgery and in conjunction with orbital radiation.

Orbital decompression surgery involves the surgical expansion of the bony orbital cavity and removal of orbital fat to reduce orbital pressure and proptosis. Combined with high-dose perioperative corticosteroids, orbital decompression surgery remains, in the view of the authors, the most effective method for the rapid and sustained reversal of visual loss associated with thyroid optic neuropathy and malignant exophthalmos. Although the authors employ orbital radiation in the management of the early inflammatory complications of Graves' disease, in the treatment of thyroid optic neuropathy, we reserve orbital radiation to those patients unresponsive to orbital decompression and patients unable to undergo surgery.[8,9]

---

*See also Chapter 25, "Evaluation and Spectrum of Orbital Diseases," in this volume.—Ed.

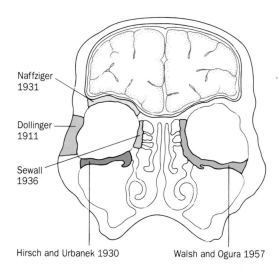

Naffziger 1931

Dollinger 1911

Sewall 1936

Hirsch and Urbanek 1930

Walsh and Ogura 1957

Figure 27-1 *Early methods of orbital decompression.*

27-2

OVERVIEW OF ORBITAL DECOMPRESSION

Orbital decompression techniques involving one, two, three, and four walls have been described in the management of Graves' ophthalmopathy. Early orbital decompression surgery involved the removal of a single orbital wall (Figure 27-1). In 1911 Dollinger described the Kronlein lateral orbitotomy approach for removal of the lateral orbital wall and is credited with the first description of orbital decompression surgery.[10] In the 1930s, Naffziger described the removal of the orbital roof; Sewall, the medial orbital wall; and Hirsch and Urbanek, the orbital floor in an attempt to correct thyroid-related proptosis.[11-13] In 1957 Walsh and Ogura described the simultaneous removal of the medial wall and orbital floor in what amounted to a combination of the Sewall and Hirsch techniques.[14] This two-walled orbital decompression remains the most common procedure today and is effective in releasing pressure on the optic nerve and reducing mild to moderate degrees of proptosis (4 mm).

Many approaches to the bony orbit are described in the literature, including transcutaneous, transconjunctival, transantral, transcranial, and transnasal. The advent of miniplate fixation and craniofacial surgery has led to the development of more extensive orbital expansion procedures.[15,16] These include advancement and outward rotation of the lateral orbital wall in an attempt to achieve a greater degree of lateral orbital expansion. In combination with traditional techniques, these procedures allow for a greater reduction in proptosis (>6 mm) and may be indicated in the management of severe exophthalmos.

Advances in endoscopic sinus surgery have recently been employed in the development of a "closed" decompression of the medial orbital wall and orbital floor. These techniques have also been used in combination with the open decompression techniques and may play a larger role in orbital decompression surgery in the future. Another relatively new approach to orbital decompression surgery is the "balanced" orbital decompression. The procedure involves the symmetric decompression of both the medial and the lateral orbital walls, with preservation of the orbital floor. This approach has a lower incidence of postoperative muscle imbalance and may be useful in patients with no preoperative diplopia. To further broaden the scope of the surgical options, Oliveri has reported good results with meticulous extirpation of intraconal and extraconal orbital fat without bone removal.[17] This fat-extirpation technique can be used in conjunction with traditional techniques to achieve greater degrees of decompression.

27-3

INDICATIONS FOR ORBITAL DECOMPRESSION

Indications for orbital decompression surgery include visual loss from compressive optic neuropathy, severe proptosis with exposure keratopathy, recurrent globe prolapse anterior to the eyelids, and cosmetically objectionable exophthalmos. Although some of the "bug-eyed" appearance of Graves' ophthalmopathy can be masked with eyelid surgery, patients with greater than 24 to 25 mm of proptosis usually require orbital decompression surgery prior to eyelid surgery to achieve acceptable cosmetic results. Improved techniques in orbital decompression surgery have led to an increase in the number of elective cases for the cosmetic correction of exophthalmos. When possible, orbital decompression surgery should be delayed until the thyroid function has been regulated and the orbitopathy stabilized, with no evidence of progression for several months. In cases of severe visual loss, such postponement may not be possible.

27-4

EVALUATION OF THE THYROID PATIENT

A multidisciplinary approach to the thyroid patient, involving an endocrinologist, a neuro-ophthalmologist, a strabismus specialist, and an orbital surgeon, is required. Preoperative evaluation of the thyroid status is imperative to avoid the risk of thyroid storm. A careful evaluation of the visual function, including visual acuity, pupillary examination, color vision evaluation, and formal visual field testing, establishes a baseline level of visual function to be used for future comparison. Slit-lamp biomicroscopy with fluorescein helps identify any corneal surface irregularities,

which can contribute to visual impairment and ocular discomfort. A detailed evaluation of extraocular muscle motility is essential and aids in predicting the extent of postdecompression motility disturbance. Preoperative computed tomography (CT) scans should include coronal sections through the orbits to identify the position of the cribriform plate, to visualize ethmoid air-cell anatomy, and to rule out preexisting sinus disease. Although orbital magnetic resonance imaging (MRI) provides excellent soft-tissue detail, it does not display the bone detail necessary for preoperative planning.

As orbital decompression is often the first step in a series of rehabilitative procedures, a thorough discussion of the treatment plan should be undertaken with the patient prior to surgery. Subsequent steps may include extraocular muscle surgery to reduce diplopia and eyelid surgery to correct significant eyelid retraction. A discussion of the surgical risks should include diplopia, abnormal globe displacement, sinusitis, infraorbital hypesthesia, nasolacrimal duct obstruction, significant blood loss requiring transfusion, cerebrospinal fluid leaks, meningitis, and visual loss.

27-5

TECHNIQUES FOR ORBITAL DECOMPRESSION

The most commonly employed orbital decompression procedures are modifications of the medial wall and orbital floor technique first described by Walsh and Ogura (Figure 27-2).[14] Various approaches to these areas have been used, including transantral, transcutaneous via subciliary or external ethmoidectomy incisions, transconjunctival, and transnasal with the aid of an endoscope.[18,19] Ophthalmologists most commonly use either the transconjunctival or the transantral approach, and some advocate a combination to maximize the benefits of these two techniques.[20]

McCord and Moses first described a lateral canthotomy, transconjunctival approach to avoid cutaneous scar formation and ectropion.[21] This is the approach most often used by the authors. Advocates of this anterior orbital approach state that better visualization of the anterior orbital structures, including the infraorbital neurovascular bundle, lacrimal sac, and inferior oblique muscle, reduces the operative morbidity. Some reports suggest that the transantral approach has a greater complication rate, including a higher incidence of strabismus, oroantral fistulas, infraorbital hypesthesia, and sinusitis.[22,23] Advocates of the transantral approach, however, believe that this approach provides better exposure of the posterior orbital floor. This may aid in a more complete posterior decompression, which is the most critical factor when dealing with compressive optic neuropathy. Good results have been achieved with both approaches, and the choice remains that of the individual surgeon.

The authors generally prefer a transconjunctival anterior technique with and without removal of the lateral orbital wall. This technique is performed under general anesthesia. Once the patient is prepped and draped in the usual sterile fashion, a small amount of 0.5% lidocaine with 1:200,000 epinephrine is infiltrated transconjunctivally into the lateral canthus and lower eyelid. The vasoconstricting effect of the epinephrine reduces intraoperative bleeding. A surgical headlight and operating loupes are essential for good visualization of the anatomic landmarks during the procedure.

A lateral canthotomy with an inferior cantholysis is completed to free the lower eyelid, exposing the inferior fornix. A unipolar electrocautery is used to divide the conjunctiva and lower eyelid retractors between the inferior tarsal border and the inferior conjunctival fornix. The fat pockets of the lower eyelid are sequentially exposed and liberally debulked; this step is similar to a transconjunctival lower eyelid blepharoplasty (Figure 27-3). Once fat has been removed back to the level of the infraorbital rim, the periosteum is incised along the inner aspect of the orbital rim. A Freer periosteal elevator is then used to elevate the periorbita from the orbital floor. The periosteum is thick and strongly adherent at the orbital rim, but dissects off the orbital floor with minimal resistance. A blunt-tipped Freer periosteal elevator or Sewall orbital retractors can be used to reflect the periorbita off the orbital floor more posteriorly (Figure 27-4).

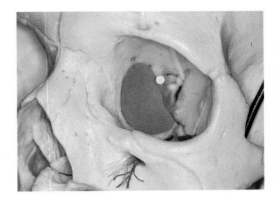

Figure 27-2 *Colored area represents bone removed from orbital floor and medial orbital wall during orbital decompression surgery.*

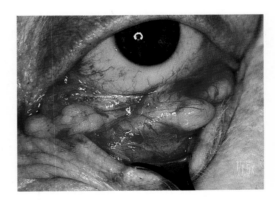

Figure 27-3 *Fat pads of lower lid are exposed and liberally debulked through transconjunctival incision.*

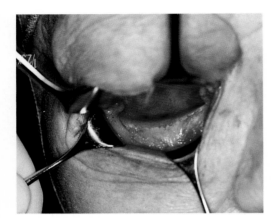

Figure 27-4 *Sewall retractors are used to reflect orbital contents superiorly, exposing orbital floor.*

Inspection of the orbital floor reveals a small elevation over the infraorbital neurovascular bundle. A curved hemostat is used to puncture a hole in the anterior orbital floor medial to the neurovascular bundle. A small bone punch is then used to remove the anteromedial orbital floor. The posteromedial orbital floor is then removed using a front-biting instrument such as ethmoidectomy forceps. The orbital floor should be removed to the posterior wall of the maxillary sinus. The posterior wall is identified by the thick, three-pronged strut of bone formed by fusion of the orbital floor, superomedial wall of the maxillary sinus, and infralateral wall of the ethmoid sinus. Although removal of this strut may be necessary in treating compressive optic neuropathy, it can result in a greater degree of postoperative muscle imbalance and diplopia. For this reason, the strut should be spared in cosmetic orbital decompression surgery without optic neuropathy.

The dissection then proceeds into the ethmoid sinus, starting posterior to the lacrimal bone. The ethmoid bone, air cells, and mucosa are removed back to, and including, the posterior ethmoid air cells. Brisk bleeding can occur as the ethmoid sinus is entered and is best controlled by the thorough extirpation of the ethmoid mucosa. Complete removal of the posterior ethmoid air cells is more critical in treating compressive optic neuropathy. The dissection is kept below the medial canthal tendon and frontoethmoidal suture to avoid inadvertent damage to the cribriform plate. Careful preoperative evaluation of the coronal CT images is essential in identifying the location of the cribriform plate relative to the ethmoid sinus. The most inferior extension of the cribriform plate is usually into the anterior ethmoid air cells, where great care should be taken to avoid cerebrospinal fluid leaks.

Removal of the posterior orbital floor and posterior ethmoid air cells back to the optic canal is essential to reduce pressure on the optic nerve. Visualization of these structures, however, can be difficult with this transconjunctival approach. Digital palpation of the orbital floor and medial orbital wall assists in identifying residual bone struts, which may hinder a complete decompression of the orbital apex. Some surgeons employ the transconjunctival approach inferiorly, combined with either an external ethmoidectomy (Lynch) approach or a transnasal endoscopic approach to the medial orbital wall. These latter approaches may provide better visualization of the posteromedial orbital wall.

For those patients with mild proptosis (<24 mm), this inferomedial orbital decompression is generally satisfactory. Patients with moderate proptosis (24 to 28 mm) usually require removal of the lateral orbital floor and lateral wall (Figure 27-5). A curved hemostat or small osteotome can be used to puncture the orbital floor lateral to the infraorbital nerve. The orbital floor is thicker in this area and slightly more difficult to puncture. Front- and back-biting instruments are then used to remove the lateral orbital floor back to the infraorbital fissure. Care is taken not to dissect into the infraorbital fissure, where damage to the infraorbital nerve and excessive bleeding can occur. The anterior portion of the infraorbital fissure extends into the midorbit and is quickly encoun-

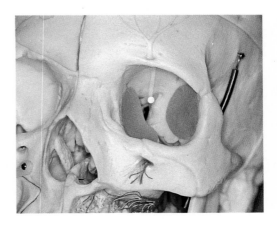

Figure 27-5 *Bone can be removed from lateral orbital wall when additional decompression is needed.*

tered when dissecting posteriorly along the lateral orbital floor. Even with maximal orbital decompression, a strut of bone should be preserved over the infraorbital nerve to prevent the globe from dropping too far inferiorly (ie, hypoglobus).

Next, the lateral canthal tendon can be disinserted and the inner aspect of the lateral orbital wall either burred away with a small, round burr on a power drill or excised with a large rongeur, leaving the orbital rim intact. Moderate lateral expansion of the orbit can be achieved by aggressive burring of the bone along the lateral orbital wall. Some authors advocate a second incision in the upper eyelid crease to assist in removing the most superior and posterior aspect of the lateral orbital wall. Other techniques of lateral orbital decompression include complete removal of the lateral orbital wall through an extended lateral canthotomy incision,[8] advancing or rotating the lateral orbital wall with miniplate fixation,[15,16] and a coronal transtemporalis approach for removal of the lateral wall while leaving the orbital rim intact.[24]

As mentioned earlier, some orbital surgeons advocate a "balanced" orbital decompression to reduce the incidence of postoperative diplopia and globe displacement. The procedure involves a symmetric decompression of the medial and lateral orbital walls while leaving the orbital floor intact. This technique may be best suited for patients with no preoperative diplopia, mild to moderate proptosis, and no evidence of optic neuropathy.

Removal of additional orbital fat can assist in a more complete orbital decompression.[17] Fat from within and around the muscle cone can be removed from the medial, inferior, and lateral orbit through this incision. A second incision in the upper eyelid crease can access the superior orbit for additional fat removal. Great care must be taken when removing intraconal and posterior orbital fat to avoid excessive bleeding and injury to vital structures.*

The advent of miniplate and microplate fixation has ushered in a new era in craniofacial surgery. These techniques have been used to develop more aggressive orbital expansion procedures.[15,16] Advancement and rotation of the lateral orbital wall expands the orbit both internally and externally, and can aid in a greater reduction in proptosis. For severe exophthalmos, some authors have advocated a neurosurgical approach to a four-walled decompression.[25,26] These four-walled decompressions allow maximal expansion of the orbital volume, resulting in a greater reduction in exophthalmos. The procedures may involve greater morbidity, however, and are best reserved for patients with severe proptosis (>30 mm). Figures 27-6 and 27-7 demonstrate examples of preoperative and postoperative CT images and clinical photographs in patients who have undergone orbital decompression surgery.

---

*Many surgeons advocate opening/slitting the periorbita to allow fat prolapse, with or without fat excision, to enhance the decompressive effect—ED.

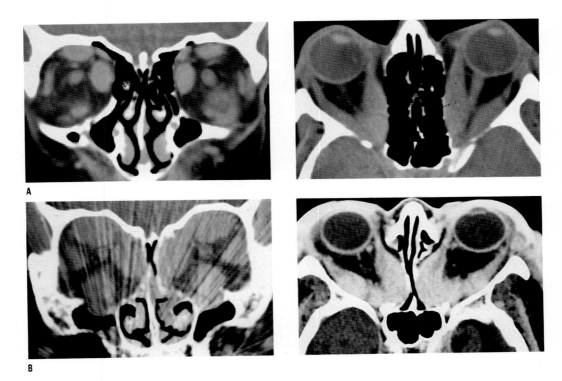

Figure 27-6 *Severe thyroid orbitopathy. (A) Preoperative CT images show massive enlargement of extraocular muscles. (B) Postoperative CT images of another patient demonstrate thorough decompression of medial orbital wall and medial two thirds of orbital floor, showing how muscles prolapse into ethmoid and maxillary sinuses.*

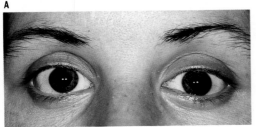

Figure 27-7 *Proptosis from Graves' disease. (A) Preoperative appearance. (B) Postoperative appearance shows substantial reduction in proptosis.*

27-6

COMPLICATIONS OF ORBITAL DECOMPRESSION

Orbital decompression surgery by any approach carries a significant risk of serious complications. These include diplopia, obstruction of the maxillary sinus ostium with secondary sinusitis, preseptal and orbital cellulitis, nasolacrimal duct obstruction, lateral canthal deformity, globe malposition (ie, hypoglobus), extensive blood loss, cerebrospinal fluid leaks and secondary meningitis, infraorbital hypesthesia, and visual loss.

Maxillary sinusitis may require placement of a nasoantral window to facilitate adequate sinus drainage. Persistent diplopia will require corrective strabismus surgery. Eyelid retraction is not specifically addressed with orbital decompression surgery, and corrective eyelid surgery may be required despite a reduction in proptosis. Numbness of the ipsilateral cheek and gums is common, usually lasts from 3 to 6 months, and in some cases is permanent. Damage to the lacrimal sac or nasolacrimal duct may lead to permanent nasolacrimal obstruction, requiring secondary dacryocystorhinostomy. Persistent or recurrent optic neuropathy can occur even after maximal orbital decompression surgery. In this event, an orbital CT scan should be obtained to rule out residual bone that may be impinging on the optic nerve. Reoperation may be necessary to remove residual bone struts near the orbital apex. In the face of failed orbital decompression surgery with no evidence of residual bony compression of the optic nerve, systemic corticosteroids and orbital radiation therapy should be instituted.

REFERENCES

1. Felig P, et al, eds: *Endocrinology and Metabolism.* 2nd ed. New York: McGraw-Hill; 1987: 440–443.

2. Trobe JD, Glaser JS, Laflamme P: Dysthyroid optic neuropathy: clinical profile and rationale for management. *Arch Ophthalmol* 1978; 96:1199–1209.

3. Neigel JM, Rootman J, Belkin RI, et al: Dysthyroid optic neuropathy: the crowded orbital apex syndrome. *Ophthalmology* 1988;95: 1515–1521.

4. Gorman CA: Temporal relationship between onset of Graves' ophthalmopathy and diagnosis of thyrotoxicosis. *Mayo Clin Proc* 1983;58: 515–519.

5. Kazim M, Trokel S, Moore S: Treatment of acute Graves' orbitopathy. *Ophthalmology* 1991; 98:1443–1448.

6. Char DH: The ophthalmopathy of Graves' disease. *Med Clin North Am* 1991;75:97–119.

7. Donaldson SS, Bagshaw MA, Kriss JP: Supervoltage orbital radiotherapy for Graves' ophthalmopathy. *J Clin Endocrinol Metab* 1973; 37:276–285.

8. McCord CD Jr: Orbital decompression for Graves' disease: exposure through lateral canthal and inferior fornix incision. *Ophthalmology* 1981;88:533–541.

9. Carter KD, Frueh BR, Hessburg TP, Musch DC: Long-term efficacy of orbital decompression for compressive optic neuropathy of Graves' eye disease. *Ophthalmology* 1991;98: 1435–1442.

10. Dollinger J: Die Druckentlastung der Augenhohle durch Entfernung der auBeren Orbitalwand bei hochgradigen Exophthalmus (Morbus Basedow) und konsekutiver Hornhauterkrankung. *Dtsch Med Wochenschr* 1911;37: 1888–1890.

11. Naffziger HC: Progressive exophthalmos following thyroidectomy: its pathology and treatment. *Ann Surg* 1931;94:582–586.

12. Sewall EC: Operative control of progressive exophthalmos. *Arch Otolaryngol* 1936;24: 621–624.

13. Hirsch VO, Urbanek GR: Behandlung eines excessiven Exophthalmus (Basedow) durch Entfernung von Orbitalfett von der Kieferhohle aus. *Monatsschr F Ohrenh* 1930;64: 212–213.

14. Walsh TE, Ogura JH: Transantral orbital decompression for malignant exophthalmos. *Laryngoscope* 1957;67:544–568.

15. Wolfe SA: Modified three-wall orbital expansion to correct persistent exophthalmos or exorbitism. *Plast Reconstr Surg* 1979;64: 448–455.

16. Wulc AE, Popp JC, Bartlett SP: Lateral wall advancement in orbital decompression. *Ophthalmology* 1990;97:1358–1369.

17. Olivari N: Transpalpebral decompression of endocrine ophthalmopathy (Graves' disease) by removal of intraorbital fat: experience with 147 operations over 5 years. *Plast Reconstr Surg* 1991;87:627–641.

18. Kennedy DW, Goodstein ML, Miller NR, Zinreich SJ: Endoscopic transnasal orbital decompression. *Arch Otolaryngol Head Neck Surg* 1990;116:275–282.

19. Anderson RL, Linberg JV: Transorbital approach to decompression in Graves' disease. *Arch Ophthalmol* 1981;99:120–124.

20. Kulwin DR, Cotton RT, Kersten RC: Combined approach to orbital decompression. *Otolaryngol Clin North Am* 1990;23:381–390.

21. McCord CD Jr, Moses JL: Exposure of the inferior orbit with fornix incision and lateral canthotomy. *Ophthalmic Surg* 1979;10:53–63.

22. Warren JD, Spector JG, Burde R: Long-term follow-up and recent observations on 305 cases of orbital decompression for dysthyroid orbitopathy. *Laryngoscope* 1989;99:35–40.

23. DeSanto LW: Transantral orbital decompression. In: Gorman CA, Waller RR, Dyer JA, eds: *The Eye and Orbit in Thyroid Disease.* New York: Raven Press; 1984:231–251.

24. Leatherbarrow B, Lendrum J, Mahaffey PJ, et al: Three wall orbital decompression for Graves' ophthalmopathy via a coronal approach. *Eye* 1991;5:456–465.

25. Maroon JC, Kennerdell JS: Radical orbital decompression for severe dysthyroid exophthalmos. *J Neurosurg* 1982;56:260–266.

26. Stranc M, West M: A four-wall orbital decompression for dysthyroid orbitopathy. *J Neurosurg* 1988;68:671–677.

Optic Nerve Sheath Decompression

Thomas C. Spoor, MD, MS
John G. McHenry, MD, MPH

Optic nerve sheath decompression (ONSD) has been described as a good operation looking for indications. The generally accepted, peer-reviewed indication for ONSD is papilledema and progressive visual loss.[1-5] Papilledema may be secondary to brain tumor, pseudotumor cerebri, cryptococcal meningitis, or any other cause of elevated intracranial pressure compressing the optic nerve fibers at the lamina cribrosa. Less than universally agreed indications include arteritic and nonarteritic ischemic optic neuropathy,[6-8] optic pits with serous retinal detachments, optic neuropathy accompanying acute retinal necrosis,[9] central retinal vein occlusions, optic nerve drusen with progressive visual loss, hydrocephalus, cryptococcal meningitis, and traumatic optic neuropathy. Only treatment of nonarteritic anterior ischemic optic neuropathy (NAION) with ONSD has undergone the scrutiny of a controlled clinical trial and surgery in this cohort of patients proved to be of no benefit and possibly detrimental to patients with NAION.

28-1

HISTORICAL BACKGROUND

Optic nerve sheath decompression for treatment of visual loss secondary to refractory papilledema was first described by DeWecker in 1872.[10] He identified the optic nerve sheath by palpation and incised it blindly with a guarded knife. Later, Carter and Müller incised the optic nerve sheath under direct visualization after disinserting the lateral rectus muscle.[11-13] In 1964, Hayreh demonstrated the effectiveness of ONSD in relieving experimental papilledema in rhesus monkeys.[14]

Clinical acceptance was enhanced after Smith, Hoyt, and Newton described relief of chronic papilledema by ONSD.[15] They

approached the optic nerve medially after performing an antecedent lateral orbitotomy to enhance exposure. That same year, Davidson described approaching the optic nerve sheath through a lateral orbitotomy.[16] In 1992, Anderson refined this approach by making a lateral eyelid crease incision and omitting the osteotomies. This approach is presently preferred by some surgeons.[3]

Galbraith and Sullivan were the first to approach the optic nerve through a transconjunctival medial orbitotomy and disinsertion of the medial rectus muscle.[17] This is the surgical approach preferred by most surgeons.[1,2,4,8]

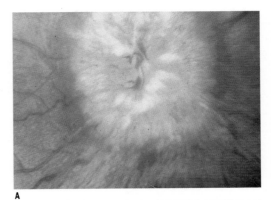

A

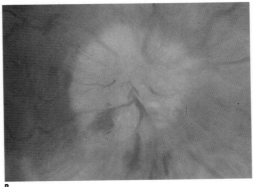

B

Figure 28-1 *High-grade, asymmetric papilledema in a patient with pseudotumor cerebri. (A) Right eye. (B) Left eye.*

28-2

INDICATIONS FOR OPTIC NERVE SHEATH DECOMPRESSION

Patients with papilledema and visual loss, especially progressive visual loss, are suitable candidates for optic nerve sheath decompression, which may effectively relieve the papilledema and restore visual function in these patients. The following case is illustrative. A 35-year-old woman presented with high-grade papilledema (Figure 28-1). Neuroimaging studies revealed no evidence of a compressive mass lesion. Intracranial pressure was markedly elevated by lumbar puncture. Visual acuity was 20/200 OD, 20/25 OS, and visual fields were markedly constricted in both eyes. ONSD was performed first on the right eye and then on the left eye 1 week later. By 6 weeks after surgery, optic disc swelling had resolved (Figure 28-2) and visual function had normalized.

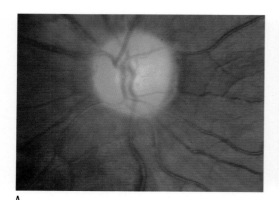

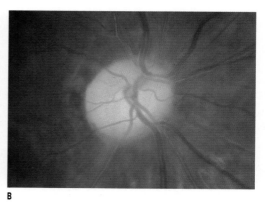

A

B

Figure 28-2 *Resolution of papilledema after successful ONSD. (A) Right eye. (B) Left eye.*

It is important to understand that after successful ONSD, the intracranial pressure may remain elevated but the optic discs may not swell again. Analogous to patients with chronic open-angle glaucoma, patients with pseudotumor cerebri must be followed up routinely with reproducible visual fields to detect evidence of recurrent visual dysfunction.[18] Visual field loss secondary to elevated intracranial pressure may be treated with systemic acetazolamide. If visual loss is progressive, secondary ONSD is technically more difficult than primary ONSD but may be performed successfully.[5] In the authors' experience, neurosurgical shunting procedures are not ideal management for patients with pseudotumor cerebri who have failed ONSD. Lumboperitoneal shunts are prone to infection, may require multiple revisions, and may fail to protect visual function.[19]

ONSD may successfully restore visual function in patients with visual loss secondary to papilledema caused by brain tumors or infections. The risks of operation must be weighed against the patient's degree of visual loss, progression of symptoms, and life expectancy. If general anesthesia is too risky or contraindicated, ONSD may be performed with a local anesthetic. Patients with visual loss secondary to cryptococcal meningitis, raised intracranial pressure, and papilledema are also candidates for ONSD.

Successful ONSD treatment of patients with acute retinal necrosis syndrome has been reported.[9] Patients were operated on if visual loss was not compatible with the retinal changes observed and there was clinical evidence of a compressive optic neuropathy; these patients are rare in most practices.

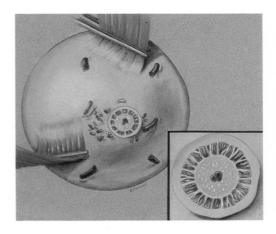

Figure 28-3 *View of posterior pole from orbit, showing increased number of short ciliary vessels temporal to optic nerve.*

28-3

TECHNIQUE OF OPTIC NERVE SHEATH DECOMPRESSION

Optic nerve sheath decompression is performed with the operating microscope via a transconjunctival medial orbitotomy. For severely ill patients in whom general anesthesia is contraindicated, ONSD may be performed with a retrobulbar, peribulbar, or infiltrative anesthetic. The medial approach is the most direct route to the optic nerve and is preferred by many surgeons. Because there are fewer short ciliary vessels, the medial approach allows access to the nerve sheath with minimal disruption of the vessels and nerves (Figure 28-3). If short ciliary vessels are violated, the resulting infarction includes peripheral nasal optic nerve and nasal retina and the visual deficits are rarely significant. Fenestration of the optic nerve sheath overlying the medial optic nerve is safer. The medial optic nerve consists of peripheral nasal fibers (Figure 28-4). Impaling or otherwise injuring these nerve fi-

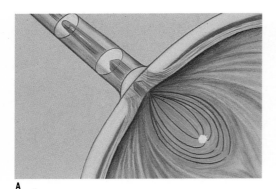

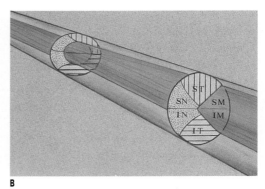

A

B

Figure 28-4 *Optic nerve fiber arrangement, demonstrating temporal section of papillomacular optic nerve fibers.*

bers causes a usually insignificant peripheral temporal visual field deficit. The lateral optic nerve contains the papillomacular bundle, and injury to these nerve fibers may cause a very significant central visual defect.

The authors presently prefer to use a local infiltrative anesthetic delivered in such a manner as to avoid elevating intraorbital pressure, which occurs in retrobulbar or peribulbar anesthetic administration. After appropriate intravenous sedation has been attained, approximately 4 to 5 cc of 2% lidocaine with hyaluronidase is administered in a modified van Lindt fashion to obviate forced eyelid closure. A speculum is then used to open the eye, and 0.5 to 1 cc of anesthetic solution is instilled under the conjunctiva with a 30-gauge needle. The anesthetic is gently spread with a cotton-tipped applicator beneath the conjunctiva. A 360° peritomy is performed with Westcott scissors. Sub-Tenon's tunnels are gently made above and below the medial rectus muscle with the scissors. Approximately 2 to 3 cc of anesthetic solution is gently instilled into each tunnel with a syringe and a blunt-

thesia is too risky or contraindicated, ONSD may be performed with a local anesthetic. Patients with visual loss secondary to cryptococcal meningitis, raised intracranial pressure, and papilledema are also candidates for ONSD.

Successful ONSD treatment of patients with acute retinal necrosis syndrome has been reported.[9] Patients were operated on if visual loss was not compatible with the retinal changes observed and there was clinical evidence of a compressive optic neuropathy; these patients are rare in most practices.

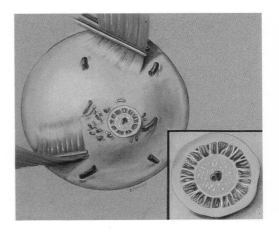

Figure 28-3 *View of posterior pole from orbit, showing increased number of short ciliary vessels temporal to optic nerve.*

28-3

TECHNIQUE OF OPTIC NERVE SHEATH DECOMPRESSION

Optic nerve sheath decompression is performed with the operating microscope via a transconjunctival medial orbitotomy. For severely ill patients in whom general anesthesia is contraindicated, ONSD may be performed with a retrobulbar, peribulbar, or infiltrative anesthetic. The medial approach is the most direct route to the optic nerve and is preferred by many surgeons. Because there are fewer short ciliary vessels, the medial approach allows access to the nerve sheath with minimal disruption of the vessels and nerves (Figure 28-3). If short ciliary vessels are violated, the resulting infarction includes peripheral nasal optic nerve and nasal retina and the visual deficits are rarely significant. Fenestration of the optic nerve sheath overlying the medial optic nerve is safer. The medial optic nerve consists of peripheral nasal fibers (Figure 28-4). Impaling or otherwise injuring these nerve fi-

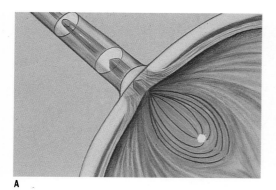

A

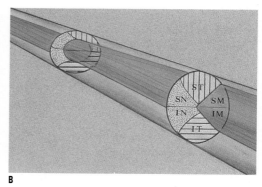

B

Figure 28-4 *Optic nerve fiber arrangement, demonstrating temporal section of papillomacular optic nerve fibers.*

bers causes a usually insignificant peripheral temporal visual field deficit. The lateral optic nerve contains the papillomacular bundle, and injury to these nerve fibers may cause a very significant central visual defect.

The authors presently prefer to use a local infiltrative anesthetic delivered in such a manner as to avoid elevating intraorbital pressure, which occurs in retrobulbar or peribulbar anesthetic administration. After appropriate intravenous sedation has been attained, approximately 4 to 5 cc of 2% lidocaine with hyaluronidase is administered in a modified van Lindt fashion to obviate forced eyelid closure. A speculum is then used to open the eye, and 0.5 to 1 cc of anesthetic solution is instilled under the conjunctiva with a 30-gauge needle. The anesthetic is gently spread with a cotton-tipped applicator beneath the conjunctiva. A 360° peritomy is performed with Westcott scissors. Sub-Tenon's tunnels are gently made above and below the medial rectus muscle with the scissors. Approximately 2 to 3 cc of anesthetic solution is gently instilled into each tunnel with a syringe and a blunt-tipped balanced salt solution cannula. Dilation of the pupil indicates that adequate analgesia and akinesia may be anticipated. The globe may be gently massaged for a few moments to allow the anesthetic to work effectively. The medial rectus is isolated and secured with a 6-0 polyglactin (Vicryl) suture, and the muscle is disinserted from the globe. Two 5-0 polyglactin sutures are passed through the medial rectus insertion and used to retract the globe laterally. Mosquito hemostats are used to attach the sutures to the drapes. It is important to intermittently release these sutures because traction increases intraocular pressure and may decrease ocular perfusion.

The medial rectus complex is retracted medially with a small malleable retractor (Figure 28-5). This maneuver exposes the vortex veins and the long ciliary arteries. The optic nerve sheath lies beneath a pad of intraconal fat between the long ciliary vessels. The surrounding fat may be retracted with cotton-tipped applicators and 0.5-inch neurosurgical cottonoids to reveal short ciliary vessels and nerves overlying the optic nerve sheath (Figure 28-6). If exposure is poor, intermittent pressure on the globe with a cotton-tipped applicator will often bring the nerve into view. If exposure is still inadequate, the retractors are removed from the orbit and the traction sutures released. After sufficient time for reperfusion has been allowed, the process is repeated until exposure is adequate.

The ciliary vessels and nerves are retracted with a 45° nerve hook to expose the optic nerve sheath. The sheath is incised with a 15° Superblade (Figure 28-7).

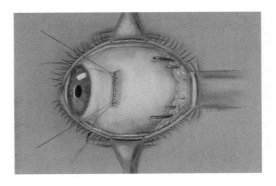

Figure 28-5 *Exposure of optic nerve sheath by retracting globe laterally with two 5-0 polyglactin sutures and medial rectus complex medially with malleable retractor. Optic nerve lies between long ciliary vessels.*

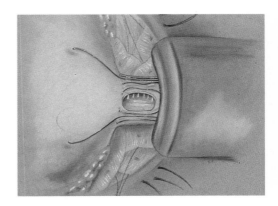

Figure 28-6 *Orbital fat may be packed away from operative field with neurosurgical cottonoids and cotton-tipped applicators.*

Figure 28-7 *Incision of optic nerve sheath with small, sharp blade.*

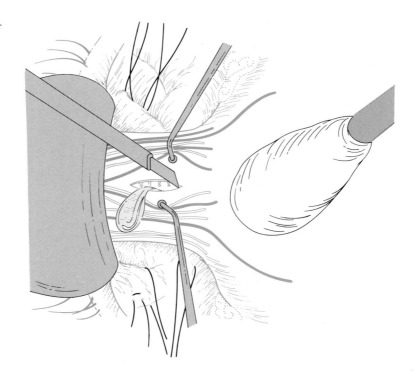

Cerebrospinal fluid will often flood the orbit when the nerve sheath is incised. The incision is enlarged by passing a nerve hook into it and elevating the dura and arachnoid from the underlying pia of the optic nerve (Figure 28-8). With the nerve sheath elevated, it may be fenestrated, or slit, safely without damage to the underlying optic nerve or pial vessels (Figure 28-9). Fenestration and slitting may be accomplished with any microsurgical scissors or the 15° Superblade. The authors prefer the DORC or Grieshaber straight microscissors used by vitreoretinal surgeons for fenestration of the dura and arachnoid. Two or three slits are routinely made, and the trabeculations between the optic nerve and its sheaths are lysed with a nerve hook or microvascular dissector (Figure 28-10). This maneuver theoretically increases the flow of cerebrospinal fluid and minimizes the chance of an early fistula closure and the need for a second operation. After the fenestrations, or slits, are made, the medial rectus is reinserted and recessed 2 mm. The conjunctiva is closed with a 7-0 polyglactin suture (Figure 28-11).

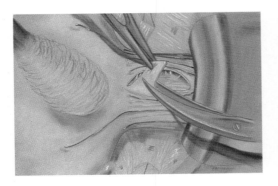

Figure 28-8 *Dura and arachnoid are elevated from underlying optic nerve with small, blunt nerve hooks.*

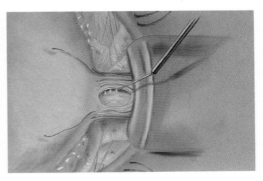

Figure 28-10 *Lysis of trabeculations between optic nerve sheath and optic nerve.*

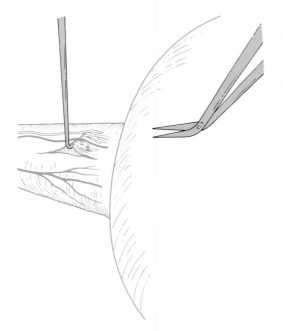

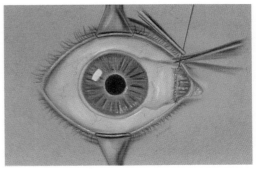

Figure 28-11 *Medial rectus is reattached and recessed 2 mm, and conjunctiva is closed.*

Figure 28-9 *Fenestration of optic nerve sheath.*

28-4

MECHANISM OF OPTIC NERVE SHEATH DECOMPRESSION

Although the mechanism of successful optic nerve sheath decompression is unknown, two possibilities have been postulated. First, the operation may create a permanent fistula, draining cerebrospinal fluid and reducing local subarachnoid pressure.[1,2,4,20] Another proposed mechanism postulates that fistula closure and glial proliferation in the subarachnoid space protect the optic nerve from high intracranial pressure.[16,21] Davidson reported two pathologic studies demonstrating postoperative occlusion of the ONSD site and the subarachnoid space by early granulation tissue.[16,21] Hayreh described similar pathologic findings in 9 monkeys with balloon-induced papilledema that had previously undergone ONSD.[14]

Keltner,[20] examining the optic nerve from a patient 39 days after ONSD, found no pathologic evidence for blockage of either the fistula or the subarachnoid space surrounding the optic nerve. The patient was, however, treated with corticosteroids and immunosuppressive drugs, hindering his fibroblastic response. Clinical observations of patients undergoing ONSD—including relief of headaches,[1-3] improvement of edema in the contralateral unoperated optic disc,[2] and complete filling of the subarachnoid space without evidence of fibrosis or obstruction of the optic nerve sheath to the back of the eye after instillation of intrathecal iopamidol[1]—support fistulization, not fibrosis, as the proposed mechanism of ONSD.

28-5

RESULTS OF OPTIC NERVE SHEATH DECOMPRESSION

Regardless of the mechanism, optic nerve sheath decompression does relieve papilledema and restore visual function in patients with visual loss due to elevated intracranial pressure. The majority of patients undergoing ONSD have papilledema secondary to pseudotumor cerebri. These patients have a chronic disease and may have elevated intracranial pressure for years regardless of treatment.[22] Although ONSD relieves the papilledema and restores the visual function in these patients, they need to be followed up routinely to detect deteriorating visual function. The authors suggest automated perimetry monthly after surgery until these patients are stable and then every 3 to 4 months. This will allow timely detection of surgical failures as manifested by recrudescences of visual dysfunction.

ONSD may fail any time after surgery, including shortly after surgery. These patients may have an initial diminution in their papilledema and improvement in their visual function, but it rapidly stagnates. Reoperation often demonstrates that the fenestration site is blocked and sealed by orbital fat. The authors also reviewed the results with patients up to 5 years after surgery. Operative failure, defined as progressive deterioration in visual field, occurred in 15% of patients 6 months after surgery. This failure rate increased to 35% at 3 years and 50% at 5 years.[18] This experience reemphasizes the need for careful long-term followup care in these patients.

Secondary ONSD is technically more difficult to perform than primary ONSD but may successfully restore visual function in patients with a failed primary procedure.[5] The technical difficulty arises from the excessive scarring and vascularization present in the orbit. Reviewing the initial experience with secondary ONSD, the authors found that 90% of the patients had stable visual function 3 months postoperatively. Reoperation is a useful therapy for progressive visual loss following initially successful ONSD in patients with pseudotumor cerebri.

Approximately 25% of the authors' patients required a second procedure or other form of therapy to obviate their visual loss. The authors' experience in performing more than two ONSDs on an eye has not been good. Although initially successful, they all failed eventually. Subsequently, we rarely offer more than two ONSDs per eye. The limited chance of long-term success is rarely worth the increased risk of operative complications.

28-6

COMPLICATIONS OF OPTIC NERVE SHEATH DECOMPRESSION

Optic nerve sheath decompression should be performed carefully, utilizing the illumination and magnification available with the operating microscope. Surgical diligence should minimize operative complications, but they do occur. Visually devastating complications such as central retinal artery occlusions and optic nerve infarctions have been reported, as have less serious consequences, like long ciliary artery occlusions.[23,24] These occlusions result from vascular compromise of the ocular circulation, possibly by excessive, prolonged traction on the globe during the operation. Therefore, the authors suggest not maintaining traction on the globe for more than 1 or 2 minutes at a time during the operation. After 1 or 2 minutes of traction, the surgery should be halted, the traction sutures released, and the eye permitted to perfuse normally for a few moments.

Less devastating complications include those of strabismus surgery, particularly the possibility of a "lost" muscle or a perforated globe when passing traction sutures or reinserting the medial rectus. These may be avoided by close attention to surgical technique.

Intraoperative hemorrhage may occur if the ciliary vessels are damaged. This can usually be managed by placing Gelfoam and a cottonoid over the bleeding site, releasing the traction sutures, and placing gentle pressure on the globe. Occasionally, bleeding may need to be controlled with a bipolar cautery, utilizing the lowest possible effective setting to minimize any potential damage to the optic nerve or its blood supply. The risk of postoperative hemorrhage may be minimized by meticulous hemostasis prior to completion of the operation.

Younger patients with good vision may complain of difficulty with near vision after surgery due to injury to the short ciliary nerves. This may also be accompanied by a tonic pupil or sector dilation of the pupil. These complaints rarely require more treatment than reassurance because they usually subside spontaneously. Postoperative diplopia is uncommon, except in patients undergoing bilateral or sequential ONSD. Aside from cases with slipped muscles and an obvious large-angle deviation, diplopia rarely requires treatment and often subsides spontaneously. Conjunctival chemosis and swelling after surgery may cause corneal dellen formation, which can be treated with aggressive ocular lubrication if necessary.

REFERENCES

1. Brourman ND, Spoor TC, Ramocki JM: Optic nerve sheath decompression for pseudotumor cerebri. *Arch Ophthalmol* 1988;106:1378–1383.

2. Sergott RC, Savino PJ, Bosley TM: Modified optic nerve sheath decompression provides long-term visual improvement for pseudotumor cerebri. *Arch Ophthalmol* 1988;106:1384–1390.

3. Corbett JJ, Nerad JA, Tse DT, Anderson RL: Results of optic nerve sheath fenestration for pseudotumor cerebri: the lateral orbitotomy approach. *Arch Ophthalmol* 1988;106:1391–1397.

4. Keltner JL: Optic nerve sheath decompression: how does it work? has its time come? *Arch Ophthalmol* 1988;106:1365–1369.

5. Spoor TC, Ramocki JM, Madion MP, Wilkinson MJ: Treatment of pseudotumor cerebri by primary and secondary optic nerve sheath decompression. *Am J Ophthalmol* 1991;112:177–185.

6. Sergott RC, Cohen MS, Bosley TM, Savino PJ: Optic nerve decompression may improve the progressive form of nonarteritic ischemic optic neuropathy. *Arch Ophthalmol* 1989;107:1743–1754.

7. Spoor TC, Wilkinson MJ, Ramocki JM: Optic nerve sheath decompression for the treatment of progressive nonarteritic ischemic optic neuropathy. *Am J Ophthalmol* 1991;111:724–728.

8. Kelman SE, Elman MJ: Optic nerve sheath decompression for nonarteritic ischemic optic neuropathy improves multiple visual function measurements. *Arch Ophthalmol* 1991;109:667–671.

9. Sergott RC, Anand R, Belmont JB, et al: Acute retinal necrosis neuropathy: clinical profile and surgical therapy. *Arch Ophthalmol* 1989;107:692–696.

10. DeWecker L: On incision of the optic nerve in cases of neuroretinitis. *Int Ophthalmol Congr Rep* 1872;4:11–14.

11. Carter RB: On retrobulbar incision of the optic nerve in cases of swollen disc. *Brain* 1887;10:199–209.

12. Carter RB: Operation of opening the sheath of the optic nerve for the relief of pressure. *Br Med J* 1889;1:399–401.

13. Müller L: Die Trepanation der Optikus-scheide: Eine neue Operation zur Heilung der Stauungspapille. *Wien Klin Wochenschr* 1916; 2:1001–1003.

14. Hayreh SS: Pathogenesis of edema of the optic disc (papilloedema): a preliminary report. *Br J Ophthalmol* 1964;48:522–542.

15. Smith JL, Hoyt WF, Newton TH: Optic nerve sheath decompression for relief of chronic monocular choked disc. *Am J Ophthalmol* 1969;68:633–639.

16. Davidson SI: A surgical approach to plero-cephalic disc edema. *Eye* 1969;89:669–690.

17. Galbraith JE, Sullivan JH: Decompression of the perioptic meninges for relief of papille-dema. *Am J Ophthalmol* 1973;76:687–692.

18. Spoor TC, McHenry JG: Long-term effectiveness of optic nerve sheath decompression for pseudotumor cerebri. *Arch Ophthalmol* 1993; 111:632–635.

19. Kelman SE, Sergott RC, Cioffi GA, et al: Modified optic nerve decompression in patients with functioning lumboperitoneal shunts and progressive visual loss. *Ophthalmology* 1991;98: 1449–1453.

20. Keltner JL, Albert DM, Lubow M, et al: Optic nerve decompression: a clinical patho-logic study. *Arch Ophthalmol* 1977;95:97–104.

21. Davidson SI: The surgical relief of papilloe-dema. In: Cant JS, ed: *The Optic Nerve*. Pro-ceedings of Second William Mackenzie Memo-rial Symposium, Glasgow, 1971. London: Kimpton; 1972;3:174–179.

22. Corbett JJ, Savino PJ, Thompson HS, et al: Visual loss in pseudotumor cerebri: follow-up of 57 patients from five to 41 years and a pro-file of 14 patients with permanent severe visual loss. *Arch Neurol* 1982;39:461–474.

23. Rizzo JF, Lessell S: Choroidal infarction af-ter optic nerve sheath fenestration. *Ophthalmol-ogy* 1994;101:1622–1626.

24. Plotnik JL, Kosmorsky GS: Operative com-plications of optic nerve sheath decompression. *Ophthalmology* 1993:100:683–690.

Periorbital and Craniofacial Surgery

James R. Patrinely, MD
Samuel Stal, MD
Randal S. Weber, MD

The spectrum of therapeutic and reconstructive possibilities in complex orbitocranial disorders has been greatly expanded through the development of craniofacial surgery and cooperative interaction among related surgical disciplines. The patient is the ultimate benefactor of this collaborative effort.*

Because the orbit represents a bridge between the face and the cranium, congenital craniofacial deformities and acquired disorders such as trauma or tumors of the orbit and ocular adnexa often require the coordinated management of a team of specialists. Over the past decade, multidisciplinary teams involving craniofacial surgeons, neurosurgeons, ophthalmologists, otorhinolaryngologists, orthodontists, geneticists, and other professionals have developed as interest and expertise in craniofacial surgery have broadened.[1-3]

Craniofacial surgery was pioneered by Paul Tessier, who developed the principles of bone reconstruction for major congenital deformities. He developed techniques of en bloc mobilization of cranial and skeletal segments and proved that large segments of the craniofacial skeleton could be temporarily devascularized and mobilized and yet survive. Tessier also showed that the orbit can be successfully moved as long as the neurovascular integrity was maintained. These techniques and principles have been applied in the correction of complex congenital, traumatic, and oncologic craniofacial deformities.[3-5] Other researchers have explored and developed en bloc craniofacial surgical techniques to resect tumors of the paranasal sinuses that involve the orbit and anterior cranial fossa.[6-7]

---

*As the realm of orbital surgery expands, it is essential that ophthalmologists and ophthalmic plastic surgeons have a working knowledge of the principles and practices of periorbital and craniofacial surgery. Thus this comprehensive overview of the subject. —ED.

29-1

PRINCIPLES OF CRANIOFACIAL SURGERY

The principles of craniofacial surgery developed from the contributions of Tessier are as follows:[4,5]

1. Adequate incisions with wide subperiosteal exposure for access and mobilization, including 360° orbital dissection

2. Use of osteotomies for access and exposure

3. Osteotomies and mobilization of skeletal segments ("monoblock") with rigid fixation of repositioned segments for better results than onlay bone grafting from another site

4. Mobilization of the "effective orbit" (anterior two thirds) with the globe while preserving ocular function

5. Use of the coronal approach as a source of bone grafts and exposure to the upper half of the orbit

6. Use of autogenous (usually cranial) bone grafts for reconstruction

7. Use of available vascular supply (ie, superficial temporal vessels) and soft tissue of the periorbital region to provide blood supply and soft tissue to remote sites (orbit)

8. Combination of several procedures and corrections into a single operation to try to maximize growth potential of facial bones, decrease the infection rate, and decrease the number of subsequent revisions

9. Soft-tissue correction after structural bone alignment

10. Exposure of the floor of the anterior cranial fossa through a bifrontal craniotomy to provide superior exposure for resecting tumors of the paranasal sinuses with intracranial extension (protection of vital neural structures is afforded by this approach)

11. Use of a pericranial flap to provide vascularized soft tissue for repair of the floor of the anterior cranial fossa and superior medial orbit (this tissue effectively sequesters the intracranial structures from the contaminated secretions of the nose and paranasal sinuses)

29-2

PREOPERATIVE EVALUATION

The preoperative evaluation is particularly important in craniofacial surgery and must be tailored to the problem at hand. Advances in diagnostic imaging, such as the three-dimensional computerized tomographic (CT) scan and magnetic resonance imaging (MRI), have greatly facilitated surgical planning and allow the surgeon to visualize complex spatial deformities of the craniofacial skeleton. Computer graphics of the three-dimensional image also allow the surgeon to preoperatively fabricate a prosthesis or template for a bone graft.[3] The limitations of three-dimensional CT scanning include increased scanning time, radiation exposure, cost, and intraorbital artifact.[3] For intraorbital disorders (late enophthalmos, tumors, etc), however, the traditional two-dimensional axial and coro-

nal CT scans with 1.5- to 3.0-mm cuts is superior to three-dimensional scans for defining bone anatomy or destruction, soft-tissue position, and other anatomic subtleties.[8] The MRI scan is excellent for central nervous system structures and is helpful in orbital soft-tissue analysis with modifications in techniques such as fat suppression. MRI is particularly useful in defining the exact location and size of a tumor within the orbit and its relationship to the optic nerve as well as intracranial extension. In congenital deformities, the plain skull radiograph (standardized at 6 feet) is useful for anthropometric measurements. Standardized full-face photographs are needed to document preoperative appearance and to analyze postoperative results and techniques.

Because extensive orbital tumors may include the anterior cranial fossa, despite "negative" CT scans, preoperative neurosurgical consultation should be sought.[8] In tumor cases, the amount of bone resected will depend on tumor type, preoperative imaging, and bone appearance at the time of surgery because frozen sections are not available on bone specimens. Posterior orbital extension and cavernous sinus involvement are best evaluated by preoperative carotid angiography. Angiography assesses cerebral contralateral blood supply and the integrity of the circle of Willis by temporary balloon occlusion of the internal carotid artery when permanent occlusion of the internal carotid artery during tumor resection is contemplated.

29-3

EXTENDED ORBITOTOMY AND ORBITECTOMY

According to the location within the orbit and local extension, some orbital tumors require extended incisions and exposure for adequate visualization and safe resection. This is particularly true for posterior orbital lesions (with or without cranium or sinus involvement) that do not lend themselves to removal by conventional orbitotomy techniques and for malignant tumors that require wide surgical margins.[9] Such malignant disorders include epithelial tumors of the lacrimal gland and sarcomas (fibrosarcoma, osteosarcoma, liposarcoma, chondrosarcoma). Sino-orbital tumors include squamous cell carcinoma or adenocarcinoma, esthesioneuroblastoma, osteosarcoma, and inverting papilloma. Cutaneous neoplasms that may invade the orbit directly or by perineural extension include basal cell carcinoma, squamous cell carcinoma, malignant melanoma, and Merkel cell carcinoma. The predominant central nervous system tumors that invade the orbit are meningioma, astrocytoma, and neurofibroma. Other disorders that may require extensive orbitotomy or orbitectomy are mucopyocele (allergic aspergillosis), mucormycosis, fibrous dysplasia, and traumatic foreign bodies.

The sections that follow describe several subtypes of extended orbitotomy or orbitectomy. Multiple modifications of these techniques exist. Each approach to the orbit has inherent advantages and limitations. The optimal approach is determined by consideration of a number of factors and then appropriately customized to the patient by the surgical team.

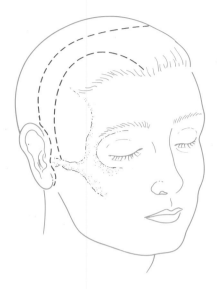

A

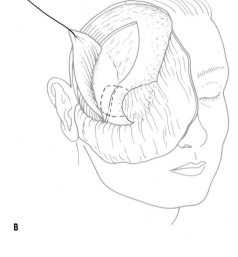

B

29-3-1 Extended Lateral Orbitotomy

Lesions located in the lateral orbital apex can sometimes be accessed by utilizing an extended lateral orbitotomy. In this approach, the standard bone flap for lateral orbitotomy is enlarged to include portions of adjacent sphenoid, temporal, or frontal bone so that a wider and more posterior area of the orbit can be accessed. Lesions that require such exposure include meningioma, lacrimal gland carcinoma, orbital apex tumors, and ophthalmic artery aneurysms.

Often these extended approaches require a large incision in the form of a coronal or hemicoronal forehead flap to provide adequate visualization (Figure 29-1). The coronal incision is an ear-to-ear incision across the vertex of the skull that may extend to the zygomatic arch in front of the ear. The scalp is incised in stages, and bleeding of the flap is controlled by

Figure 29-1 *Coronal and hemicoronal incisions. (A) Coronal incision (posterior dashed line) extends across vertex of skull and exposes entire upper anterior cranium and upper orbits. Hemicoronal incision (anterior dashed line) provides sufficient unilateral orbital access. (B) With hemicoronal scalp flap reflected, temporalis muscle insertion can be divided to expose extended lateral orbit.*

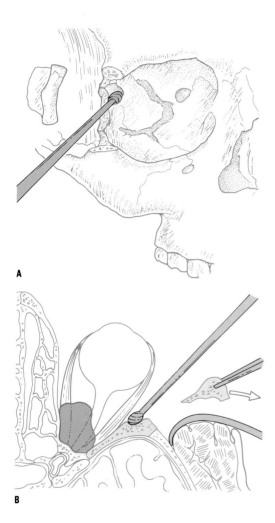

A

B

Figure 29-2 *Extended lateral orbitotomy. (A) High-speed cutting burr is used to remove bone from greater wing of sphenoid posterior to standard lateral orbitotomy. (B) Bone can be removed back to dura of middle cranial fossa to gain additional exposure to orbital apex.*

preinjection of dilute epinephrine, tourniquet sutures, hemostats, or Raney clips. The temporalis fascia and muscle are carefully preserved to minimize deformity and to be available for vascularized tissue transfer for reconstruction. The dissection is carried inferiorly toward the orbital rim in the subgaleal plane until about 1 or 2 cm above the orbital rim, where the periosteum is incised and raised with the flap.[8] The temporalis muscle may also be disinserted and reflected from its fossa to expose the entire lateral orbital wall. The hemicoronal forehead flap (Dandy-type neurosurgical flap) can also be utilized for unilateral exposure to minimize the surgical wound area, but there may be transient upper-forehead paralysis postoperatively as well as more visible alopecia.[10,11] The zygomatic arch can be divided anteriorly and posteriorly, leaving the masseter muscle attached. The bone remains vascularized and is retracted inferiorly, providing further exposure of the lateral and posterior orbit as well as the infraorbital fissure and pterygomaxillary fossa. The remote coronal or hemicoronal incisions can sometimes be used for the standard lateral orbitotomy to avoid the surgical scar from the direct approach.

The standard lateral orbitotomy can be extended by removing additional bone of the greater wing of the sphenoid bone more posteriorly than the normal margin of dissection. This bone becomes thicker posteriorly, as the middle cranial fossa is approached. The bone can be burred away to permit access to the deep lateral portion of the muscle cone (Figure 29-2). The dissection can be extended to expose the anterior, temporal, or frontal dura for visualization of the deep orbital apex.[12-15]

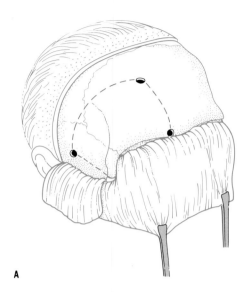

A

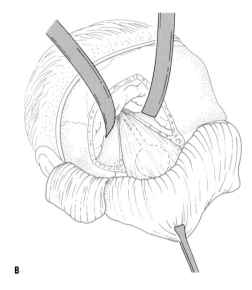

B

The vascular bone in this area may require frequent applications of bone wax.

Extended lateral-wall bone flaps with adjacent temporal or parietal bone can be used to gain access to the deep lateral and superior orbital compartment. In these dissections, the inferior osteotomy is made near the base of the lateral orbital wall or into the lateral inferior orbital rim. The other osteotomies include a portion of the temporalis fossa and the inferior frontal bone (Figure 29-3). The intraorbital osteotomy may extend back to the superior orbital fissure so that the entire lateral wall and the majority of the orbital roof can be removed in a single bone segment. The cranial bone cuts are made by either a high-speed bone scalpel, a craniotome, or a Gigli saw using preplaced burr holes. Once the tumor is removed, bone defects are reconstructed with split calvarial bone grafts, and the bone flap is wired or plated back into position.

Figure 29-3 *Extended superolateral orbitotomy. (A) Osteotomies through frontal, temporal, and parietal bones can be combined with superior and lateral orbital osteotomies to allow removal of single bone segment for full superolateral orbital exposure. (B) With frontal lobe retracted, entire orbit can be unroofed for exposure.*

29-3-2 Extended Superior Orbitotomy

Extended exposure to the superior orbit is obtained through a frontal or temporal frontal craniotomy, as previously described. The transcranial orbitotomy allows excellent exposure of the superior, posterior, and medial portions of the orbit and cribriform plate. It also allows for a complete exploration of the optic nerve, orbital apex, and superior orbital fissure. The superior orbitotomy is particularly valuable for medial apex lesions with intracranial extension. A variety of disorders may require the extended superior orbitotomy.[13,14,16,17] These include meningioma, cholesterol granuloma of the frontal bone, eosinophilic granuloma with bone erosion, neurofibromatosis, fibrous dysplasia, lacrimal gland carcinoma, frontal sinus carcinoma, esthesioneuroblastoma, primary optic nerve glioma or meningioma, and encephalocele. Malignant orbital tumors without intracranial extension should not be exposed to the cranial cavity by transcranial exploration.[8,18] In these cases, orbital exenteration may be necessary. Traumatic indications include optic canal decompression, foreign body, or orbital roof fracture.

Transcranial orbitotomy is performed through a coronal incision, and either a frontal or a frontotemporal bone flap, as previously described, is utilized. The frontal osteotomy bone cut is made 2 cm above the orbital rim in an attempt to avoid the frontal sinus (Figure 29-4). A one-to-one frontal sinus plain x-ray will provide a precise template of the frontal sinus configuration. If the frontal sinus is entered, it should be obliterated by drilling out the mucosal lining and packed with Gelfoam, fat, temporalis muscle, or bone, with the goal of closing off the nasofrontal duct and inducing sinus fibrosis. For malignant tumors, the authors prefer to cranialize the frontal sinus by removing the posterior wall and using vascularized pericranium to separate the anterior fossa from the nose.[19] A pericranial or galeal flap is sometimes used to further seal the opening and minimize postoperative infection.[16,17] The frontal lobe can be retracted after decreasing its volume with intravenous hyperosmotic agents. If the tumor has invaded the cranium or if optic canal exposure is needed, the dura is opened and the frontal lobe is retracted superiorly.

If the tumor is confined to the orbit, the dissection is extradural, with the dura elevated from the roof of the orbit to the anterior clinoid process and the sphenoid ridge.[17] An extradural approach is preferred for unroofing the orbit and optic canal in trauma repair. A high-speed drill is used to remove the orbital roof. The orbital lesion can be directly approached from above after the periorbita is opened. Gentle traction is applied to the frontal nerve and the levator–superior rectus muscle complex. Occasionally, it is necessary to section the levator at its origin or to open the annulus of Zinn, usually superomedially (to avoid the innervation of the muscles) to gain additional exposure.[13,16,17,20] The orbital roof is replaced with a bone graft or an alloplastic implant, and the wound is closed in layers in standard fashion. For malignant tumors, bone grafting is avoided and the pericranial flap

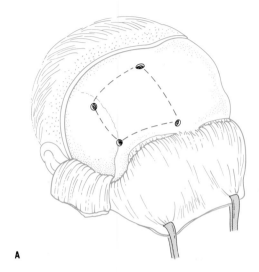

A

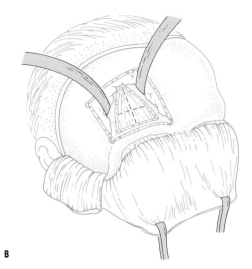

B

provides adequate support for the brain to prevent herniation into the nasal fossa or orbit.[19]

29-3-3 Extended Inferior Orbitotomy

Inferiorly positioned orbital tumors can be accessed by lateral orbitotomy or transconjunctival dissection according to the nature and location of the tumor. Occasionally, there is adjacent sinus involvement (or orbital involvement of a primary sinus malignancy) or additional working space is required, making transorbital approaches suboptimal. Maxillary sinus cancers extending superiorly into the orbital floor require inferior orbitotomy. If the periorbita is not invaded, the orbital contents can often be preserved. Such disorders include primary maxillary sinus malignancies, inferior orbital apex tumors, or deep orbital dissection for repair of late enophthalmos.

The Caldwell-Luc transantral approach through the gingival–buccal sulcus will allow exposure of the inferior orbit back

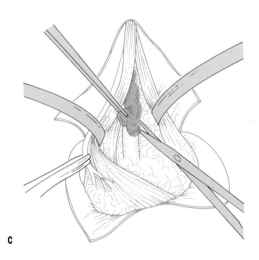

C

Figure 29-4 *Extended superior orbitotomy. (A) Burr holes outline frontotemporal bone flap. (B) Supraorbital ridge and frontal sinus are left intact, and orbit is unroofed. (C) Periorbita is opened and levator–superior rectus muscle complex is retracted to expose optic nerve.*

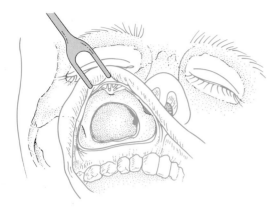

Figure 29-5 *Caldwell-Luc transantral approach to inferior orbit.*

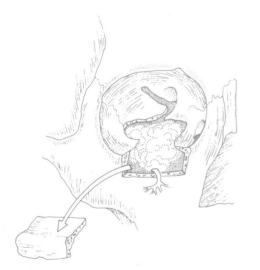

Figure 29-6 *Inferior orbital marginotomy.*

to within 7 mm of the optic canal (Figure 29-5). The posterior wall of the maxillary sinus is approximately 5 to 7 mm anterior to the optic foramen, so exposure to the deep apex is not possible. Additional exposure can be gained by removing a trapezoid-shaped fragment of the inferior orbital rim back to the inferior orbital fissure while preserving the infraorbital neurovascular bundle (Figure 29-6). This facilitates deep dissection and exposure of the orbital floor and maxillary sinus.[21] The floor is then reconstructed with bone grafts, and the osteomized rim segment is refixated. With malignant tumors, a skin graft is used. The orbital floor can later be reconstructed with vascularized bone grafts or with micromesh titanium or Vitallium plates.

29-3-4 Maxillectomy

Malignant tumors of the maxillary and ethmoid sinuses can invade the orbit by direct extension along pre-existing pathways such as nerves, blood vessels, and neural foramina. Invasion also occurs through direct invasion and destruction of the lamina papyracea and orbital floor. Chronic inflammatory disease of the sinuses and benign neoplasms may extend into the orbit through pressure erosion of bone. Surgical planning must take into account the histology and the anatomic sites involved. Approaches for benign and malignant disease often differ and, for the latter, the overriding concern is complete extirpation of the tumor. Constricted surgical access may result in incomplete tumor excision, injury to the orbital contents, or inadvertent entrance into the cranial cavity.

For staging malignant tumors, the maxillary sinus can be divided into two regions, a suprastructure and an infrastructure, by an imaginary line (Ohngren's line) drawn from the medial canthus of the eye to the angle of the mandible. Tumors of the maxillary suprastructure not only have a worse prognosis but are more likely to extend into the orbit or ethmoid sinus. Suprastructure malignancies destroy the infraorbital plate or gain access by extension along the infraorbital nerve. These tumors frequently extend superomedially into the ethmoid sinus, medial orbit, and cribriform plate.

The surgical approach is influenced by tumor location and histology. For malignant lesions, the Weber-Ferguson incision, which extends from the nasofacial crease through the upper lip, provides excellent exposure to the entire maxillary sinus, ethmoid, and medial orbit. Through this incision, visualization of the entire maxilla and the medial and lateral orbital walls is possible (Figure 29-7). The orbit may be exenterated if tumor invasion of the periorbita is found at the time of surgery. For mucopyoceles and benign neoplasms such as inverted papillomas, requiring medial maxillectomy, the midfacial degloving procedure allows access to the medial nasal wall, maxillary sinus, and orbital floor.[22] The procedure requires sublabial and intranasal incisions, which permit elevation of the soft tissues over the maxillae and nasal dorsum. Because all of the incisions are hidden, the cosmetic result is excellent; however, exposure to the medial orbit is poor but can be remedied with the addition of a Lynch (frontoethmoid) incision.[23]

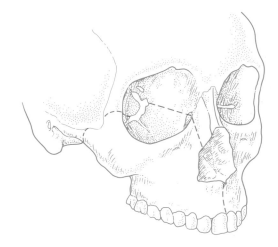

Figure 29-7 *Bone cuts for maxillectomy.*

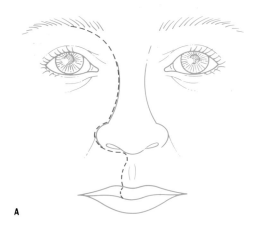

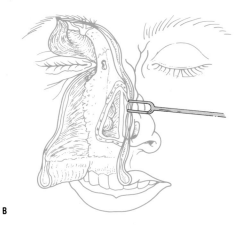

A

B

Figure 29-8 *Lateral rhinotomy incision. (A) Lateral rhinotomy and medial orbital (Lynch) incision follows natural facial contours. (B) Nose is reflected to expose entire hemi-midface.*

29-3-5 Extended Medial Orbitotomy

Exposure to the medial orbit is difficult because the globe and adjacent bony structures cannot be retracted. The combined medial and lateral orbitotomy described by McCord and Cole[24] can be utilized for small apex lesions, but other disorders may require wider visualization and exposure.* These conditions include ethmoid sinus carcinoma, esthesioneuroblastoma, midline meningoencephalocele, juvenile nasopharyngeal angiofibroma, mucormycosis, and sometimes optic canal trauma. The lateral rhinotomy and Lynch incisions will widely expose the medial orbit and paranasal sinuses (Figure 29-8). The incision follows the natural contour of the nasofacial angle on one side, extends around the medial canthus, and is well concealed postoperatively. The incision al-

*See also Chapter 26, "Surgical Exploration of the Orbit," in this volume.—ED.

lows the nose to be mobilized and swung to one side, with the nasofacial angle on the other side acting as a hinge. Soft-tissue dissection of the medial orbital margins on both sides with antral inspection is then possible.[25]

A transfrontal craniotomy may also be utilized to widely expose the medial orbit. Resection of the cribriform plate and the ethmoid sinus offers a panoramic view of the entire superomedial orbit.[19]

29-4

ORBITAL TRANSLOCATION

In vertical orbital dystopia, one orbit and globe is higher than the other in a vertical plane. The horizontal correlate of vertical orbital dystopia is orbital hypertelorism, in which the orbits are displaced on the horizontal plane.[1] Orbital hypertelorism is a physical finding, not a syndrome, and is distinguished from telecanthus (lateral displacement of the medial canthal tendons) by radiographic evidence of increased distance between the medial orbital walls (interdacryon) on posteroanterior cephalograms.[26]

Conditions that cause vertical or horizontal orbital dystopia include craniosynostosis (eg, Crouzon's syndrome, plagiocephaly), orbitofacial clefting syndromes (eg, hemifacial microsomia, Goldenhar's syndrome), posttraumatic events (fractures, radiation in children), or neoplasia (fibrous dysplasia, neurofibromatosis, Romberg's disease, encephalocele). Table 29-1 summarizes the more common congenital craniofacial syndromes. Figures 29-9 through 29-15 illustrate the craniosynostosis and clefting syndromes listed in the table.*

The craniosynostosis syndromes occur when one or more cranial sutures close prematurely. These conditions affect the orbit because a rapidly growing brain distorts the skull with a closed suture causing an overexpansion in the area of normal sutures. Because the midfacial structures are attached to the undersurface of a cranial vault, alterations in the growth of the anterior cranium (inferior displacement of the anterior cranial fossa with anterior expansion of the middle cranial fossa) affect the developing orbits and face (maxillary hypoplasia, dental malocclusion, shallow orbits with exophthalmos, orbital dystopia).[26,27] Generally, the closed cranial suture will need to be released ("strip craniectomy") and the skull reshaped before the child is 1 year old. Psychosocial considerations play an important role in the timing of subsequent midfacial and orbital correction.

---

*For additional information on congenital anomalies and craniofacial deformities, see Chapter 7, "Embryology and Anomalies of the Eyelid, Orbit, and Lacrimal System," in Volume 1 of Ophthalmology Monograph 8, published in 1993.—ED.

TABLE 29-1

Congenital Craniofacial Syndromes

Craniosynostosis Syndromes	Pathophysiology	Common Ophthalmologic Findings	Other Features	Hallmarks
Crouzon's (Figure 29-9)	Premature closure of cranial suture (especially coronal and sagittal) with faciosynostosis	Shallow orbits; proptosis; V exotropia; hypertelorism; "parrot beak" nose; lagophthalmos	Midface hypoplasia; steep forehead; relative prognathism; flattened occiput; arched palate; autosomal dominant	Facial appearance and lack of extremity involvement
Apert's (Figure 29-10)	Same	Same as Crouzon's but more severe proptosis and hypertelorism; supraorbital ridge	Same as Crouzon's but more severe midface hypoplasia; retardation; dental/palatal abnormalities; nasal airway obstruction; turribrachycephaly; autosomal dominant	Syndactyly of hands and feet
Pfeiffer's (Figure 29-11)	Same	Same as Crouzon's but less severe proptosis	Same as Apert's but milder; normal intelligence; can be associated with muscular torticollis; autosomal dominant	Long, broad thumbs and toes; variable soft-tissue syndactyly of hands and feet
Plagiocephaly (Figure 29-12)	Closure of any single cranial suture	Orbital dystopia; possible strabismus	Normal intelligence; suture = palpable ridge; skull flat on affected side → prominent (bossing) on opposite side; skull obliquity; chin deviated to affected side	"Harlequin" eyes on anteroposterior x-ray

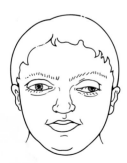

Figure 29-9
Crouzon's syndrome.

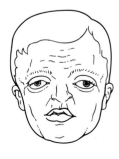

Figure 29-10
Apert's syndrome.

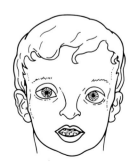

Figure 29-11
Pfeiffer's syndrome.

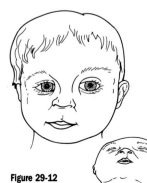

Figure 29-12
Plagiocephaly.

TABLE 29-1 *(cont.)*

Congenital Craniofacial Syndromes

Clefting Syndromes	Pathophysiology	Common Ophthalmologic Findings	Other Features	Hallmarks
Treacher Collins (Tessier clefts 6,7,8) (Figure 29-13)	Neural crest cell migration failure vs local ischemia; M = F; bilateral common	Lower lid notching and lash hypoplasia (medial two thirds); antimongoloid palpebral fissure obliquity	Hypoplastic mandible and zygoma; external and middle ear malformation; macrostomia; abnormal dentition (anterior open bite); malocclusion; pretragal fistula; normal intelligence; micrognathia; conductive hearing loss; autosomal dominant	Antimongoloid slant; sideburns = marker
Goldenhar's (Tessier cleft 7) (Figure 29-14)	Same; bilateral rare	Corneoscleral dermoids; subconjunctival and anterior lipodermoids; upper lid coloboma; strabismus	Unilateral facial hypoplasia; mandibular ramus abnormality; microtia; preauricular skin tags; micrognathia; vertebral abnormalities (hemivertebrae)	Corneoscleral dermoids
Hemifacial microsomia (Tessier cleft 7) (Figure 29-15)	Same; M > F; bilateral rare	Orbital dystopia; upper lid coloboma; strabismus; lateral canthal dystopia	Microtia; macrostomia; asymmetric mandible; maxillary hypoplasia; CN VII involvement; micrognathia; malocclusion (chin deviated to affected side)	Facial asymmetry

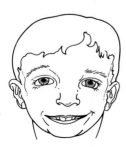

Figure 29-13
Treacher Collins syndrome.

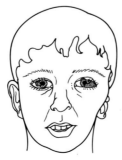

Figure 29-14
Goldenhar's syndrome.

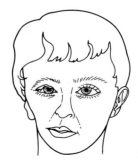

Figure 29-15
Hemifacial microsomia.

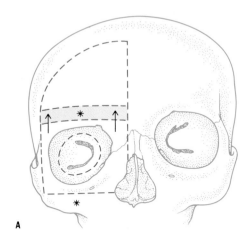

A

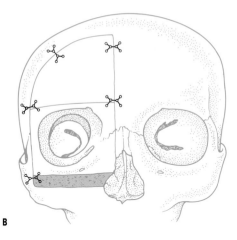

B

Figure 29-16 *Vertical orbital translocation. (A) Inner and outer orbital circumferences are osteotomized and segment of frontal bone is removed. (B) Orbit is translocated superiorly and some of frontal bone is grafted inferiorly.*

Tessier pioneered orbital translocation surgery by utilizing a circumferential orbital osteotomy around the orbital rims and inside the orbital cavity behind the equator of the globe. By mobilization of the outer half of the orbit, the globe can be secondarily repositioned. The orbits are moved as "boxes," with the apex and fissure structures unaffected.[4] Depending on the deformity, various procedures are employed as outlined below.

29-4-1 Vertical Orbital Translocation

Vertical orbital translocation is accomplished by moving the circumferential orbit, except for the apex. A limited exposure frontal craniotomy allows osteotomies of the orbital roof. A predetermined width of frontal bone removed to allow elevation of the orbit and the frontal bone segment is grafted inferiorly to fill the resultant void in the maxilla (Figure 29-16).[28]

29-4-2 Horizontal Orbital Translocation

Most patients with hypertelorism have orbitofacial clefts or encephaloceles. This correction utilizes a neurosurgical frontal osteotomy with preservation of the supraorbital rims (frontal bar). The orbits are outlined by box-like osteotomies through coronal and lower eyelid incisions. The periorbita is elevated circumferentially back to the posterior one third of the orbit, and a 360° intraorbital osteotomy is made in the anterior half of the orbit. The enlarged ethmoid cells are exenterated from the exposed interorbital space once the median segment is removed. The orbits are then translocated with rigid interosseous fixation, and bone grafts are inter-

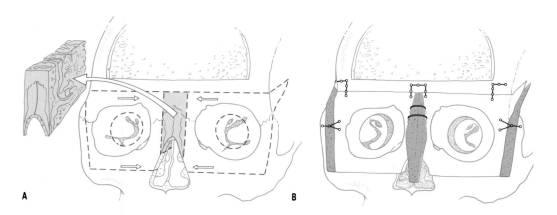

A   **B**

posed in the gaps formed in the lateral walls in the zygoma to maintain the medial position of the orbits (Figure 29-17). The resultant midline soft-tissue excess is sometimes more problematic than the skeletal correction. Various midline resections, nasal reconfigurations, and medial canthoplasties are employed to augment the final effect.

The bipartition procedure separates the face in two vertical segments and is considered in all hypertelorism corrections, although it is usually reserved for the most severe cases. This technique was introduced by Tessier and J. C. Van der Meulen. The geometric concept is ideal as it can satisfy many goals, such as bringing the orbits together, enlarging the maxilla, and leveling the palate. The procedure can also be used as an access approach to the nasal pharynx for correcting subcranial tumors and treating choanal atresia.

Bipartitioning is usually performed in patients with either Apert's syndrome or a midline cleft.[29] The hard palate is split in the midline or along the margins of the facial cleft. Access from the alveolus and

Figure 29-17 *Horizontal orbital translocation. (A) Both orbits are osteotomized; midline ethmoid cells and nasal bone are removed. Frontal craniotomy, sparing supraorbital rims (frontal bar), is also performed. (B) Orbits are translocated medially; bone grafts are used to fill resulting defects and help reconstruct nose.*

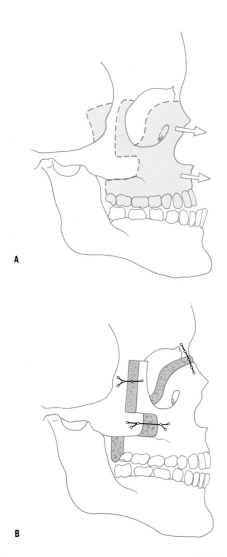

A

B

Figure 29-18 *Le Fort III advancement. (A) Osteotomies are performed to allow mobilization of midface. (B) Nasomaxillary complex is advanced forward and bone grafts are used to fill in resulting defects.*

the hard palate is from above to keep the palate mucosa intact. Multiple bone grafts are then used to fill the periorbital defects and to reconstruct the nose. Fixation is obtained with plates and screws. The orbital complexes are de-rotated by bending the orbital frontal complex immediately so that the facial width can be reduced. Because of the extensive dissection and exposure required, the morbidity of an infection is significant.

Hypotelorism is more unusual and its correction is basically the hypertelorism repair in reverse.

29-4-3 Anterior Orbital Translocation

The exophthalmos present in the craniosynostosis syndromes is directly related to diminution in orbital volume, which is usually shallow in the anteroposterior dimension. There may also be a medial displacement of the lateral wall. Procedures to effectively deepen the orbit and correct the exophthalmos include anterior advancement of the midface and inferior orbital rims and forward movement of the supraorbital rims. Depending on the characteristics and severity of the deformity, various intracranial and extracranial procedures are employed.[26]

A Le Fort III osteotomy to advance the midface may be accomplished by an extracranial approach or combined with an intracranial or frontal bone (supraorbital rim) advancement. Advancement of the frontal bone and the midface as a single segment is termed a *monoblock advancement*.[26] The Le Fort osteotomy is performed through scalp and buccal incisions. The osteotomy configurations are outlined in Figure 29-18. Rigid interosseous fixation is required for stabilization of advanced naso-maxillary complex and bone grafts placed in the resulting defects. When a brow and orbital roof advancement is also needed, the Le Fort III advancement is combined with a frontal bone advancement through a combined intracranial approach (Figure 29-19). Despite the total midface advancement, the growth rate of the maxilla often lags compared to the mandible, and secondary orthognatic surgery (Le Fort I) is almost always required.

29-5

ORBITAL RECONSTRUCTION

Craniofacial surgical principles are also applied to complex orbital reconstruction for trauma or tumor defects. Traumatic repair should be undertaken early to restore and maintain the normal anatomy of the craniofacial skeleton. Secondary soft-tissue corrections are also more successful when performed early, prior to cicatrization contracture. Adaptation of the principles and techniques of rigid internal skeletal fixation in primary bone grafting permits a stable anatomic reconstruction of most traumatic orbital deformities.

In contrast to early traumatic repair, reconstruction for malignant tumor defects should be delayed for 12 to 24 months, until recurrence has been ruled out. If the tumor recurs early after an extensive reconstruction, fewer reconstructive options will be available following the resection. Also, if postoperative irradiation is planned, vascularized tissue (flaps, microvascular grafts, etc) will be needed to prevent necrosis of bone grafts.

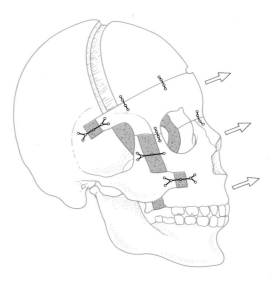

Figure 29-19 *Frontal bone and midface (Le Fort III) advancement.*

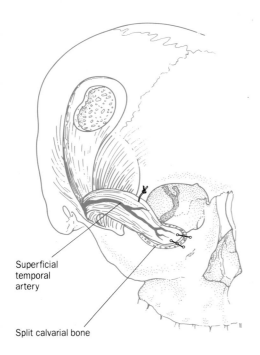

Superficial
temporal
artery

Split calvarial bone

Figure 29-20 *Vascularized cranial bone graft.*

29-5-1 Bone Grafts

Advances in primary bone grafting have added a new dimension to the treatment of complex orbital defects. These techniques allow one-stage restoration of the normal orbital three-dimensional anatomy. Free autogenous bone grafts are the optimal material to replace skeletal defects. Cortical or corticocancellous bone is able to bear stress and resist deformation. Eventually, there is substitution and appositional bone formation so that the graft becomes incorporated into the facial skeleton. Rigid fixation of the graft promotes a better osteogenic response and more rapid vascularization with less resorption. Nonetheless, there still is some unpredictable resorption of onlay and intraorbital bone grafts. Bone grafts can be safely used to cover exposed sinus cavities, and they do not necessarily have to be removed in cases of postoperative wound infection.[30-33]

With the coronal incision, the donor site of cranial bone is readily available, usually from the parietal area, and can be split from the cranial surface with a curved osteotome or obtained by splitting a full-thickness piece of calvaria that has been removed from the operative site.[30-33] The main disadvantage of cranial bone is that it is rigid and will not bend easily to reconstruct the orbital floor contour. Contouring may be facilitated by leaving the periosteum or outermost cortical layer intact, thus allowing microfractures of the bone graft to accomplish curvature and yet maintain a single piece. Rib grafts can be easily split, curved, and contoured; they are useful in deep orbital reconstruction, but may demonstrate more resorption when used as onlay grafts on the facial skeleton. The iliac crest can provide large amounts of corticocancellous bone in large segments, but these grafts are less elastic and are associated with considerable pain at the donor site postoperatively.[33]

Microvascular surgical advances have made vascularized bone grafts, composite flaps, and free tissue distal flaps (deltopectoral, sternomastoid) available to increase bone graft coverage and survivability in selected cases. The superficial temporal artery can be anastomosed for blood supply in free grafts or used with a temporoparietal flap to carry a vascularized cranial bone graft (Figure 29-20).[34]

Interosseous wire fixation has been the mainstay of fracture fixation and is still useful in the absence of comminuted fractures or bone deficiencies. In the late 1960s, orthopedic screws and plates were used in Europe to rigidly fixate fractures and osteotomies of the face. This led to the development of thin custom plates and small screws that could be used on the craniofacial skeleton.[33,35,36] This approach has become popular in the United States since the early 1980s. Unlike wire, screws and plates provide a firm three-dimensional fixation of bone segments. Also, the rigid immobilization provided by the plates and lag screws allows early revascularization of the bone and eliminates shearing motion. Newer materials such as titanium and Vitallium have increased the strength and ductility of the plates while decreasing corrosion and size. Currently, the trend is toward the smaller ("micro"), lower-profile plates around the orbit to minimize palpable deformities.[35,36] The plates can be left in place indefinitely or removed later during a secondary procedure.

REFERENCES

1. Fries PD, Katowitz JA: Congenital craniofacial anomalies of ophthalmic importance. *Surv Ophthalmol* 1990;35:87–119.

2. Schafer ME: Craniofacial surgery: its evolution and application. *Neurol Clin* 1985;3:331–357.

3. Toth BA, Di Loreto DA, Stewart WB: Multidisciplinary approach to the management of complex bony and soft tissue orbitocranial disorders. *Ophthalmology* 1988;95:1013–1026.

4. Tessier P, Hervouet F, Lekieffre M, et al: *Plastic Surgery of the Orbit and Eyelids.* New York: Masson Publishing Co; 1981.

5. Wolfe SA: Application of craniofacial surgical precepts in orbital reconstruction following trauma and tumour removal. *J Maxillofac Surg* 1982;10:212–223.

6. Ketcham AS, Wilkins RH, Van Buren JM, Smith RR: A combined intracranial facial approach to the paranasal sinuses. *Am J Surg* 1963;106:698–703.

7. Cheesman AD, Lund VJ, Howard DJ: Craniofacial resection for tumors of the nasal cavity and paranasal sinuses. *Head Neck Surg* 1986;8:429–435.

8. Jackson IT, Laws ER, Martin RD: A craniofacial approach to advanced recurrent cancer of the central face. *Head Neck Surg* 1988;5: 474–488.

9. Jackson IT: Orbitectomy. In: Hornblass A, ed: *Oculoplastic, Orbital, and Reconstructive Surgery*. Baltimore: Williams & Wilkins; 1990: 1249–1259.

10. Stewart WB, Levin PS, Toth BA: Orbital surgery: the technique of coronal scalp flap approach to the lateral orbitotomy. *Arch Ophthalmol* 1988;106:1724–1726.

11. Patrinely JR, Cech DA: Hemicoronal flap approach for lateral orbitotomy. *Arch Ophthalmol* 1989;107:1421–1422.

12. Jones BR: Surgical approaches to the orbit. *Trans Ophthalmol Soc UK* 1970;90:269–281.

13. Maroon JC, Kennerdell JS: Surgical approaches to the orbit: indications and techniques. *J Neurosurg* 1984;60:1226–1235.

14. Rootman J: *Diseases of the Orbit: A Multidisciplinary Approach*. Philadelphia: JB Lippincott Co; 1988:579–612.

15. Viale GL, Pau A: A plea for postero-lateral orbitotomy for microsurgical removal of tumours of the orbital apex. *Acta Neurochir* (Wien) 1988;90:124–126.

16. Housepian EM: Intraorbital tumors. In: Schmidek HH, Sweet WH, eds: *Current Techniques in Operative Neurosurgery*. New York: Grune & Stratton; 1977:143–160.

17. Schucart W: Transcranial approach of the orbit. In: Hornblass A, ed: *Oculoplastic, Orbital, and Reconstructive Surgery*. Baltimore: Williams & Wilkins; 1990:1261–1264.

18. Mohr C, Schettler D, Heesen J: The surgical approach to orbital space-occupying lesions. *J Craniomaxillofac Surg* 1989;17:149–154.

19. Blacklock JB, Weber RS, Lee YY, Goepfert H: Transcranial resection of tumors of the paranasal sinuses and nasal cavity. *J Neurosurg* 1989;71:10–15.

20. Leone CR Jr, Wissinger JP: Surgical approaches to diseases of the orbital apex. *Ophthalmology* 1988;95:391–397.

21. Tessier P: Inferior orbitotomy: a new approach to the orbital floor. *Clin Plast Surg* 1982;9:569–575.

22. Maniglia AJ: Indications and techniques of midfacial degloving: a 15-year experience. *Arch Otolaryngol Head Neck Surg* 1986;112:750–752.

23. Baredes S, Cho HT, Som ML: Total maxillectomy. In: Blitzer A, Lawson W, Friedman WH, eds: *Surgery of the Paranasal Sinuses*. Philadelphia: WB Saunders Co; 1985:317–329.

24. McCord CD Jr, Cole HP: Surgical approaches to the orbit. In: McCord CD Jr, Tanenbaum M, Nunery WR, eds: *Oculoplastic Surgery*. 3rd ed. New York: Raven Press; 1995:504–507.

25. Bridger GP: Radical surgery for ethmoid cancer. *Arch Otolaryngol* 1980;106:630–634.

26. McCarthy JG: Craniofacial surgery. In: Hornblass A, ed: *Oculoplastic, Orbital, and Reconstructive Surgery*. Baltimore: Williams & Wilkins; 1990:826–845.

27. Dufresne CR, Jelks GW: Classification of craniofacial malformations. In: Smith BA, Della Rocca RC, Nesi FA, Lisman RD, eds: *Ophthalmic Plastic and Reconstructive Surgery*. St Louis: CV Mosby Co; 1987;2:1185–1237.

28. McCarthy JG, Jelks GW, Valauri AJ, et al: The orbit and zygoma. In: McCarthy JG, ed: *Plastic Surgery*. Philadelphia: WB Saunders Co; 1990:1574–1670.

29. Salyer KE: *Techniques in Aesthetic Craniofacial Surgery*. Philadelphia: JB Lippincott Co; 1989.

30. Tessier P: Autogenous bone grafts taken from the calvarium for facial and cranial applications. *Clin Plast Surg* 1982;9:531–538.

31. Zins JE, Whitaker LA: Membranous versus endochondral bone: implications for craniofacial reconstruction. *Plast Reconstr Surg* 1983; 72:778–785.

32. Levin PS, Stewart WB, Toth BA: The technique of cranial bone grafts in the correction of posttraumatic orbital deformities. *Ophthalmic Plast Reconstr Surg* 1987;3:77–82.

33. Antonyshyn O, Gruss JS: Complex orbital trauma: the role of rigid fixation and primary bone grafting. *Adv Ophthalmic Plast Reconstr Surg* 1987;7:61–92.

34. McCarthy JG, Cutting CB, Shaw WW: Vascularized calvarial flaps. *Clin Plast Surg* 1987; 14:37–47.

35. Munro IR: The Luhr fixation system for the craniofacial skeleton. *Clin Plast Surg* 1989; 16:41–48.

36. Luhr HG: Indications for use of a microsystem for internal fixation in craniofacial surgery. *J Craniofac Surg* 1990;1:35–52.

PART VIII

The Anophthalmic Socket

CHAPTER 30

Enucleation and Evisceration

Mark R. Levine, MD
Steven Fagien, MD

Removal of an eye and management of the anophthalmic socket have always been challenges to the ophthalmologist and the ocularist working closely with the ophthalmic surgeon. The surgeon strives to produce dynamic and static symmetry between the normal side and the anophthalmic side, along with the best possible motility—goals that are not always directly compatible.

Characteristics of the ideal anophthalmic socket are as follows:[1]

1. A centrally placed, well-covered, buried implant of adequate size, fabricated from an inert material

2. Deep unobstructed conjunctival fornices

3. An inferior eyelid and fornix that can adequately support the prosthetic eye

4. A superior eyelid that is symmetric with the normal eyelid in contour and function

5. A supratarsal eyelid fold that is symmetric with the supratarsal fold of the normal eyelid

6. Anophthalmic socket soft tissues that are not displaced inferiorly when compared to the normal side

7. Normal position of the lashes

8. Eyelid and prosthetic movement that approaches the normal side

No single procedure answers all these requirements, as evidenced by the variety of surgical techniques advocated over the years. However, modifications with newer materials and designs show promise in achieving a natural postoperative appearance, symmetry, motility, and little socket discharge. The purpose of this chapter is to present indications and techniques for enucleation, evisceration, and dermis–fat grafts, designed to give satisfactory cosmetic and functional results with a minimum of postoperative complications.

30-1

ENUCLEATION

It is not clear when the first enucleation took place. As early as 500 BC, Egyptians wore ocular prostheses, which were placed in situ over phthisic globes as external cosmetic coverings for disfigured globes and held in place with an adhesive substance or thong.

Johannes Lange, in 1555, was the first to mention the removal of the eye but he gave no details. In 1855, Cretchett reported the use of enucleation for numerous nonmalignant ocular conditions. Frost, in 1886, was the first to use an ocular implant within Tenon's capsule following an enucleation. Over the years, various enucleation techniques and implant materials have come and gone. More recently, in 1972, Soll reported the placement of a spherical implant posterior to the posterior layer of Tenon's capsule, within the fatty tissue of the muscle cone.[2] This reduced the extrusion rate, allowed for a larger ocular implant to minimize enophthalmos, and enhanced motility with the placement of a large centrally placed implant. Today hydroxyapatite and polyethylene materials hold promise.

Enucleation has been an acceptable therapeutic modality for intraocular tumors, severely traumatized eyes, and blind, painful, cosmetically disfigured eyes. However, absolute indications for enucleation have diminished in recent years. Improved techniques of radiation have led to an alternative therapy for retinoblastoma.[3] Use of corticosteroids and other immunosuppressant agents has diminished the risk of sympathetic ophthalmia. Recent studies cast doubt on the role of enucleation in preventing metastatic spread of malignant melanoma.[4]

Many variations on the basic theme of enucleation are known to yield superior results. Each change in technique is designed as an improvement, but as with many advances, something is sacrificed in order to achieve a different goal. For instance, buried implants with attachments for muscles are designed to give better movement of the prosthesis and less enophthalmos; however, some of the implants extrude or migrate. Integrated implants are supposed to give improved movement over the buried implants, but extrusion increases significantly.[5]

30-1-1 Indications for Enucleation

Five major indications exist for enucleation:

1. An extensively traumatized globe, with prolapse of uveal tissue or loss of both light projection and perception (enucleation is done to avoid the possibility of sympathetic ophthalmia)

2. An irritated, blind, painful, deformed, or disfigured globe (although some surgeons may suggest topical corticosteroids or a trial fit of a scleral shell if the globe is not painful prior to enucleation), usually secondary to absolute glaucoma, retinal detachment, or chronic inflammation

3. A globe without useful vision that is producing sympathetic ophthalmia, or a blind eye that may excite sympathetic inflammation

4. Intraocular tumors that are nontreatable by another means

5. Patients who are not candidates for evisceration because they fear the risk of sympathetic ophthalmia[6]

30-1-2 Classification of Implants

Orbital implants can be classified as integrated or nonintegrated.[7] Nonintegrated implants have no direct attachments to the extraocular muscles and are usually single spheres of inert material (silicone or methylmethacrylate) buried beneath the conjunctiva and Tenon's capsule in the muscle cone. The rectus muscles may or may not be incorporated into the soft-tissue closure anterior to the implant. Implants may be inserted posterior to the posterior layer of Tenon's capsule within the fatty tissue of the muscle cone.

Integrated orbital implants may be further classified as buried or exposed. Buried implants may have either a spherical or an irregular shape. The spherical implants may be wrapped in sclera, fascia lata, or lyophilized dura to which the extraocular muscles can be sutured. The spherical implants may be left unwrapped, and the muscles sutured directly to the implant material, such as a wire-mesh covered spherical implant. In buried integrated orbital implants with an irregular surface, muscle attachment is achieved by passing the muscles through tunnels in the implant (Allen implant) or through grooves in the implant created by mounds on the anterior aspect (Iowa and Universal implants).

In exposed integrated implants, the muscles are directly attached to the implant and a portion of the implant is exposed to the outside environment. The exposed portion is in the form of a projection or an indentation, which permits the implant to be directly coupled to a prosthetic eye with its posterior projection. Although these implants give excellent motility, this benefit is outweighed by their disadvantage of chronic infections and extrusion. The exposed integrated implant violates two basic surgical principles: (1) a wound must be completely epithelialized to avoid breakdown; and (2) a foreign body left partly exposed will eventually extrude or become infected.

The enucleation of an eye necessitates the replacement of the equivalent spherical volume of 6 ml. An 18-mm ball has a volume of 3.1 ml. This is approximately 3 ml short of the 6 ml lost by removing the globe. The average prosthesis must then be 2 ml or more to make up the difference. The natural globe weighs 7.5 g, and an average prosthetic eye weighs

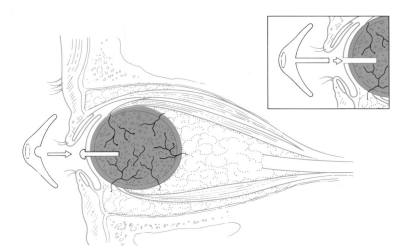

Figure 30-1 *Hydroxyapatite sphere well vascularized, with stem drilled into middle of sphere. Motility implant with ball and socket coupled to prosthetic eye. Ball is projected onto stem, which couples with indentation onto prosthesis for quick, darting movements.*

20 g. Obviously, the advantage of using a large implant is to keep the prosthesis lightweight. This will reduce the incidence of lower eyelid inferior displacement by gravitational force on the prosthetic eye.

Over the years, there have been many implant materials, the first being glass. Many materials have followed, including cartilage, fat, bone, cork, aluminum, wood, silk, ivory, and paraffin.[8] Presently, acrylic and silicone materials are most commonly used, with the most common configuration being spherical. The most promising implant materials today are hydroxyapatite and polyethylene. Hydroxyapatite is an inorganic salt of calcium phosphate similar to the inorganic portion of normal human bone (Figure 30-1). There are several advantages to these orbital implants. First, the material may develop complete fibrovascular ingrowth, which may be enhanced by making drill holes in the implant. Second, when the

implant is exposed, it becomes covered by the surrounding fibrovascular tissue and then by epithelium. This makes it ideal for use as a buried integrated motility implant.

In 4 to 6 months, after vascularization of the implant as determined by a computed tomography (CT) scan with contrast, a magnetic resonance imaging (MRI) scan with gadolinium, or a technetium 99m bone scan, a hole can be drilled through conjunctiva into the buried implant. This hole becomes lined by fibrous tissue and conjunctival epithelium. A peg with a spherical head can be placed in the drilled hole. A ball/socket coupling then will allow movement of the implant to be directly transferred to the prosthetic eye. Moreover, the orbital implant-peg integration takes weight off the lower eyelid and fornix, with less sagging or rounding.[7,8]

30-1-3 Enucleation Technique

During the preoperative evaluation, the patient is advised of the advantages and disadvantages of having an enucleation, followed by fitting and wearing of a prosthesis. The prosthesis is generally fit 4 to 8 weeks after the surgery, to allow the edema to subside and maximize the correct sizing of the prosthesis. Aspirin, anti-inflammatory medications, and anticoagulants are discontinued at least 7 to 14 days preoperatively.

The operation may be performed under general or attended local anesthesia, with supplemental intravenous sedation. A retrobulbar injection of 2% lidocaine with 1:100,000 epinephrine, 0.75% bupivacaine, and Wydase is given with a long, blunt retrobulbar needle. This combination may be supplemented with a frontal nerve block and an infraorbital block in attended local cases. The injection is useful with general anesthesia, as the epinephrine may improve hemostasis and the bupivacaine may provide a longer postoperative period of analgesia.

The procedure is begun by making a 360° peritomy at the limbus with the preservation of as much conjunctiva as possible. Each of the rectus muscles is isolated and left attached to Tenon's capsule (Figure 30-2). Before the muscle has been separated from the globe, an absorbable suture such as 6-0 polyglactin (Vicryl) is threaded through the muscle a few millimeters from the insertion, with one of the sutures extending on each side of the muscle. Then the muscle is separated from the globe. The muscles are cut from the globe, leaving stumps of insertion at the medial and lateral rectus muscles; 4-0 silk sutures are attached to these muscle stumps for fixation or rotation of the globe at a later time.

The superior oblique muscle tendon is cut, and the muscle is allowed to retract. The inferior oblique muscle is cut close to the globe and may be attached to the inferior border of the lateral rectus. This gives support to the orbital implant and enhances motility. If allowed to retract, it will most likely settle near the inferior rectus muscle since there is a sheath common to each. When all muscles are disinserted, Tenon's capsule should be bluntly dissected from the globe as far posteriorly as possible. This will eliminate adhesions that might remain attached to the globe after the optic nerve is cut. Adhesions may be difficult to find once the nerve is cut, because of occasional profuse bleeding. Once Tenon's capsule is dissected from the globe, a curved hemostat is placed over the optic nerve and vessels, and is closed. This crushing pressure remains in place for 5 minutes to diminish bleeding after enucleation. The hemostat is removed and the enucleation scissors are used to palpate the optic nerve from the temporal or nasal approach. The 4-0 silk sutures placed in the lateral and medial rectus muscle stumps can be used to prolapse the globe anteriorly to facilitate more optic nerve removal (Figure 30-3). In most cases, 2 to 4 mm of optic nerve

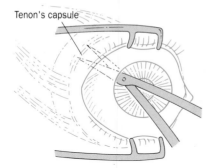

Tenon's capsule

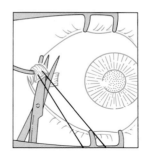

Figure 30-2 *Tenon's capsule is separated from globe between rectus muscles, but is left attached to muscles. Double-armed 6-0 polyglactin suture is placed through distal rectus muscle, and muscle is disinserted from globe.*

Figure 30-3 *Cutting of optic nerve. (A) Traction sutures are placed through insertion of medial and lateral rectus stumps. (B) Close-up of scissors cutting nerve as posterior as possible, leaving significant amount attached to globe. (C) With anterior traction, scissors are placed behind globe temporally, and (D) optic nerve is cut.*

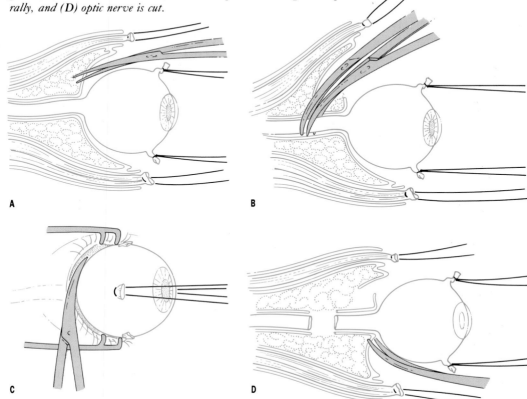

A

B

C

D

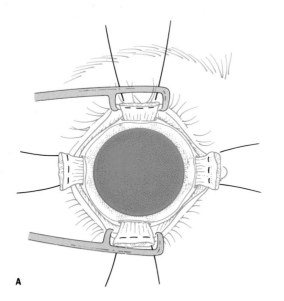

A

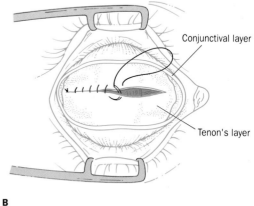

Conjunctival layer

Tenon's layer

B

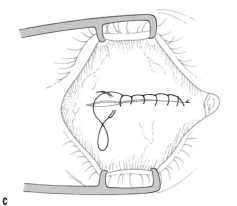

C

Figure 30-4 *Placement of ocular implant. (A) Methylmethacrylate sphere is placed within muscle cone. (B) Anterior aspect of Tenon's capsule is closed with interrupted 6-0 polyglactin suture. (C) Conjunctiva is closed with running, locking 6-0 chromic catgut suture.*

stump on the globe is sufficient. If a retinoblastoma is present, 10 mm of optic nerve should be removed. Bleeding may be controlled either by pressure from a test tube wrapped in a gauze pad or by direct visualization and cauterization of bleeding sites. Once bleeding is controlled, the implant is inserted within the muscle cone.

Selection and placement of an ocular implant provide an opportunity for great variation in technique. If an 18- to 20-mm spherical implant is placed within the muscle cone without closing Tenon's capsule, migration of the implant inferotemporally or superotemporally is common (Figure 30-4). On the other hand, centralization of the implant within the muscle cone by closing the posterior rent in Tenon's capsule (with a pursestring suture) necessitates the use of a smaller implant,

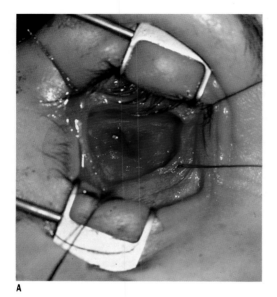

A

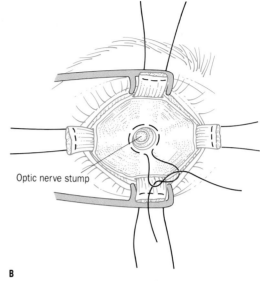

Optic nerve stump

B

16 to 18 mm in size, which may produce some enophthalmos but may enhance motility and anterior positioning of the implant (Figure 30-5).* This can sometimes be remedied by the ocularist with a larger prosthesis. The muscles may then be attached in the following manner: the medial rectus is approximated and tied loosely to the lateral rectus muscle in front of the sphere, and the superior rectus muscle is gently advanced and loosely attached to the inferior rectus muscle. Too much advancement and tight closure, especially of the superior rectus, may lead to implant migration or upper eyelid ptosis. Anterior Tenon's is closed with 6-0 poly-

Figure 30-5 *Rent in posterior Tenon's capsule, where optic nerve was cut. (A) Photograph. (B) Drawing.*

---

*The surgeon should choose the largest implant that can be placed without undue tension over the layers to be closed and without loss of the conjunctival fornices and compromise of eyelid closure.—ED.

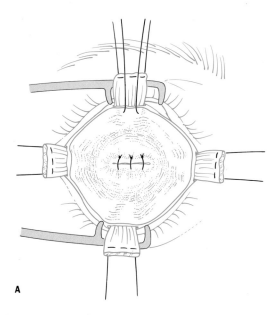

A

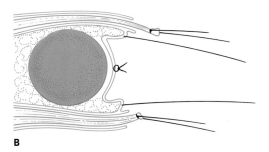

B

Figure 30-6 *Placement of implant in muscle cone.*
(A) Posterior Tenon's capsule from around optic nerve is sutured over sphere with nonabsorbable 4-0 nylon sutures after implant is placed within muscle cone deep to posterior Tenon's fascia.
(B) Running, locking 6-0 chromic catgut sutures close anterior Tenon's capsule.

glactin interrupted sutures, and conjunctiva is closed with a running 6-0 chromic catgut suture.

An alternative technique is wrapping an 18- to 22-mm sphere in autogenous fascia lata or preserved sclera. The wrapped implant is inserted into the muscle cone and each of the rectus muscles is sutured to the fascia lata or sclera in four quadrants with the 5-0 polyglactin sutures that are already attached to the rectus muscles. Care should be taken in the advancement and attachment of the superior rectus muscle to avoid a postoperative ptosis. Tenon's anterior to the extraocular muscle is closed with interrupted 6-0 polyglactin sutures, and the conjunctiva is closed with a running 6-0 chromic catgut suture.

Another alternative, and the authors' preferred method for insertion of a spherical implant, is to place the sphere posterior to the posterior layer of Tenon's capsule within the orbital fat (Figure 30-6).[9] This technique allows for larger implants of 20 to 22 mm, which reduces the volume deficit and subsequent enophthalmos. Also, the use of larger implants deeper in the muscle cone decreases the incidence of migration, and the incidence of extrusion is decreased as the anterior and posterior layers of Tenon's are closed over the implant. The posterior layer of Tenon's capsule from around the optic nerve is sutured over the sphere with 4-0 nylon or 4-0 polyglactin. Anterior Tenon's and conjunctiva are closed as separate layers. Interrupted sutures are preferred in Tenon's fascia. A running, locking 5-0 chromic catgut suture is employed in the conjunctiva. Movement should be adequate with this type of closure since the muscles will continue to function and therefore move the fornices. It is the movement of the fornices that pushes the prosthesis in the appropriate direction. A transparent medium-sized conformer with drainage perforations is placed to maintain the fornices.*

The size of the conformer is important so as to place little tension on the wound. Two 4-0 silk suture tarsorrhaphies are done nasally and temporally. This is accomplished by taking the double-armed 4-0 silk, going through skin and orbicularis of the lower eyelid 4 mm from the lashes and exiting through the meibomian gland orifices, then going through the orifices of the meibomian glands of the upper eyelid and exiting 4 mm back of the lashes through the skin and orbicularis. Cotton bumpers are placed under the loop in the lower and upper eyelid. Antibiotic ointment and a pressure patch are employed. The patch and tarsorrhaphy sutures may remain in position for 48 to 72 hours, to minimize postoperative edema and assure conformer retention.

The technique of the placement of an integrated implant such as the Iowa or Universal implant is one of isolating each of the rectus muscles from adjacent Tenon's capsule and the intramuscular septa. A 4-0 chromic suture placed at the insertion of each rectus muscle is passed through central holes in the Universal implant (1 of 5 sizes). These are then tied and secured to each other. Proper and complete closure of Tenon's capsule is the most important factor in the retention of

the implant. Proper closure prevents dehiscence over the mounds and potential extrusion. Tenon's is closed completely with interrupted 5-0 polyglactin and the conjunctiva is closed with a running 6-0 chromic suture.

At this writing, the newest advance in technique for a buried integrated implant is the porous hydroxyapatite orbital implant developed by Arthur Perry. In Perry's implant technique, posterior Tenon's capsule is not closed. The size of the porous hydroxyapatite implant is determined by placing an acrylic or silicone sphere into the muscle cone. A 20- to 22-mm implant can usually be accommodated. When sclera or fascia lata is used to wrap the implant, there is an increase in diameter of 1.5 to 2 mm; therefore, if a 22-mm silicone implant fits well, a 20-mm hydroxyapatite wrapped implant is the equivalent.[7,8]

If sclera preserved in Neosporin and 70% isopropyl alcohol is to be used, it is soaked in saline and Neosporin solution for 20 minutes. If autogenous fascia lata is used, antibiotic-soaked fascia is discretionary. Multiple drill holes are made in the porous hydroxyapatite to encourage more rapid vascular ingrowth, and sclera or fascia lata is wrapped around the sphere and sutured in a baseball fashion with 5-0 polyglactin. The anterior and posterior poles of the wrapped implant are marked with a pen, and a window is cut out of the fascia or sclera about 5 to 8 mm from the anterior pole, corresponding to the muscle insertions (Figure 30-7). Small windows are made in the posterior pole and slightly

---

*This maneuver is critical in all enucleations and eviscerations, as it is with other socket reconstructions, to aid in maintenance of the conjunctival culde-sac during healing.—ED.

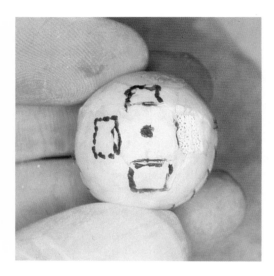

Figure 30-7 *Hydroxyapatite sphere wrapped in sclera, with windows in sclera for attachment of rectus muscles.*

posterior to the equator. Many of the windows correspond to the drill holes, with both techniques encouraging vascularization of the implant.*

The rectus muscles are sewn to the sclera by passing the double-armed 5-0 polyglactin through the anterior lip of the scleral window. Anterior Tenon's is sutured with interrupted 6-0 polyglactin, with every third suture incorporating anterior Tenon's capsule, fascia, or sclera. The conjunctiva is closed with a running 6-0 chromic catgut suture. Antibiotic ointment and a medium-sized conformer are placed, and care is taken to ensure that the conformer does not put pressure on the closure of the conjunctiva and Tenon's capsule. Two intermarginal temporary tarsorrhaphy sutures of 4-0 silk are placed in the nasal and temporal one third of the eyelid, and two patches are applied for 2 to 3 days. The tarsorrhaphy sutures are removed in 2 to 3 days, and an antibiotic corticosteroid drop is applied twice a day. The socket is ready for a prosthesis fitting in approximately 6 weeks.

The implant is generally vascularized in approximately 6 months, and can be assessed with a technetium 99m bone scan, CT scan with contrast, or MRI with gadolinium. Drilling the hole for the motility prosthesis is done with retrobulbar anesthesia. The area on the surface of the conjunctiva to be drilled is marked with a

---

*Many surgeons prefer to place the hydroxyapatite implant without enwrapping, to avoid the risk of transmissible diseases through use of banked sclera or to avoid an additional donor site. Plastic drapes cut in strips serve as an efficient temporary wrap to introduce the implant into the soft-tissue socket and then are slid out from behind the implant.—ED.

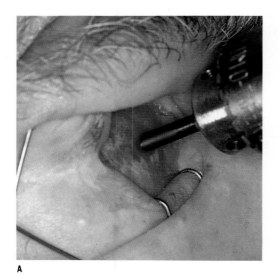

A

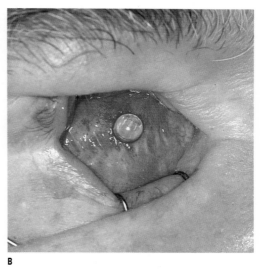

B

pen. This can be facilitated by having the ocularist make a template of the patient's prosthetic eye. In the area of the pupil, a through-and-through hole is made through the template to allow the conjunctiva to be marked for the correct location for drilling. An eyelid speculum is placed between the eyelids, and the marked conjunctiva is lightly cauterized with a battery-heat cautery. With the conjunctiva grasped by toothed forceps, a hole 3 mm in diameter and 10 to 13 mm deep is drilled. Making a perpendicular hole is critical, so alignment must be carefully defined. The peg hole is irrigated with antibiotics and a flat-headed peg 2.5 mm in diameter and 10 mm long is placed in the drilled hole. The patient's prosthetic eye is worn over the flat peg and in 3 to 4 weeks the flat peg is changed for a ball-headed peg that is 13 mm long. This peg is then coupled to a hemispheric indentation in the back of the patient's prosthetic eye (Figure 30-8). The 3- to 4-week inter-

Figure 30-8 *Peg placement. (A) Drill hole is made into hydroxyapatite, 13 mm in length. (B) Placement of stem with ball attached, presenting externally to conjunctiva, which will articulate with prosthesis.*

val allows for vascularization of the drilled hole. This implant is truly a buried integrated implant, with extraocular muscles attached and a fibrovascular ingrowth that imparts excellent motility.*

30-1-4 Treatment of Extruding Orbital Implants

Despite the proper choice of implant and careful surgical technique, some implants may extrude completely or may slowly become exposed. This problem seems to be characteristic of tantalum mesh implants, which gradually cut their way through tissue over a number of years and are now rarely used (Figure 30-9). Extrusion of implants can occur early or late in the postoperative course. Early extrusion is secondary to infection, edema, hemorrhage, too large an implant, or poor technique. Late extrusion is usually related to tissue erosion from a rough prosthesis and subsequent infection or epithelialization of the socket and contraction.[10] It is important to wrap the hydroxyapatite implant, preferably in fascia lata, as the coarse nature of its surface may lead to breakdown of conjunctiva and Tenon's capsule over it.

---

*Motility with this implant may actually cause displacement of the prosthesis from the cul-de-sac. Translation of fine, rapid ocular movements to the prosthesis is also enhanced and important for helping to create a "natural" look to the prosthesis. Volume replacement because of the light weight of the hydroxyapatite implant is also quite good and is another reason for its use.—ED.

Treatment choice depends on the cause. Infection requires removal of the implant. Systemic and topical antibiotics must be used. Antibiotic-soaked gauze, based on culture and sensitivity test results, is used to pack the socket for 5 to 7 days. Once the infection has cleared, a secondary implant is placed. If the socket is clean and the extrusion is less than 50% (5 to 10 mm of exposure), the surgeon can patch the exposed area. Merely undermining and reapproximating the tissue is inadequate, as the wound will dehisce. Ingrowth of the epithelial fibrovascular tissue occurs and can line the implant cavity. It must be excised as part of the reconstructive procedure. The patch may be either donor sclera or autologous fascia lata. Donor sclera is easily obtained from an eye bank. Care must be taken to remove all uveal tissue. Viral transmission such as HIV remains possible and is evaluated. After the scleral patch is soaked in antibiotic solution for 20 minutes, an oversized scleral patch (to allow for shrinkage) is centered over the exposed implant. A 360° pocket is dissected between Tenon's and conjunctiva. Excessive dissection of the conjunctiva can severely limit the cul-de-sac.

Six double-armed 5-0 polyglactin sutures are used to bring the ends of the patch into the depth of the pocket, and the knots are tied over conjunctiva in the fornices (Figure 30-10). Conjunctiva is then closed with 6-0 chromic gut over the patch, without tension. If necessary, sclera may be left bare and it will epithelialize by migration of conjunctiva within 6 weeks. This method provides good vascular supply to both sides of the graft.[11,12]

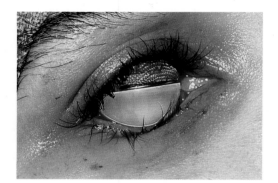

Figure 30-9 *Extrusion of implant that is half mesh and half methylmethacrylate.*

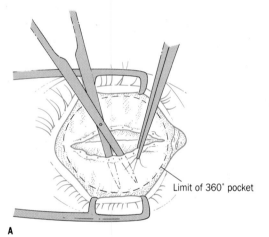

Limit of 360° pocket

A

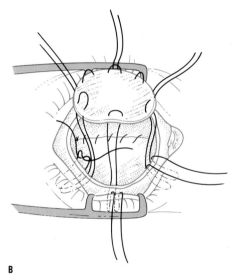

B

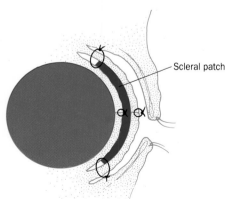

Scleral patch

C

Figure 30-10 *Use of scleral patch graft. (A) Dissection of conjunctiva and Tenon's over exposed implant. (B) Scleral patch is placed in position over exposed defect, with sutures placed through sclera and out through conjunctiva and Tenon's, (C) then tied externally.*

Sometimes it is difficult to dissect conjunctiva from Tenon's. In these cases, a 360° pocket may be formed between the implant and its surrounding tissues. The graft is placed similarly into the pocket; the conjunctiva–Tenon's layer is then closed externally to the graft. Autogenous fascia lata can also be used.

After placement of the patch, an appropriately sized conformer is placed. The conformer must be large enough to prevent contracture and loss of the cul-de-sac, but should not create tension on the wound. Two 4-0 silk suture tarsorrhaphies are completed and left in place for 2 to 3 days with a firm pressure dressing to reduce postoperative edema and hemorrhage.

Extrusions greater than 50% require removal of the implant. Placement of a smaller secondary implant alone is possible, but it may extrude again or lack adequate orbital volume. Another approach is to envelop a 16- to 18-mm implant in donor sclera or autogenous fascia lata (Figure 30-11). Autogenous fascia lata is thick and pliable, and forms a strong, well-vascularized barrier to extrusion.[13] Extraocular muscles are easily attached to it. The conjunctiva is carefully dissected from the orbital contents, noting and not injuring the rectus muscles. If the procedure takes place within 2 to 3 weeks after extrusion, a cavity may be found within the muscle cone. The muscle cone, however, is often found to be a shrunken fibrotic mass. Epithelial fibrovascular ingrowth lining the extrusion site and socket must be identified and excised. Sharp dissection in the oblique meridian will avoid damaging the rectus muscles, which may not be visualized. Excision of scar tissue and posterior dissection continue until Tenon's capsule and extraocular muscles can be easily stretched over the implant without tension.

The fascia lata is obtained from the lateral thigh and is wrapped around a 14- to 18-mm implant like a baseball. The fascia adds 2 mm of diameter to the implant. Double-armed 4-0 polyglactin sutures are placed in each quadrant of the fascia-enveloped sphere. The implant is then placed within the cavity. The sutures are brought out between the rectus muscles and tied externally, positioning the implant. Tenon's capsule posterior to the recti is sutured over the ball with 5-0 polyglactin interrupted sutures, taking a bite of the fascia lata with each suture. This fixes the implant centrally and creates a barrier. The recti are then approximated gently with 5-0 polyglactin, and anterior Tenon's is closed with 6-0 polyglactin. Conjunctiva is closed with running 6-0 chromic catgut, and an appropriate conformer is placed (Figure 30-12). Suture tarsorrhaphies are completed and a pressure patch is applied for 3 days.

An alternative method for a secondary implant is the dermis–fat graft. The vascularity of the conjunctiva and anterior ciliary arteries markedly decreases the incidence of fat atrophy. The dermis–fat graft is also indicated as a primary orbital implant, especially in cases of burns and trauma. The dermis–fat graft is valuable as a spacer when the fornices are compromised due to surgical trauma (retinal detachments), chemical burns, or immunologic insults such as Stevens-Johnson syndrome or cicatricial pemphigoid. The dermis–fat graft can serve to increase the surface area of the fornices as well as increasing the volume of the orbit. These grafts do not migrate or extrude and have excellent motility from attachment to the extraocular muscles. Motility of the prosthesis is achieved by movement of the fornices, as well as the interface of the prosthesis and dermis–fat graft, but results can be unpredictable. The techniques of harvesting and placing dermis–fat grafts are discussed later in the chapter.

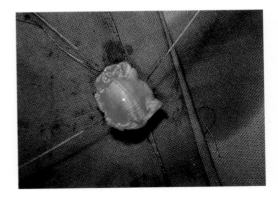

Figure 30-11 *Sphere wrapped in fascia lata, with three 4-0 polyglactin sutures coming in different directions, which will come out through conjunctiva and Tenon's externally between rectus muscles to position implant centrally.*

30-2

EVISCERATION

Evisceration involves the surgical removal of the intraocular contents through an incision or opening in the cornea or sclera. The procedure can be performed with or without the removal of the cornea. The optic nerve, sclera, extraocular muscles, and periorbita are left virtually intact in most cases. The first report of an evisceration has been credited to James Beer in 1817. While he was performing an iridectomy for acute glaucoma, an expulsive suprachoroidal hemorrhage occurred. During this surgical procedure, the remaining contents within the scleral shell were removed and the final cosmetic result was reportedly good. In 1874, Noyes performed the first planned surgical evisceration. He published a review of the evisceration procedure that he used in cases of severe intraocular infection and reported good cosmetic results. Interestingly, there were no reported cases of sympathetic ophthalmia. In 1884, Graefe advocated

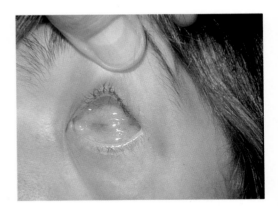

Figure 30-12 *Postoperatively healed socket, following placement of sphere (wrapped in fascia lata) into muscle cone, with good fornices and centrally placed implant.*

evisceration in the presence of a severe panophthalmitis to prevent intracranial spread via the incised dura. The same year, Mules reported placing a spherical glass implant within the scleral shell after evisceration. Although the grass sphere was originally used for the evisceration procedure, Frost adapted it for use in enucleation. His fear was that patients undergoing evisceration could develop sympathetic ophthalmia. Therefore, he chose enucleation over evisceration. Now, about 175 years after its first description, some surgeons still reserve evisceration only for cases of suppurative endophthalmitis,[14] while others consider evisceration their procedure of choice.[15] The theoretic possibility of sympathetic ophthalmia remains one of the most controversial topics in ophthalmology.

Evisceration has several distinct advantages over enucleation. The primary advantage is the final cosmetic result (including motility) after fitting the ocular prosthesis. Many adaptations of the enucleation procedure have attempted to surgically duplicate the evisceration procedure, while still removing the entire globe and its connection to the extraocular muscles, optic nerve, and periorbita. Obviously, if it were not for the fear of sympathetic ophthalmia, evisceration would likely be the procedure of choice in many instances.

Because evisceration, for the most part, is intraocular surgery, as opposed to enucleation, which is orbital surgery, evisceration minimally affects orbital contents with regard to anatomic distortion, resorption of orbital fat, and the like. The orbital fat and the suspensory attachments to the conjunctival fornices are relatively undisturbed, making late enophthalmos and superior sulcus deformities less likely to occur. The orbital volume is minimally changed from its original state, which allows the placement of a relatively thin cosmetic prosthetic shell. In cases of endophthalmitis, evisceration allows intraocular extirpation and removal of the infection without the potential spread to the subarachnoid space, where the possibility of intracranial infection or meningitis is real.[14] The patient also may be more willing, psychologically, to undergo a procedure that avoids removal of the entire eyeball. In most surgeons' hands, the procedure is quicker and possibly better tolerated by elderly, debilitated patients. The incidence of extrusion of the orbital implant appears to be less than that of enucleation.[16]

Evisceration also has several well-known disadvantages and contraindications. These include the potential for, or documented presence of, an intraocular tumor and the risk of sympathetic ophthalmia or adverse reaction to treatment for ophthalmia (eg, poorly controlled diabetic patients who could not tolerate systemic corticosteroids). Other situations that could contraindicate evisceration include penetrating ocular injuries with prolapse of uveal tissue and eyes that have undergone multiple surgical procedures, such as vitrectomy and scleral buckling, which may make the surgery more difficult and increase the threat of sympathetic ophthalmia.[17] Severely phthisic eyes have also been regarded as poor candidates for standard evisceration; however, recent innovations may make evisceration possible in these instances.[18-20] Pain may also persist after the evisceration.[21] Finally, if a thorough pathologic examination of the globe contents is indicated, evisceration should not be performed.

30-2-1 Evisceration Technique

The procedure can be performed either with attended local anesthesia or under general anesthesia. In view of the typical psychological burden placed on the patient, general anesthesia is usually preferred. If general anesthesia is not used, a retrobulbar anesthetic of 0.75% bupivacaine mixed with 2% lidocaine with 1:100,000 epinephrine is typically the anesthetic of choice. The surgery may be performed with or without a keratectomy.

30-2-1-1 Evisceration Without Keratectomy   If the cornea is to be retained, a modification of the procedure described by Hughes is utilized.[22] The greatest advantage of evisceration with corneal preservation is the ability to place a larger spherical implant than would otherwise be possible. An incision is made through conjunctiva and Tenon's capsule 4 mm posterior to the limbus. The superior rectus muscle is identified, a 5-0 polyglactin suture is placed across its insertion site, and the muscle is disin-

serted. Approximately 2 mm above the insertion site, a transverse sclerotomy is performed through sclera only. The incision is made circumferentially for approximately 160° (Figure 30-13). A long cyclodialysis spatula is passed forward between the choroid and sclera to lyse the attachments of the uveal tissue at the level of the scleral spur. An evisceration spoon is then placed into this plane, and the remaining intraocular contents are removed.

Significant bleeding can be encountered secondary to interruption of vortex vessels and the central retinal artery. The bleeding can usually be controlled by direct pressure, by inserting a warmed or iced test tube, or by packing the scleral shell with thrombin-soaked gauze for several minutes. If the bleeding continues, the artery may be identified using gentle irrigation and suction and cauterized (preferably with bipolar cautery). After the bleeding has stopped completely, the internal scleral cavity is cautiously inspected and meticulously cleansed with moistened gauze. The cavity is then thoroughly swabbed with small gauze sponges moistened with absolute alcohol. This ensures that all uveal pigment is removed or denatured as much as possible, to limit the small potential risk for sympathetic ophthalmia, as well as destroying and removing nerves. The corneal endothelium is then addressed, either removing or de-

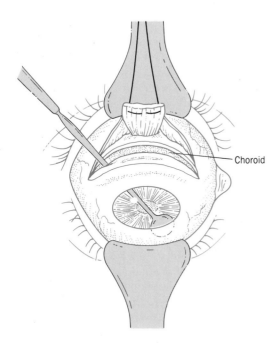

Choroid

Figure 30-13 *Sclerotomy is made 2 mm above superior rectus insertion, through sclera but not choroid, extending 160° around upper part of globe. Evisceration spoon is swept around to break all scleral spur attachments and is rotated 360° to separate choroid posteriorly.*

briding the posterior surface of the cornea at the level of the endothelium and Descemet's membrane to cause scarification.

If endophthalmitis had been present, the scleral cavity should be lavaged with the antibiotic solution indicated by previous culture and sensitivities (preferably nonpreserved for intravenous use). If a severe suppurative infection had been present, the scleral shell may be additionally lavaged with povidone-iodine solution. The wound may then be packed with antibiotic-soaked gauze and allowed to heal by secondary intention. If necessary, volume augmentation surgery is performed after the infection has cleared. If the infection is less severe, the sclera is packed but closed later (delayed primary wound closure), after placement of an alloplastic implant or a dermis–fat graft. If the corneal stroma is infected or necrotic, keratectomy should be performed.[14]

If the cornea has been preserved during evisceration, the wound opening is typically enlarged to accommodate an implant 14 to 18 mm in diameter. Some techniques describe an overlapping of the scleral wound to reinforce wound closure and prevent extrusion.[14] Typically, a 5-0 polyglactin suture is used for single interrupted or horizontal mattress wound closure without tension. The superior rectus muscle is reattached to its insertion site with the preplaced suture (Figure 30-14). Conjunctiva and Tenon's are then closed with a 6-0 chromic suture.

30-2-1-2 Evisceration With Keratectomy The surgical procedure is similar when the cornea is excised (in cases of severe corneal disease and/or endophthalmitis). The procedure is begun with an initial 360° peritomy and the cornea is removed. The contents of the globe are evacuated as described above. The conjunctiva and Tenon's capsule are then reflected posteriorly (fornix-based) to allow incisions to be made in the sclera at the 10:30- and 4:30-o'clock positions. These incisions are made to avoid injury to the rectus muscles. The enlarged sclera opening permits placement of the sphere, which is usually 12 to 16 mm. If the scleral pouch is too small to allow for an adequate-sized implant, radial expansion sclerotomy incisions are most effective (Figure 30-15). Closure of the sclera is performed using interrupted or horizontal mattress 5-0 polyglactin sutures without tension. Tenon's capsule is closed separately from conjunctiva, with interrupted 6-0 polyglactin sutures. The conjunctiva is approximated with a continuous 6-0 chromic suture. It is often helpful to close the conjunctiva and Tenon's capsule in a different axis than the scleral closure.[23]

An antibiotic or a corticosteroid–antibiotic combination ophthalmic ointment is placed in the conjunctival fornices. Usually, when the cornea is preserved, an acrylic conformer is not necessary. However, a conformer or symblepharon ring may be used in cases where the cornea is excised. An intermarginal suture can also be used. The pressure bandage is removed after 3 to 5 days. The fitting of the prosthesis may begin as early as 3 weeks after surgery. Patients can have a considerable amount of postoperative discomfort following evisceration. A short course of systemic corticosteroids is most helpful.

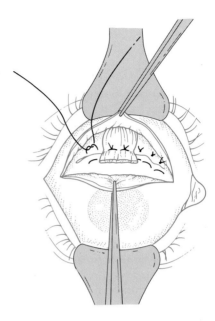

Figure 30-14 *Spherical implant is inserted into scleral shell. Conjunctiva is closed with running 6-0 chromic catgut suture. Wound edges are overlapped and sutured together with multiple horizontal mattress sutures, using 5-0 polyglactin to imbricate wound edges. Superior rectus muscle is reattached at its original position.*

Figure 30-15 *Expansion sclerotomies to accommodate larger implant for evisceration surgery. Courtesy Charles M. Stephenson, MD.*

30-2-2 Implant Materials

A multitude of materials have been used, including glass, gold, tantalum, silicone, and silicone mesh.[24] Most recently, dermis–fat grafts and hydroxyapatite or polyethylene implants have shown promising results. The type of spherical implant is the surgeon's choice. The glass sphere has been the standard for many years, but there is some concern about possible shattering. Silicone implants have been well tolerated, but recent Federal Drug Administration policies regarding silicone implants may make these more difficult to use in the future. Hydroxyapatite spheres, which have been more popularly used after enucleation, may improve motility even more if at a later date the eviscerated orbit containing a hydroxyapatite sphere is drilled for placement of a peg, as is done in enucleation surgery. A recent advance in spherical implants is the use of a porous polyethylene material that has been well tolerated for use in other aspects of cosmetic and facial plastic surgery.[18-20,25,26]

Compared to enucleation, evisceration appears to yield a more favorable cosmetic result. With evisceration, the motility of the prosthesis is typically superior to other procedures performed for reconstruction of the anophthalmic socket after primary removal of a blind, painful eye. As with any surgical procedure, a thorough educational discussion with the patient should occur prior to scheduling surgery. The risks of sympathetic ophthalmia (albeit very rare) should be mentioned. The patient's expectations are best met when good rapport is established between surgeon, patient, and ocularist.

30-3

DERMIS–FAT GRAFTS

Historically, composite dermis and free fat grafts have been used extensively by plastic and reconstructive surgeons.[27,28] Free fat grafts had been generally abandoned after unsatisfactory results were obtained because of significant fat resorption.[29,30] Leaf and Zarem reported good success with soft-tissue reconstruction of the face using lipodermal grafting.[31] Barraquer, in 1901, was the first to describe autogenous fat grafting to the orbit.[32] There were few descriptions in the literature of dermis–fat grafts to the orbit until Smith and Petrelli, in 1978, described the first use of a composite dermis–fat graft in the orbit for an extruding orbital implant.[33] Then Hawtof used strips of composite dermis–fat grafts to correct supratarsal and superior sulcus deformities, and others described its use to correct both anophthalmic patients and trauma-induced deformities in sighted patients.[34] Many variations have since evolved for the use of lipodermal grafts in the treatment of the anophthalmic socket.[35-38]

Unlike free grafts, the composite dermis–fat graft is more resistant to resorption and serves as an excellent replacement for the extruded orbital implant, as it is a natural integrated socket expander. The proximity of the fat to dermis is vital for fat survival in the composite graft.[35] The anophthalmic soft-tissue socket has a rich blood supply, supported by the conjunctiva and anterior ciliary vessels, which contributes to the success of composite grafts. There is little potential for extrusion or rejection.

Dermis–fat grafts have been used most frequently after extrusion or migration of an orbital implant following enucleation. The graft has also been used to expand orbital volume, to treat partly contracted sockets, to augment socket volume after enucleation without implant, to repair extrusion of an evisceration implant, and to augment superior suclus deformities in anophthalmic patients.[18,39,40] Recently, the dermis–fat graft has been repopularized as a primary implant after enucleation and evisceration.[18-21,36]

Secondary dermis–fat grafts have been more popular than primary dermis–graft surgery, but paradoxically the rate of fat resorption is significantly greater after secondary implantation.[41] It is an ideal source for orbital augmentation after significant trauma and tissue loss due to chemical or thermal injuries, but these situations are believed to be the primary cause of graft ulcerations[18] and graft–fat atrophy.[36] The lipodermal grafted socket also has excellent motility, especially when the extraocular muscles are attached to the edge of the dermis graft, as described in Smith and Petrelli's paper.[33] The excellent socket motility, however, is often not directly transmitted to the prosthesis.

Distinct disadvantages have included an unpredictable rate of absorption, with resulting superior sulcus deformity and volume deficiency. Eyelid retraction has been noted and is thought to be second-ary to the adherent rectus muscles retracting on the fat graft with shrinkage. The posterior pull of the muscles is transmitted to the levator complex and the inferior rectus (and attachments to the lower eyelid retractors), resulting in eyelid retraction.[36] It may also follow that the retraction of the muscles and the posterior pull of the dermis–fat graft add to enophthalmos and apparent volume depletion, requiring a larger ocular prosthesis and additional volume augmentation surgery. Nunery's experience showed a 3-year reoperative rate of approximately 60%. Two thirds of his patients required major changes in their ocular prosthesis within 1 year, due to a change in the socket anatomy from fat reabsorption.[36]

30-3-1 Grafting Technique

Most surgeons prefer to perform dermis–fat grafting with the patient under general anesthesia, although a local anesthetic can be used if general anesthesia is contraindicated. The site of the donor graft may be the lower abdomen or the thigh, according to the surgeon's preference.[42] These non-weight-bearing sites may be less tender in the postoperative period and less likely to develop wound dehiscence. This also allows the patient to remain supine during the entire surgical procedure. Alternatively, the inferomedial buttocks region (near the inner gluteal fold)[38,40] or an area inferior to the level of the lateral iliac crest at the region overlying the greater trochanter may be chosen. The patient's head is placed in a standard position, and the lower body is rotated to the opposite side of the orbit undergoing surgery. A pillow is placed between the legs, and the ipsilateral flexed lower extremity is crossed over the opposite knee, exposing the buttocks well, while keeping the head in primary position.

If dermis–fat grafting is performed primarily after enucleation or evisceration, the globe (or its contents) is removed in a manner of the surgeon's choice. Meticulous hemostasis must be maintained, without overzealous cautery (preferably bipolar).

30-3-1-1 Grafting in the Enucleated Patient
The extraocular muscles are isolated and a double-armed 5-0 polyglactin suture is threaded through the distal end prior to disinsertion, as in strabismus surgery. Tenon's fascia may be opened in all four quadrants of the intermuscular membrane.[36] This allows orbital fat to come into contact with the graft fat, enhancing graft viability. Other authors, however, have suggested "minimal" dissection, believing that deep dissection beneath the conjunctiva and Tenon's layer creates a potential space for dehiscence and loss of socket vascularity with resulting increased fat atrophy.[39] However, the authors of this chapter prefer opening the Tenon's capsule to allow fat-to-fat contact and enhanced graft survival.

30-3-1-2 Grafting in the Eviscerated Patient
An evisceration with keratectomy is performed, as previously described. The scleral shell must be opened significantly to allow fat vascularization and to minimize fat atrophy, resulting enophthalmos, and superior sulcus deformity. This allows the procedure to be performed on phthisic eyes. Large radial scleral incisions are performed from the limbus to the optic nerve in the quadrants between the rectus muscles, to allow orbital fat to be exposed to the graft. Alternately, the posterior sclera may be fully excised.[20]

30-3-1-3 Grafting for an Extruding Implant After Enucleation
The dermis–fat graft has been most heralded as a secondary implant in patients who have had extruded orbital implants, whether after enucleation or after evisceration. A horizontal incision is made, with either a sharp blade or a fine-tip needle cutting cautery, in the area of the exposure and is extended medially and laterally. This allows minimal risk of injury to the levator–superior rectus complex. At this point, the standard extruding implant will usually present itself. A glistening pseudocapsule is often seen, which must be excised. In cases of integrated orbital implants (tantalum mesh or hydroxyapatite), extensive dissection may be necessary to remove the implant. Hemostasis must be meticulously maintained, but cautery should be minimized (sometimes, packing the socket for a few minutes is all that is necessary). The intraconal space and extraocular muscles should be identified and isolated, as they will later be sewn to the edge of the dermis–fat graft. If the muscles cannot be easily identified, an attempt should be made to identify the

muscle remnants. Attachment of these remnants to the dermis edge not only aids in motility, but enhances graft survival.

30-3-1-4 Grafting for an Extruding Implant After Evisceration

Conjunctiva, Tenon's, and sclera are opened over the area of extrusion and undermined. The implant is removed. The sclera is incised posteriorly in four quadrants to expose the orbital fat, if this was not done in the original procedure.

30-3-2 Harvest of the Dermis–Fat Graft

A circle 20 to 25 mm in diameter (conveniently the size of a balanced salt solution bottle) is traced over the abdominal region or buttock. Historically, the area has been dermabraded by either a wire brush or a dental burr,[33] but some surgeons have found postoperative epithelial inclusion cysts and keratinization, which they attributed to inadequate removal of the epidermis.[18,20] Therefore, the authors recommend split-thickness sharp excision of the epidermis and superficial dermis. This should be performed in vivo, before complete excision of the graft. There is less graft manipulation and nonperfusion time if the epidermis is removed prior to excision of the cylindrical graft. A split-thickness skin graft can be obtained with a No. 15 Bard-Parker blade or dermatome. A sharp blade or scissors are then used to incise subcutaneous tissue and fat to a depth of 10 to 15 mm. Careful attention should be paid to directing the incision circumferentially, with the most posterior edge of the graft at least as wide as the dermis to prevent conization of the dermis–fat graft, which would limit potential volume. It is not unusual for the area to appear much smaller after the excision than when it was demarcated.

After complete composite graft excision, the graft is brought to the orbital surgical field without delay (Figure 30-16). This minimizes handling and manipulation of the tissue, as well as potential contamination. Hemostasis at the donor site can be achieved with unipolar cautery. The wound is packed with gauze moistened with a local anesthetic solution containing epinephrine. Attention is then directed to the socket.

30-3-3 Implantation of the Dermis–Fat Graft

The enucleated or eviscerated socket is now ready for implantation of the dermis–fat graft. Excising small triangular sections from equispaced quadrants of the dermis, followed by suture closure, promotes a more convex surface to the graft, which may aid in the socket–prosthesis interface and thus motility.[38] The edge of the dermis is sewn to the rectus muscles, via the preplaced sutures (or to the anterior scleral ring in evisceration) in the respective quadrants. Tenon's capsule is approximated to the dermis circumferentially with multiple interrupted 5-0 polyglactin sutures—conjunctiva and Tenon's are advanced over the peripheral dermis in evisceration (Figure 30-17). After several cardinal sutures are placed, excess fat may be trimmed. An overcorrection of approximately 20% to 30% should allow for typical graft atrophy, resulting in satisfactory

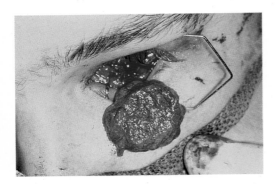

Figure 30-16 *Implant has been removed, and dermis–fat graft placed next to socket.*

orbital volume. If there is ample conjunctiva after undermining, the conjunctiva may be approximated over the graft. Most often, however, the conjunctiva is sewn over the peripheral dermis for several millimeters and the central dermis is left to spontaneously epithelialize. An acrylic conformer (symblepharon ring) that is centrally open is placed to enhance the fornices without adding undue pressure to the graft. Antibiotic ointment is applied, followed by a light pressure dressing of two eye patches.

The donor site wound is closed with multiple deep 4-0 polyglactin sutures for the deep wound, 5-0 polyglactin sutures for the superficial subcutaneous closure, and a near-far/far-near type of vertical mattress closure of 4-0 silk for the skin. A pressure dressing consisting of fluffs and foam tape is also applied to the donor site for several days. Prophylactic intravenous intraoperative antibiotics (Cefzol 1 gram) for extruding implants are preferred.

The orbit dressing may be removed on the first postoperative day to inspect the graft. Routinely, oral and topical antibiotics are used for 1 week. The skin sutures at the donor site should remain for at least 10 days. Full epithelialization of the dermis occurs within 1 month. A prosthesis may be fitted in 4 to 6 weeks.

30-3-4 Complications and Results

Minor complications include conjunctival cysts and granulomas, graft ulcers, socket keratinization, and retention of cilia (Figure 30-18). These can all be managed in an office setting with local or topical anesthesia.[41] Fat atrophy and resulting loss of volume are variable.[36,41] This usually re-

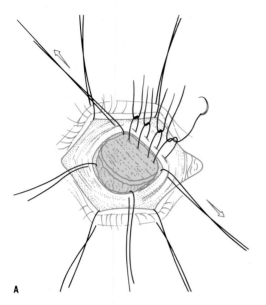

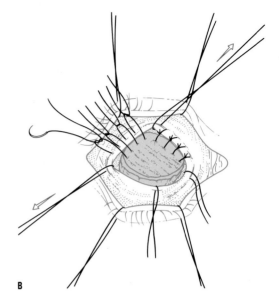

quires more major surgical efforts, including a secondary dermis–fat graft or other alloplastic volume augmentation methods. Early reports of dermis–fat grafting for implant extrusion in enucleation patients showed good, long-lasting results in more than 80%.[43] Failures have been primarily attributed to the inability to isolate and attach the extraocular muscles to the dermis and compromised orbital vascular supply after radiation treatment or chemical injury. Other causes implicated in failure have been advanced age, infection, graft trauma from manipulation, inadequate-size graft (too large or too small), excessive cautery, or inadequate hemostasis.[41] The authors would also add that the underlying health and habits of the patient play a significant role. Vascular disease, diabetes, and the use of cigarettes or alcohol may affect the graft viability. Finally, particular

Figure 30-17 *Placement of dermis–fat graft. (A) Dermis–fat graft being sutured into position with four rectus muscles aligned and attached to dermal edge. (B) Progression of suturing.*

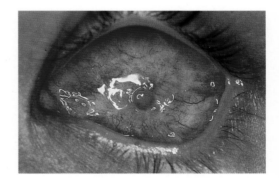

Figure 30-18 *Well-healed dermis–fat graft with epithelial inclusion cyst.*

attention to prosthetic fit is necessary to obtain a good cosmetic result.[44] Ophthalmologist and ocularist communication is essential for a satisfactory outcome.*

---

*For more information, see Chapter 33, "Overview of Ocular Prosthetics," and Chapter 34, "Management and Care of Ocular Prostheses," in this volume.—ED.

REFERENCES

1. Gougelmann H: Enucleation, evisceration and exenteration: an ocularist's point of view. In: Hornblass A, ed: *Tumors of the Ocular Adnexa and Orbit*. St Louis: CV Mosby Co; 1990:305–319.

2. Soll DB: Enucleation surgery: a new technique. *Arch Ophthalmol* 1972;87:196–197.

3. Reese AB: *Tumors of the Eye*. Hagerstown, MD: Harper & Row; 1976.

4. Zimmerman LE, McLean IW, Foster WD: Statistical analysis of follow-up data concerning uveal melanomas, and the influence of enucleation. *Ophthalmology* 1980;87:557–564.

5. Stone W Jr: Complications of evisceration and enucleation. In: Fasanella RM, ed: *Management of Complications in Eye Surgery*. Philadelphia: WB Saunders Co; 1965:388–425.

6. Schaefer DP, Della Rocca RC: Enucleation. In: Smith BC, ed: *Ophthalmic Plastic and Reconstructive Surgery*. St Louis: CV Mosby Co; 1987:1278–1299.

7. Perry AC: Advances in enucleation. In: Nunery W, ed: *Ophthalmic Plastic and Reconstructive Surgery*. Philadelphia: WB Saunders Co; 1991:173–182.

8. Perry AC: Integrated orbital implants. In: Bosniak SL, Smith BC, eds: *Advances in Oph-thalmic Plastic and Reconstructive Surgery*. New York: Pergamon Press; 1990:75–81.

9. Soll DB, ed: *Management of Complications in Ophthalmic Plastic Surgery*. Birmingham, AL: Aesculapius Publishing Co; 1976.

10. Oberfeld S, Levine MR: Diagnosis and treatment of complications of enucleation and orbital implant surgery. In: Bosniak SL, Smith BC, eds: *Advances in Ophthalmic Plastic and Reconstructive Surgery*. New York: Pergamon Press; 1990:107–117.

11. Helveston EM: A scleral patch for exposed implants. *Trans Am Acad Ophthalmol Otolaryngol* 1970;74:1307–1310.

12. Helveston EM: Human bank scleral patch; for repair of exposed or extruded orbital implants. *Arch Ophthalmol* 1969;82:83–86.

13. Levine MR: Extruding orbital implant: prevention and treatment. *Ann Ophthalmol* 1980; 12:1384–1386.

14. Shore JW: Evisceration. In: Levine MR, ed: *Manual of Oculoplastic Surgery*. New York: Churchill Livingstone; 1988:189–194.

15. Baylis H, Shorr N, McCord CD, et al: Evisceration, enucleation and exenteration. In: McCord CD, Tanenbaum M, eds: *Oculoplastic Surgery*. New York: Raven Press; 1987: 313–327.

16. Raflo GT: Enucleation and evisceration. In: Duane TD, Jaeger EA, eds: *Clinical Ophthalmology*. Philadelphia: Harper & Row; 1986;5.

17. Stephenson CM: Evisceration. In: Hornblass A, ed: *Oculoplastic, Orbital, and Reconstructive Surgery*. Baltimore: Williams & Wilkins; 1990:1194–1199.

18. Archer KF, Hurwitz JJ: Dermis-fat grafts and evisceration. *Ophthalmology* 1989;96:170–174.

19. Borodic GE, Townsend DJ, Beyer-Machule CK: Dermis fat graft in eviscerated sockets. *Ophthalmic Plast Reconstr Surg* 1989;5:144–149.

20. Bosniak SL: Dermis-fat grafts and evisceration. *Ophthalmology* 1989;96:1276.

21. Illiff CE, Iliff WJ, Iliff NT: *Oculoplastic Surgery*. Philadelphia: WB Saunders Co; 1979.

22. Hughes WL: Evisceration. *Arch Ophthalmol* 1960;63:36–40.

23. Meltzer MA, Schaefer DP, Della Rocca RC: Evisceration. In: Smith BC, ed: *Ophthalmic Plastic and Reconstructive Surgery*. St Louis: CV Mosby Co; 1987.

24. Soll DB: The anophthalmic socket. *Ophthalmology* 1982;89:407–423.

25. Dresner SC, Braslow RA, Goldberg RA: Porous high-density polyethylene: a new orbital implant. Presented at 22nd Annual Scientific Symposium of American Society of Ophthalmic Plastic and Reconstructive Surgeons. Anaheim, CA: October 12, 1991.

26. Stephenson CM: Evisceration of the eye with expansion sclerotomies. *Ophthalmic Plast Reconstr Surg* 1987;3:249–251.

27. Peer LA: The neglected free fat graft. *Plast Reconstr Surg* 1956;18:233–250.

28. Boering G, Huffstadt AJ: The use of derma-fat grafts in the face. *Br J Plast Surg* 1967;20:172–178.

29. Wheeler JM: Enucleation of the eye with implantation of the patient's fat into the cavity. *Am J Surg* 1917;31:167–168.

30. Peer LA: Loss of weight and volume in human fat grafts with postulation of a "cell survival theory." *Plast Reconstr Surg* 1950;5: 217–230.

31. Leaf N, Zarem HA: Correction of contour defects of the face with dermal and dermal-fat grafts. *Arch Surg* 1972;105:715–719.

32. Barraquer J: Enucleation con ingerto cle tejido adiposo con la capsula de tenon. *Arch Oftalmol Hisp-Am* 1901;1:82.

33. Smith B, Petrelli R: Dermis-fat graft as a movable implant within the muscle cone. *Am J Ophthalmol* 1978;85:62–66.

34. Hawtof D: The dermis fat graft for correction of the eyelid deformity of enophthalmos. *Mich Med* 1975;74:331–332.

35. Bullock JD: Autogenous dermis-fat "baseball" orbital implant. *Ophthalmic Surg* 1987; 18:30–36.

36. Nunery WR, Hetzler KJ: Dermal-fat graft as a primary enucleation technique. *Ophthalmology* 1985;92:1256–1261.

37. Smith B, Bosniak SL, Lisman RD: An autogenous kinetic dermis-fat orbital implant: an updated technique. *Ophthalmology* 1982;89: 1067–1071.

38. Migliori ME, Putterman AM: The domed dermis-fat graft orbital implant. *Ophthalmic Plast Reconstr Surg* 1991;7:23–30.

39. Lisman RD, Smith BC: Dermis-fat grafting. In: Smith BC, ed: *Ophthalmic Plastic and Reconstructive Surgery*. St Louis: CV Mosby Co; 1987:1308–1320.

40. Della Rocca RC, Garber PF: Socket reconstruction. In: Levine MR, ed: *Manual of Oculoplastic Surgery*. New York: Churchill Livingstone; 1988:235–243.

41. Shore JW, McCord CD Jr, Bergin DJ, et al: Management of complications following dermis-fat grafting for anophthalmic socket reconstruction. *Ophthalmology* 1985;92: 1342–1350.

42. Wilkins RB, Kulwin DR, McCord CD Jr, et al: Skin and tissue techniques. In: McCord CD, Tanenbaum M, eds: *Oculoplastic Surgery*. New York: Raven Press; 1987:1–39.

43. Guberina C, Hornblass A, Meltzer MA, et al: Autogenous dermis-fat orbital implantation. *Arch Ophthalmol* 1983;101:1586–1590.

44. Przybyla VA, La Piana FG, Bergin DJ: Fitting of the dermis-fat grafted socket. *Ophthalmology* 1981;88:904–907.

CHAPTER 31

Exenteration of the Orbit

Peter S. Levin, MD
Jonathan J. Dutton, MD, PhD

Exenteration of the orbit involves removal of the eyelids, eye, and varying amounts of orbital contents. In its most extensive form, exenteration includes removal of all orbital tissues, including periorbita, and in some cases resection of adjacent bone.

31-1

INDICATIONS FOR EXENTERATION

Orbital exenteration is most commonly indicated for life-threatening malignancies where more conservative modalities of treatment have failed or are inappropriate.[1,2] Squamous cell carcinoma of the paranasal sinuses, skin, and conjunctiva with deep orbital invasion accounts for the majority of orbital exenterations in published reports. Other malignancies well represented in published series of orbital exenteration include malignant melanoma of the skin and sinuses, basal cell carcinoma, and sebaceous adenocarcinoma. Exenteration has been advocated for the management of orbital mucormycosis in immunosuppressed or diabetic patients, although less radical surgery has been successful in some situations. Orbital exenteration may also be necessary to eliminate severe deformity or orbital pain associated with progressive orbital processes such as sclerosing pseudotumor, neurofibromatosis, lymphangioma, or socket contracture (Table 31-1).

31-2

PATIENT EVALUATION

The surgeon must obtain a complete medical evaluation and advise the patient of the nature of the disease process and the prognosis for cure with medical and/or surgical therapy. The need for definitive tissue diagnosis with permanent histopathologic sections prior to making the decision to perform exenteration cannot be overemphasized. Frozen-section readings of tissues obtained intraoperatively are preliminary determinations, usually based on the observations of a single observer with limited capacity to stain tissues. Accurate diagnosis of malignancy may require special studies or consultations. In general,

TABLE 31-1

*Comparison of Orbital Exenteration at Six Institutions**

	Wilmer Institute	University of California at San Francisco	University of Kansas	Mayo Clinic	University of Naples	Duke University
	1927–1953 (N = 48)	1940–1971 (N = 48)	1951–1964 (N = 31)	1967–1986 (N = 102)	1976–1986 (N = 39)	1969–1988 (N = 99)
Squamous cell carcinoma	4	6	3	33	7	32
Skin	3	2	1	NA[†]	6	12
Sinus	1	0	2	NA	1	13
Conjunctiva	0	3	0	NA	0	6
Tear sac	0	1	0	NA	0	1
Basal cell carcinoma	11	14	11	21	9	8
Sebaceous carcinoma	0	1	0	6	0	6
Other epithelial tumors	6	8	5	9	10	15
Malignant melanoma	12	8	7	16	8	18
Conjunctiva	3	5	NA	NA	1	10
Sinus	0	0	NA	NA	0	3
Choroid	9	2	NA	8	7	1
Other	0	1	NA	NA	0	4
Rhabdomyo-sarcoma	2	5	2	2	2	2
Infectious	1	0	0	1	0	6
Other	12	6	3	14	3	12

*At Wilmer, University of California at San Francisco, and University of Naples, only exenterations performed by ophthalmology departments were surveyed; at University of Kansas, Mayo Clinic, and Duke University, all exenterations were reported, regardless of the department performing the operation.
[†]NA indicates no data available.

Source: Levin PS, Dutton JJ: A 20-year series of orbital exenteration. Am J Ophthalmol *1991;112:496–501. Published with permission from The American Journal of Ophthalmology. Copyright by The Ophthalmic Publishing Company.*

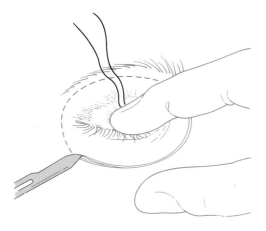

Figure 31-1 *Incision of skin and underlying orbicularis muscle is made just inside orbital rim. If skin is not infiltrated by tumor, incision may be made just outside lash lines.*

the decision to proceed with orbital exenteration should be based on finalized pathologic interpretation.

A comprehensive evaluation for metastatic disease is usually indicated. The regional nodes in the preauricular, submental, neck, and supraclavicular areas should be assessed. The parotid gland should be evaluated for inflammation or fullness. Chest x-rays, liver function tests, and bone scans may be indicated. The presence of regional spread of disease is usually an indication for additional surgery in the involved areas or for postoperative irradiation. The presence of widespread metastasis would often lead to palliative procedures such as radiation therapy or surgical debulking.

31-3

STANDARD EXENTERATION TECHNIQUE

General anesthesia is preferred. The eyelids are sewn together using an intermarginal suture of 4-0 silk to protect the cornea and conjunctiva from artifactual damage and to provide a means of traction. An incision line is marked around the orbit just inside the orbital rim. If the tumor involves the skin, a clear margin of at least 3 to 5 mm must be allowed around the lesion. Local anesthesia containing 1:100,000 epinephrine is infiltrated along the incision line for hemostasis.

The incision is made along the marked line with a scalpel blade (Figure 31-1). The authors have found no advantage to preserving the eyelid margins, although preservation of eyelid skin may be helpful in later reconstruction. In the latter case, the incision is placed just proximal to the lash line in both eyelids, and the skin is dissected from the underlying orbicularis muscle to the level of the orbital rims. Subcutaneous tissues are transected around the rim to the level of the bone using a cutting cautery. The periosteum is cut just outside the arcus marginalis along the bony rim.

A Freer or similar elevator is used to dissect the periosteum from the orbital rim and along the orbital walls toward the apex (Figure 31-2). This layer separates easily except along the inferior and superior orbital fissures, at the trochlea, at the lateral orbital tubercle, and at the origin of the inferior oblique muscle where it is firmly attached to bone. The surgeon must be particularly careful during dissection along the medial orbital wall, as the thin lamina papyracea is easily violated. Penetration into the sinuses may result in sinus–orbit fistulization. The nasolacrimal duct is transected at its entrance to the bony nasolacrimal canal. Cauterization is often helpful to establish hemostasis. If tumor involves the lacrimal sac and duct, the anterior wall of the duct is removed with rongeurs and the duct is dissected to its termination in the inferior nasal meatus.

With the periorbita freed to the apex, enucleation scissors, Metzenbaum scissors, or a wire snare is passed across the apical stump of the orbital contents (Figure 31-3). The specimen is excised and the orbit is packed with cottonoid strips soaked in epinephrine or thrombin. After 5 to 10 minutes, the packs are slowly removed and the ophthalmic artery and any residual bleeding points are cauterized. Bone wax may be necessary for any bleeders that perforate the orbital walls. Apical

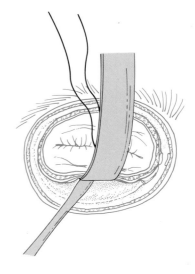

Figure 31-2 *Periorbita is freed from bony orbital margins back to orbital apex.*

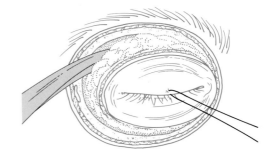

Figure 31-3 *Orbital contents are removed after severing optic nerve and other apical tissues. Empty orbital cavity may be allowed to heal by granulation, by application of split-thickness skin graft, or by regional or distant flaps/grafts.*

tissues may require additional resection with scissors or a scalpel blade.

The exenteration cavity is inspected for residual diseased tissue. Frozen-section examination of any suspect tissue at the apex, lacrimal duct, or cutaneous margins is an excellent means of judging the adequacy of resection. Additional resection is performed if necessary. If residual apical tumor cannot be completely removed—for example, at the superior orbital fissure—intraoperative cryoablation with liquid nitrogen, intracranial exploration, or postoperative radiotherapy should be considered.

Based on the particular clinical requirements, the standard orbital exenteration may be modified to less extensive or more radical procedures. A limited, anterior exenteration, in which tissues at the mid-orbit and apex are preserved, may be indicated for some invasive malignancies that have spread only into the anterior orbit or immediate retrobulbar space. In extended exenteration procedures, the entire orbital soft-tissue compartment is excised, along with adjacent structures such as orbital bones or paranasal sinuses.

31-4

RECONSTRUCTIVE OPTIONS

Orbital reconstruction following exenteration may or may not be indicated, depending on the nature of the disease process. The decision to use local, regional, or distant flaps or grafts for filling the defect and to apply an orbital prosthesis must be made on an individual case basis.

The surgeon will have to decide on local, regional, or distant procedures for cosmetic rehabilitation of the orbital defect (Table 31-2).[3] The simplest technique is to pack the orbit with iodine-impregnated gauze and allow the socket to granulate. Daily irrigation with 2% hydrogen peroxide solution or with running water from the shower head is continued until the process is complete in about 6 to 8 weeks. This option results in a deep cavity with only a relatively thin cover that usually allows detection of recurrent tumor at an early stage. During the final healing period, some contracture of the orbital margins occurs that may displace the periorbital skin and structures, such as the brow, toward or even over the orbital rim. The resulting cavity is easily covered with a black patch, and can usually be fitted with a silicone oculofacial prosthesis unless the orbital rims are significantly distorted.

Alternatively, the socket may be covered with a split-thickness skin graft. The graft is sewn to the marginal skin edges using absorbable sutures, and the orbit is packed with Xeroform gauze to provide firm apposition to the bony walls for 10 to 14 days. This technique allows more rapid healing and rehabilitation than does granulation and prevents the marginal contracture sometimes seen with the latter. Like granulation, it avoids covering the orbit with thick tissue that might mask tumor recurrence.

In the absence of malignant disease or after a suitable disease-free interval, regional flaps or distant myocutaneous flaps or grafts may be used. These have the advantage of making the orbital cavity shallow to provide a more acceptable contour for patients who choose not to wear a patch or prosthesis. Such flaps may be mobilized and rotated from the head or neck. One common example is the temporalis muscle flap. In this procedure, the anterior half of the temporalis muscle is dissected from the temporalis fossa and laid into the orbit through a defect created in the lateral orbital wall. A full- or split-thickness skin graft is then placed over the muscle or fascial flap. This procedure effectively makes the orbital cavity shallow; however, a visible depression may result in the temporal fossa. Alternatively, the superficial temporoparietal fascia of the scalp can be mobilized and rotated into the orbit along with its nutrient superficial artery. A full- or split-thickness skin graft may be placed over the fascia. The orbital cavity is filled without compromise to the hair or skin of the face or a notable temporal fossa depression.[4]

Alternatively, the orbit and, if necessary, the contiguous exposed sinus and/or intracranial cavities can be covered with distant tissue grafts, such as the latissimus dorsi, using microanastomotic techniques. Soft-tissue reconstruction may need to be

TABLE 31-2

Reconstruction of the Exenterated Socket

Local Solutions

Granulation

Split-thickness skin graft

Regional Solutions

Temporalis muscle transfer

Temporoparietal fascial flap

Distant Solution

Latissimus dorsi free flap

combined with bone grafting when bone is resected as part of the extirpative procedure.*

*See also Chapter 29, "Periorbital and Craniofacial Surgery," in this volume.—ED.

31-5

PROSTHETIC OPTIONS

The standard black patch is an acceptable cosmetic solution for many patients. A patch of appropriate size can entirely cover the exenteration cavity. The fear that some patients have about patches partially dislodging can be alleviated by inserting gauze into the socket or by wearing a flesh-colored silicone moulage beneath the patch.

Oculofacial prostheses may provide excellent aesthetic results in many patients. Contemporary devices consist of a custom-molded silicone appliance colored to match adjacent facial skin tones. It contains a methylmethacrylate ocular prosthesis painted to match the other eye, and lashes are inserted into the silicone eyelid margins. Such prostheses lack motility and the eyelids remain fixed in position. With time, discoloration from sun and wind exposure may be a problem. Also, excessive perspiration may make wearing such devices difficult in hot weather, since they are usually applied with a skin adhesive. Nevertheless, many patients wear such devices successfully. It is the authors' practice to discuss with patients the pros and cons of the various cosmetic options and allow them to make the final decision.

More recently, osseointegrated titanium brackets have been introduced, allowing direct coupling of the oculofacial prosthesis to the orbital bones.[5] This procedure is not FDA-approved and has not yet gained wide acceptance. However, it may ultimately prove to be a valuable alternative in the cosmetic rehabilitation of the exenteration patient.†

†See also Chapter 33, "Overview of Ocular Prosthetics," in this volume.—ED.

REFERENCES

1. Bartley GB, Garrity JA, Waller RR, et al: Orbital exenteration at the Mayo Clinic: 1967–1986. *Ophthalmology* 1989;96:468–473.

2. Levin PS, Dutton JJ: A 20-year series of orbital exenteration. *Am J Ophthalmol* 1991;112:496–501.

3. Levin PS, Ellis DS, Stewart WB, Toth BA: Orbital exenteration: the reconstructive ladder. *Ophthalmic Plast Reconstr Surg* 1991;7:84–92.

4. Ellis DS, Toth BA, Stewart WB: Temporoparietal fascial flap for orbital and eyelid reconstruction. *Plast Reconstr Surg* 1992;89:606–612.

5. Nerad JA, Carter KD, LaVelle WE, et al: The osseointegration technique for the rehabilitation of the exenterated orbit. *Arch Ophthalmol* 1991;109:1032–1038.

Deformities of the Anophthalmic Socket

Janet L. Roen, MD
Orkan George Stasior, MD

The anophthalmic socket is subject to two major deformities: enophthalmos and contraction. In enophthalmos, the ocular prosthesis and orbital soft tissues have a sunken-in appearance. In contraction, the socket will accommodate only a substandard-sized prosthesis or no prosthesis at all. Understanding these two disfigurements and their treatments is the goal of this chapter.

32-1

ENOPHTHALMOS

Enophthalmos is an acquired retrodisplacement of the globe or prosthesis (in the case of anophthalmic enophthalmos) within the bony orbit. Alone, enophthalmos may cause varying degrees of disfigurement. Often, enophthalmos, particularly anophthalmic enophthalmos, is exaggerated by a constellation of secondary or associated eyelid and orbital soft-tissue defects.

A deficit of orbital tissue volume causes enophthalmos. This volume deficit may be absolute or relative. Orbital soft-tissue volume may be lost due to tissue atrophy, fibrosis, or herniation of tissue through an orbital fracture into a sinus cavity. The orbital contents may remain constant, but the orbit itself may be expanded, as in an inferiorly displaced saucer type of orbital floor fracture. In such a case, the ratio of orbital soft-tissue volume to orbital volume has decreased, producing a relative tissue deficit and enophthalmos.

In the anophthalmic socket, 6 ml of tissue is removed by enucleation. Although an orbital implant may replace 2 to 4 ml of volume, and a conformer/prosthesis may replace 1 to 2 ml, a volume deficit of 1 to 3 ml may persist. Fat and muscle atrophy secondary to the enucleation procedure or antecedent trauma may further reduce the amount of soft tissue in the anophthalmic orbit.

Because of surgically altered orbital soft-tissue structure when the globe is absent, the orbital implant may migrate, orbital fat may move inferiorly and anteriorly, and the levator–superior rectus muscle complex may move inferiorly. These changes give rise to eyelid and conjunctival fornix abnormalities. Fewer changes occur when an intraconal implant is present. Severe alterations will produce a contracted socket, incapable of retaining a normal-sized or any prosthesis.

32-1-1 Diagnosis

History-taking should direct the ophthalmologist toward the cause of the patient's enophthalmos. The physician should inquire concerning previous ocular history, trauma, and general medical conditions including nutrition, endocrine disease, and neoplasia. Trauma is the most common cause of enophthalmos; such trauma may include ocular, orbital, and facial injuries as well as surgical trauma, particularly when anophthalmic enophthalmos exists. Other causes of enophthalmos must be recognized. These include scirrhous carcinoma of the breast metastatic to the orbit, starvation, radiation effects, maxillary sinusitis, and paranasal sinus carcinomas. Enophthalmos may be distinguished from contralateral exophthalmos or pseudo-exophthalmos by ruling out Graves' disease, neoplasia, glaucoma, buphthalmos, and high myopia. Finally, pseudoenophthalmos caused by microphthalmos, orbital hypoplasia, or hemifacial atrophy must be considered.

The ophthalmologist often recognizes enophthalmos by observing the patient laterally, from above, and en face, comparing the position of each globe within each orbit. If the lateral orbital rims are normal, the examiner can use a Hertel-type exophthalmometer. If the rims are not normal, a Naugle exophthalmometer can be used to quantitate the disparity in anterior projection between the two globes. The ophthalmologist must search for characteristic eyelid malpositions such as pseudoptosis of the upper eyelid, deep superior sulcus, flattened or concave lower eyelid contour, shortened or narrowed palpebral fissure, and stretched lower eyelid. The eyelid alterations usually accompany and exaggerate enophthalmos, although they may mimic enophthalmos. The examiner must also identify bony abnormalities of the orbit or facial bones and inferior globe or prosthesis displacement (hypo-ophthalmos).

32-1-2 Treatment

Treatment of enophthalmos may be surgical or nonsurgical.* Properly placed volume augmentation to the orbital soft tissue will decrease enophthalmos. Surgery to correct eyelid abnormalities may ameliorate those secondary changes of enophthalmos.

Nonsurgical management is limited to the revision of the prosthetic eye in an anophthalmic patient or the placement of a

---

*For more information about enophthalmos treatment, see also Chapter 37, "Late Repair of Posttraumatic Deformities," in this volume.—ED.

cosmetic shell overlying a small or phthisic eye to add volume and improve appearance (Figure 32-1). Ocular prostheses can be enlarged or designed with a shelf-like edge; these can restore volume and lift the upper eyelid outward and upward, treating a pseudoptosis (Figure 32-2). To accommodate a large prosthesis, fornices must be adequate. (See below regarding a forniceal reconstruction.) Magnifying lenses before a nonfunctioning eye or a prosthesis may make a narrow palpebral fissure look larger. Minifying or astigmatic lenses, as well as prisms, may also be useful.*

32-1-2-1 Surgery   The goal of surgery is to increase intraorbital volume or to create the illusion of minimal or no enophthalmos. In adding volume to the orbital cavity, the ophthalmic surgeon may place an implant within the orbit, reduce herniated orbital tissue, or both. In the anophthalmic socket, volume replacement surgery is performed with the best prosthesis in place; the prosthesis may subsequently be refitted, if indicated. Implants for volume augmentation or camouflaging procedures may be alloplastic or autogenous.

Many of the best materials are alloplastic, inert, readily available, and easy to handle. Frequently used are spheres (12 to 20 mm in diameter) of silicone as intraconal implants, silicone chips, room temperature vulcanizing silicone, and sheets of Supramid (0.1 to 0.6 mm in thickness) or silicone (0.5 to 4.0 mm in thickness), Teflon plates, and methylmethacrylate.†

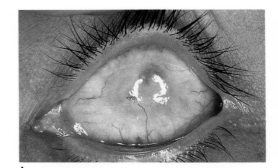

A

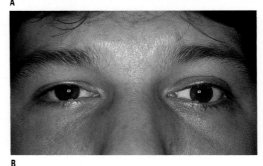

B

Figure 32-1 *Nonsurgical management of enophthalmos with scleral shell. (A) Blind eye with neovascularization and corneal scarring. (B) Scleral shell improves appearance of superior sulcus deformity.*

---

*See also Chapter 33, "Overview of Ocular Prosthetics," in this volume.—ED.

†The use of silicone is presently controversial due to problems that have occurred with breast implants.—ED.

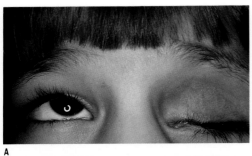

A

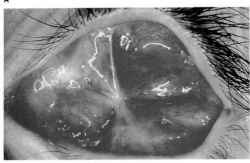

B

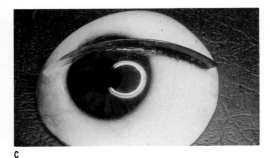

C

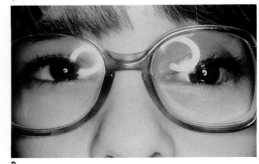

D

Figure 32-2 *Nonsurgical management of enophthalmos with prosthesis. (A) Anophthalmos with
contracted socket and neurogenic ptosis, after
enucleation and resection of orbital teratoma.
(B) Contracted socket. (C) Prosthesis with shelf
to elevate ptotic upper lid. (D) After mucous
membrane grafting, with prosthesis in place elevating upper lid.*

Titanium plates and Vitallium mesh with
anterior projections (biplanar), fixed to the
orbital rims in fracture repair, are also useful. Supramid sheets and Gortex fabric
patches have been helpful in forniceal
reconstruction.

Coralline hydroxyapatite, a porous, inorganic salt of calcium phosphate, can
allow ingrowth of fibrovascular tissue.
Wrapped in sclera, fascia, or Mersilene
sheeting, it is placed as an ocular implant.
A porous alloplastic material, polyethylene
(Medpor) or ePTFE also allows ingrowth
of fibrous tissue; Medpor is available as
blocks, plates, and spheres.

Nonautogenous tissue, such as irradi-
ated fascia lata, bone, cartilage, and
sclera, is available from tissue banks. Autogenous grafts include fascia lata, cartilage, buccal mucous membrane, dermal

fat, and iliac and calvarial bone. Fascia lata is removed from the lateral thigh where two layers of transverse fibers are reinforced by a central band of longitudinal fibers called the *iliotibial tract* or *band*.* This band runs from the gluteus maximus muscle over the greater trochanter to the tibia. A good donor site for dermal fat is the lateral buttock, between the level of the lateral iliac crest and the level of the greater trochanter. A cylinder 25 mm in diameter and 25 mm deep may be harvested en bloc for the anophthalmic socket. The epidermis is removed by scraping with a scalpel blade or mechanical dermabrasion. The fat is trimmed as necessary to fit into the socket as an intraconal implant.[†]

When a recent orbital fracture and anophthalmos coexist, the surgeon may reposit any herniated orbital soft tissue as a first step in restoring volume. A delayed repair is more difficult than early repair, because of significant scarring of the prolapsed soft tissues at the facture site. Imaging studies of the orbit, especially CT scans, are important in the presence of enophthalmos to diagnose bony derangements. The surgeon may choose to repair the bone defect, particularly an orbital floor or large medial wall fracture, with an implant. The fracture site is approached through the subperiosteal space. Prolapsed tissue is gently reposited into the orbit.

When placing an orbital implant to add volume, the surgeon works in the subper-iosteal, intraconal, or sub-Tenon's surgical space. In the anophthalmic socket, when a previously placed implant is extruding or displaced, the sub-Tenon's and intraconal spaces are used.

An implant may extrude because of poor wound closure or poor healing, tissue erosion by a large or migrating implant, and at times be combined with infection. If an infection is present, the surgeon must remove any alloplastic implant. Any epithelial lining or capsule must also be removed, whether or not infection exists. In the presence of infection, the surgeon may defer immediate implantation of an alloplastic socket implant or use an autogenous implant, which can resist infection, at the time that the extruding implant is removed. Dermal fat has become a useful autogenous implant for volume augmentation in secondary implantation and when orbital infection is present (Figure 32-3). Hydroxyapatite and porous polyethylene, which permit vascular ingrowth and may therefore migrate less than an acrylic or silicone sphere, are also useful for replacement of an extruding implant.

For a secondary implantation of an intraconal implant in the anophthalmic socket, the conjunctiva is incised horizontally, midway between the fornices or at

---

*For illustrations of the technique for obtaining fascia lata, see Figure 16-7 in Volume 2 of Ophthalmology Monograph 8, published in 1994.—ED.

[†]See also Chapter 30, "Enucleation and Evisceration," in this volume.—ED.

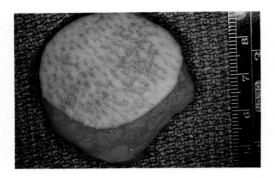

Figure 32-3 *Dermal fat graft.*

any central dimpling that identifies a site of extraocular muscle activity. Tenon's capsule is then incised horizontally or vertically. Any previous implant is removed with its tissue cover. A larger implant (alloplastic, alloplastic wrapped in sclera, or dermal fat) may be placed within Tenon's capsule if intact. The surgeon may cut a relaxing incision in the posterior Tenon's capsule, if needed, to permit placement of the enlarged implant. Alternatively, the implant may be placed through an incision in the posterior Tenon's, within the muscle cone. The four rectus muscles may be sutured directly to sclera, fascia, or polyglactin mesh or other covering of a porous implant. Tenon's capsule should be securely sutured anterior to any alloplastic implant. Tenon's may be sutured directly to a sclera-covered implant and circumferentially to the dermis of a dermal fat graft (Figure 32-4). Whenever possible, conjunctiva should also be closed using absorbable sutures.

The depth of the fornices should not be compromised by a very tight conjunctival closure because a good prosthesis cannot be fit when fornices are inadequate. The surgeon can avoid shallow fornices by two techniques: recessing the conjunctiva, which will grow over autogenous tissue (eg, dermal fat) in several weeks; or spacing two to four double-armed absorbable (4-0 chromic gut) sutures from the deep fornix through the eyelid to decrease conjunctival contracture. A firm conformer, almond-shaped or doughnut-type, should be inserted at the end of surgery and left in place for several weeks to maintain the fornices. A suture tarsorrhaphy may also be helpful.

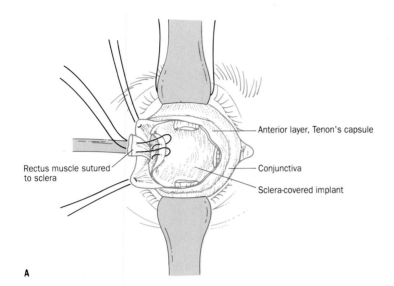

Anterior layer, Tenon's capsule

Rectus muscle sutured
to sclera

Conjunctiva

Sclera-covered implant

A

Figure 32-4 *Scleral cover over intraconal implant. (A) Four rectus muscles are sutured to edge of scleral transplant with mattress sutures. (B) Anterior layer of Tenon's capsule is closed without imbrication over surface of scleral transplant. (C) Conjunctiva is closed.*

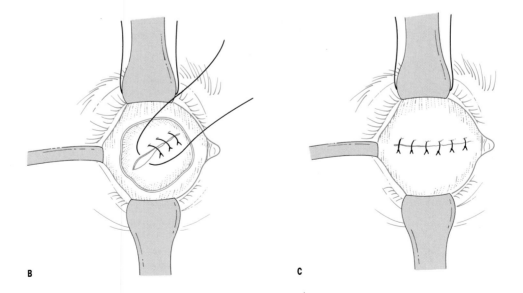

B

C

The inferolateral approach to the subperiosteal space offers good access to the posterior orbit where an implant can support the orbital tissues and advance the prosthesis anteriorly. The best-fitting prosthesis is left in the socket during surgery. A subciliary eyelid incision or lower forniceal incision is made to expose the inferolateral orbital rim. Alternatively or in combination, a lateral canthotomy may be extended to the lateral orbital rim. The periosteum is exposed, incised along the inferior orbital rim, and reflected with periosteal elevators. The surgeon then places the implant (Supramid sheets, plicated fascia, room temperature vulcanizing silicone, preformed methylmethacrylate, etc) into the subperiosteal pocket, while noting the position of the prosthesis. The periosteum is closed once satisfactory volume addition is obtained. The deep tissues and skin are closed in two layers and, if needed, a lateral canthoplasty is performed.

32-1-2-2 Postoperative Complications   The complications of implant surgery are numerous. Alloplastic implants are more prone than autogenous implants to extrude, migrate, become infected, or cause foreign-body inflammation. Migration and extrusion may occur months to years after surgery. Autogenous implants can resorb, unlike alloplastic implants. Any implant may compress or directly injure major orbital blood vessels, thereby producing orbital hemorrhage. Strict hemostasis is mandatory. If significant hemorrhage occurs postoperatively, the surgeon should be prepared to drain it. Implant surgery is not universally useful in cicatricial enophthalmos. Following orbital fracture, the fibrosis, disruption, and displacement of the orbital soft tissue and normal fibrous septa (which extend from Tenon's capsule to the periorbita) may tether the globe or remaining orbital tissue in the anophthalmic socket. When a globe is present, a preoperative forward traction test will identify such restriction and predict that implant surgery will probably not improve the enophthalmos. The test is performed by grasping the insertions of the medial and lateral rectus muscles and determining if the globe can be moved anteriorly.

32-1-2-3 Eyelid Malposition   In creating the illusion that little or no enophthalmos exists, the surgeon ameliorates or de-emphasizes eyelid malpositions and contour abnormalities. In the anophthalmic socket, eyelid surgery, like implant surgery, is performed with the best possible prosthesis present. The lower eyelid may require horizontal shortening to correct ectropion or entropion, especially in an anophthalmic socket where the prosthesis must be supported by the lower eyelid. The palpebral fissure may be expanded vertically and/or horizontally. Pseudoptosis or true ptosis of the upper eyelid may be improved by surgically elevating the eyelid. A tarsomüllerectomy or small moni-

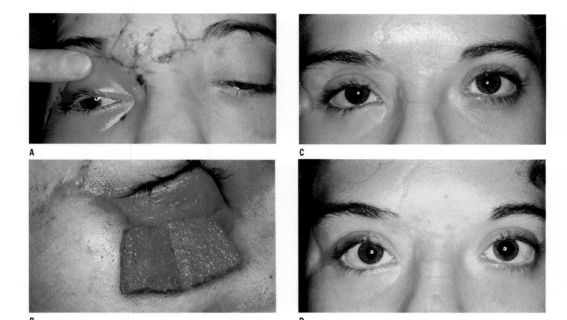

A

B

C

D

tored levator resection may be utilized (Figure 32-5).*

Laxity of the medial or lateral canthal tendons requires repair.† In a medial canthal tendon plication, a curvilinear incision 1.5 cm is made 8 to 10 mm nasal to the medial commissure. The incision is deepened to expose the medial canthal tendon; the tendon is then skeletonized superiorly and inferiorly. With scissors, a subcutaneous tunnel in the lower eyelid is made to

Figure 32-5 *Staged repair of lid malposition. (A) Orbital fractures with hypoglobus and enophthalmos. (B) Iliac bone graft used as subperiosteal implant. (C) Globe position improved, but pseudoptosis remains. (D) Improved appearance after ptosis repair.*

---

*For more information about eyelid malposition, and ptosis in particular, see Chapters 14, 15, 16, and 24 in Volume 2 of Ophthalmology Monograph 8, published in 1994.—ED.

†For discussion and illustration of medial and lateral canthal repair, see Chapter 22, "Reconstruction of Canthal Defects," in Volume 2 of Ophthalmology Monograph 8, published in 1994.—ED.

expose the deep and superficial heads of the pretarsal orbicularis muscle extending temporally toward the region of the lower punctum. A 4-0 nonabsorbable suture (eg, Prolene or Mersilene) on a half-circle needle (Ethicon OPS-5) is passed through the periosteum beneath the tendon insertion, through the tendon, and through the deep medial pretarsal orbicularis. Care is needed so that the lower canalicular system is not compromised. The suture is tied before a second suture is placed. The sutures are placed to advance the orbicularis. The lateral canthus may also be tightened by suturing tarsus to the periosteum of the lateral orbital rim directly or with tendinous, periosteal, or tarsal strips. The lower eyelid may further be supported by a fascial sling, anchored to the medial and lateral orbital rims.

32-1-2-4 Contour Abnormalities Contour abnormalities may result from bone defects and/or soft-tissue atrophy and scarring. These include posterior and inferior displacement of the lateral orbital rim, flattening of the malar bone, deep superior sulcus, and lower eyelid concavity. Bone grafts and implants of custom-molded silicone, Proplast, fascia, Medpor, or dermal fat may be placed between orbicularis and septum or just anterior to the orbital rim to compensate for either bone or soft-tissue anomalies.

In considering reconstructive procedures for enophthalmos, the prudent surgeon discusses with the patient the limits of surgery as well as the risks of implant surgery. The goal of surgery is improvement. Although perfection is elusive, one should always strive for it.

32-2

CONTRACTURE

The contracted socket is an enophthalmic socket that will not hold a prosthesis or a satisfactory prosthesis. Eyelid, conjunctival, or deep orbital tissue abnormalities reduce the retropalpebral space and prevent a normal (1 to 2 ml) prosthesis from staying in the socket.

The pathogenesis of socket contracture is incompletely understood. Factors that predispose a socket to contracture include the following:

1. Severe trauma prior to enucleation, including chemical or thermal burns

2. Poor wound healing, often associated with poor vascular supply

3. Infection

4. Cicatrizing conjunctival disease

5. Postenucleation trauma, such as radiation therapy

6. Absent or poor-fitting conformer or prosthesis

7. Absence of an intraorbital implant

The type of implant may play a role. Extrusion, much more frequent with alloplastic materials than with autogenous grafts, is associated with socket contracture. The presence of an intraorbital implant reduces orbital tissue migration inferiorly and reduces the tendency toward a shortened inferior fornix. The surgeon should take great care to maintain the inferior fornix during enucleation surgery and postoperatively to enhance the socket surface area. A conformer or prosthesis will stretch the conjunctival fornices and maintain them.

32-2-1 Diagnosis

The patient with a contracted socket may be wearing no prosthesis at all, or the prosthesis may readily fall out of the socket. The ophthalmologist will observe lack of conjunctiva, a small palpebral fissure vertically and horizontally, vertically shortened fornices, and atrophy of eyelid tissue and orbital fat. There may be no orbital implant palpable, but firm fibrous cicatrix may be palpable. Symblepharon, infectious conjunctivitis, or other conjunctival inflammation or scarring may be present. Severely contracted sockets may have a very small palpebral aperture.

32-2-2 Treatment

The goal is to permit the patient to wear an ocular prosthesis in comfort. Medical treatment can limit or reverse socket contracture. Any infectious conjunctivitis, blepharoconjunctivitis, or deeper socket infection must be treated aggressively with topical and possibly systemic antibiotics. A socket conformer, however small, should be placed if possible when the patient's prosthesis is lost or falls out of the socket. Allergic conjunctivitis in an anophthalmic socket may require topical antihistamines, decongestants, systemic antihistamines, cromolyn, lodoxamide tromethamine, or topical or systemic corticosteroids.

Care of the ocular prosthesis is essential. Prostheses should be cleaned at least weekly, with removal of any deposits. Yearly or twice yearly polishing will maintain the smooth surface of the prosthesis; this smooth surface limits giant papillary conjunctivitis and inflammation.*

32-2-2-1 Surgery   Correction of socket contracture generally requires the surgeon to augment the conjunctival surface area and often to excise cicatrix or fibrous tissue. Mild to moderate contraction may be treated with inferior fornix reconstruction. Severe socket contraction will require extensive reconstruction with autografts.

Surgery should be restricted to noninflamed and noninfected sockets. Because scarring can normally progress over 12 months after trauma, whether accidental or surgical, the surgeon should wait at least that long after previous trauma or surgery before intervening surgically.

Rebuilding the inferior fornix in its simplest form may involve deepening the fornix. The surgeon may place three or four double-armed 4-0 chromic sutures full-thickness through the lower eyelid from the conjunctival fornix, at its desired depth to the eyelid skin. These sutures

---

*For more information, see also Chapter 33, "Overview of Ocular Prosthetics," and Chapter 34, "Management and Care of Ocular Prostheses," in this volume.—ED.

create an adhesion to maintain the fornix. This deepening may be modified by attaching the inferior forniceal conjunctiva to the periosteum of the inferior orbital rim. A conformer should be placed immediately to keep the conjunctiva on stretch. A temporary tarsorrhaphy will add further stretch.

Conjunctiva may be increased in the inferior fornix by borrowing from the conjunctival "face." Incising the central conjunctiva transversely, releasing it from underlying attachments, excising scar tissue, and recessing the conjunctiva into the inferior fornix will accomplish this aim. Although typically this conjunctivoplasty is performed at the time of a dermal fat graft (as a secondary orbital implant), with scleral, tarsal, or palatal grafts, the same procedure can be performed with an alloplastic spacer, such as Supramid sheeting or Gortex, sutured over the bare orbital fibrous tissue and fat with multiple nonreactive (Prolene) sutures. The spacer remains in place for 4 to 6 weeks while new conjunctiva grows to cover the denuded orbital tissue. Again, a conformer is placed at the completion of the surgery. The spacer may be removed in 4 to 6 weeks. A prosthesis is fitted when there is minimal socket edema and inflammation, usually 6 to 8 weeks postoperatively.

Mucous membrane may be added to conjunctiva to enlarge the socket surface area. Buccal mucous membrane, full-thickness, is an excellent substitute for conjunctiva. Mucous membrane may be harvested under local anesthesia from the inner cheek as an ellipse beginning just anterior to Stensen's duct and extending just posterior to the mucocutaneous junction at the lip. An assistant should evert the cheek. Care must be taken not to incise the cheek deeply into fat and muscular layers. A running 4-0 chromic catgut suture will close the donor site. The zone of shallow inferior fornix is incised transversely and deep scar bands are excised, leaving a vascularized bed. The graft is thinned, trimmed, and placed mucosal side outward in the socket bed. Running or interrupted 5-0 polyglactin (Vicryl) sutures and placement of a conformer will secure the graft. Prosthesis refitting may be considered when healing appears quiescent, after 2 to 3 months.

Full- or split-thickness labial mucous membrane grafts are an alternative to full-thickness buccal mucous membrane. Full-thickness mucous membrane is more advantageous, when available, because shrinkage is less than with split-thickness mucosa. Patients have less postoperative discomfort in the donor site with full-thickness mucous membrane than with partial-thickness if the donor site is closed primarily.

A severely contracted socket must be repaired with extensive mucous membrane grafting. In the authors' experience, suturing a conformer into the orbital rims has been the most successful approach to date. General anesthesia is usually used.

The conjunctival face is incised transversely and the conjunctiva is undermined. Flaps are developed to recess the conjunctiva onto the inferior and superior palpebral surfaces. Anterior orbital scar tissue is excised. Two incisions are made centrally over the upper and lower orbital rims to the periosteum, which is reflected from the anterior rim toward the orbit. Two drill holes are placed from the anterior rim to the orbital floor and/or roof.

A previously designed and sized cup-shaped or C-shaped conformer with positioning holes superiorly and inferiorly is wrapped with mucous membrane, full-thickness or partial-thickness. Partial-thickness mucous membrane is harvested as follows.* The lower lip is expanded with injection of normal saline until the lip is firm. Xylocaine plus epinephrine may be used for hemostasis. With the assistant everting the lip, manually or with towel clips, a Castroviejo mucotome is set at 0.3 or 0.6 mm depth and a rectangle of mucous membrane is "shaved" transversely between the zone just inferior to the mucocutaneous junction and the superior labial frenulum. A tag suture is placed to identify the mucosal side. The graft is wrapped around the conformer with the mucosal side facing the conformer. Polyglactin sutures are used to suture the graft to itself. The conformer is secured to the orbital rims with a Supramid suture, 2-0 or 3-0, or with Prolene passing through the holes of the conformer, the graft, and the bone. The suture is tied to itself on the anterior orbital rim (Figure 32-6). The

---

*For discussion and illustration of split- and full-thickness mucous membrane grafts, see Chapter 9, "Management of Conjunctival Diseases and Chalazion," especially Figures 9-4 and 9-9, in Volume 1 of Ophthalmology Monograph 8, published in 1993.—ED.

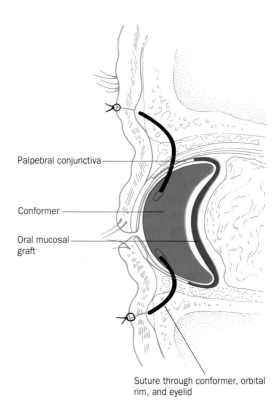

Palpebral conjunctiva

Conformer

Oral mucosal graft

Suture through conformer, orbital rim, and eyelid

Figure 32-6 *Socket reconstructed with large C-shaped conformer sutured to orbital rims.*

fitting, the prosthetic eyes are custom-painted, yielding a highly satisfactory cosmetic result.

Plastic prosthetic eyes offer advantages over the glass prostheses. Plastic can be fabricated into any design or shape, which allows for a precise fit to the tissues of the socket. Plastic eyes are relatively unbreakable; even if chipped, they can be repaired or refit. They can be polished if scratched or to remove mucus deposits, salts, and imperfections of the surface thereby ensuring comfortable blinking.[3] The average useful life expectancy of a plastic eye is 5 to 7 years, although it may be shorter in diabetic patients because their acetone level, which can affect plastic, is higher.

33-1

PATIENT CONSULTATION

Because patients are often misinformed by well-wishers, family, and friends, it is advisable to have the patient contact the ocularist for a prefitting consultation prior to enucleation or several weeks after enucleation. During this visit, much of a patient's apprehension can be dispelled by receiving basic information on the procedure, especially the fact that a temporary spacer, called a *conformer*, will be inserted behind the lids at the time of surgery. This type of information will help create a more relaxed patient at fitting appointments. Questions about care, wearing, placement, motility, and eyelid shape can be raised and resolved.

A healing time of 6 to 8 weeks is usual following enucleation. Fitting a prosthesis earlier generally requires additional adjustment or refitting later due to further healing.

33-2

CONFORMERS

A conformer is routinely placed in the eye socket at the time of enucleation or evisceration. Its purpose is to protect the suture line, maintain the fornices, prevent contracture, and provide wearing comfort to the patient. A conformer also keeps the eyelids in better shape and prevents eyelashes from entering the socket and causing irritation. With no conformer in place, the eye socket will contract; then as the prosthetic eye is worn, contracture will diminish, and refitting of the prosthesis will be necessary.

Many surgeons prefer to use silicone conformers at the time of surgery. A pair of scissors is all that is necessary to properly shape and size a silicone conformer. Another advantage is that suture material can be easily passed through the conformer. A silicone-rubber conformer does not absorb water and can be autoclaved or gas-sterilized without damage. Because the surface is not as smooth as acrylic, silicone is not as comfortable for the patient and quite often is replaced with an acrylic conformer after 2 weeks postoperatively. However, acrylic conformers are best sterilized by use of gas, as autoclave temperatures can greatly damage their shape.

An important consideration in selecting a conformer is to ensure that it is not so large as to put pressure on the suture line or overextend into the fornices. Oversizing can stretch tissues and create a lax lower lid. It is also important in fitting a conformer not to encourage necrosis over the implant by placing pressure on the anterior surface of the socket.

33-3

CONGENITAL ANOPHTHALMOS AND MICROPHTHALMOS

In the treatment of congenital underdevelopment, the objective is not to regain what was lost as in the case of acquired postsurgical anophthalmos, but to perform the larger task of encouraging the development of orbital tissue and the bony orbit itself. It is best undertaken at an early age as most of a child's growth takes place during the first three years of life. By the age of 4 years, 70% of the adult size of the globe is said to have been attained.[5] Because the growth of the globe significantly influences bony orbital growth and development, the object is to increase the size of the orbit by gradually increasing the size of conformers. Only gentle pressure is required with this sequence of conformers. Oversizing can actually create

entropion of eyelid lashes. However, oversizing is sometimes necessary to create useful space, especially in severe cases of microphthalmos and in anophthalmos. The entropion can be surgically repaired after orbital bone growth has been completed.

When the first conformers are placed, it is usually a week before these can be replaced with larger conformers. Much of the early space gained is a result of soft-tissue expansion. With time, the interval of placement will increase to once every 3 to 4 months, allowing time for orbital growth rather than soft-tissue expansion. In some cases, consideration should be given to opening the lateral canthi or to surgical placement of an ocular implant to further fill the orbit. The former will allow for a larger conformer to be placed through the palpebral fissure, and the latter will enhance volume to the orbit so that a smaller conformer can be used. Once near-symmetry is obtained, work can continue with the use of custom-fit ocular prostheses of increasing size (Figure 33-1).

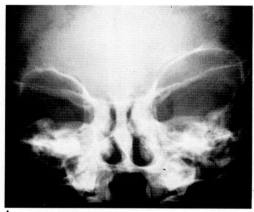

A

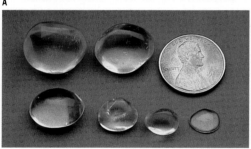

B

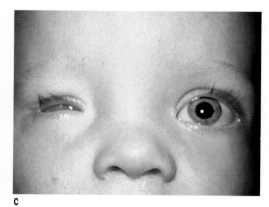

C

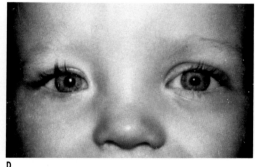

D

Figure 33-1 *Congenital anophthalmos. (A) Small orbital size OD. (B) Sequence of custom conformers from impression to stimulating growth.(C) Child 6 months old. (D) Child 1.5 years old, following 12-month course of increasingly larger conformers.*

33-4

CONTRACTED SOCKET

Conformers and, at times, pressure conformers are used to help maintain, if not increase, the socket's contracted tissue. Contracture is often seen following severe trauma, orbital fractures, alkali burns, thermal burns, radiation therapy, and infection. The removal of the conformer in these instances can cause further contraction.

A pressure conformer consists of a conformer with a peg attached to the anterior surface, extending outward between the eyelids. A patch or tape can be applied to place pressure on the peg and conformer back into the fornices of the socket. With time, larger conformers or pressure conformers can be placed.[6]

It is rarely a good course of action to allow the wearer of a prosthetic eye or a conformer to wear nothing at all for an extended period of time. This is especially true when an infection is present or after enucleation, mucosal grafting, chemical burns, or radiation therapy. Many times, contraction due to scarring occurs, and socket volume is lost. If the prosthesis itself is infected, a conformer should be placed in the socket and the prosthetic eye gas-sterilized.

33-5

FABRICATING OCULAR PROSTHESES

After the ophthalmologist and ocularist are both satisfied that the patient's socket is in satisfactory condition, a prosthetic eye can be made. Fabrication of the prosthetic eye can be accomplished in several ways. Although methods and philosophies involved in creating prosthetic eyes differ in style, form, and ways of fabrication, many of them produce excellent results in the hands of a skilled professional.

At first, ocularists fashioned plastic eyes after the shape of glass eyes; then others took impressions of eye sockets in a similar fashion to that of taking impressions in fitting dentures. The impression was translated directly into plastic. Still other ocularists copied the shape of the impression in wax, altered the shape for comfort and to improve cosmesis, and then trans-

lated the wax shape into plastic. The last method has been further developed and has been part of the training of apprentice ocularists since 1953.[7-9] This method is currently recognized as the *modified impression* method.

There are four basic ways to fit prosthetic eyes:

1. A stock eye is selected from whatever collection is available. Since stock eyes are intended to fit everyone, they fit no one as well as desired. Although obsolete for the most part in the United States, stock eyes are still currently used in other parts of the world (Figure 33-2).

2. A piece of hard wax or paraffin is formed into a shape resembling a glass eye prosthesis. A space is left on the front of the wax to accept an already prepared plastic cornea–iris piece, which is then fastened in place with melted wax. The prosthesis is smoothed (for comfort), rubbed with a paper towel, and polished with a small cloth saturated with cold water. The final form is placed in the socket and evaluated for comfort and cosmesis. It is removed from the socket and any necessary changes are made. This is done as often as necessary to achieve a satisfactory result. The shape of the wax pattern is duplicated in plastic (Figure 33-3).

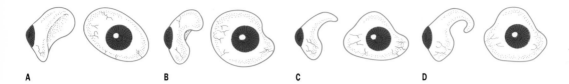

A   B   C   D

Figure 33-2 *Common shapes of Snellen Reform types of prosthetic eyes. (A) Long oval. (B) Rounded, with trochlear cut. (C) Triangular for deep, pointed superior fornix. (D) Mixed shape, with posterior horn for special support.*

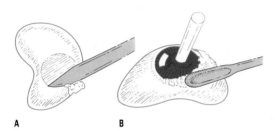

A   B

Figure 33-3 *Wax pattern shaped like traditional prosthesis, with deeply hollowed posterior surface. (A) Knife blade making space for iris–cornea piece. (a) Hard wax or paraffin. (B) Iris–cornea piece being attached to pattern. (a) Prepainted iris. (b) Melted wax being blended from cornea to pattern. (c) Stainless-steel dental wax spatula.*

3. An acceptably colored stock plastic eye is selected, an alginate impression cream is inserted around and behind it, and the prosthesis is placed in the socket. When the cream has set to a firm consistency, the form is removed from the socket, a two-piece stone mold is made in a bronze flask, the impression material is removed from the back of the prosthesis, and the impression cream is replaced with methyl-methacrylate resin. When undesirable surface irregularities have been removed and the prosthesis has been thoroughly polished, it is placed in the eye socket and evaluated. The great difficulty with this method is that if anything more than a very minor modification is necessary, removal of material from the front surface may necessitate cutting into the color so that the prosthesis must go through an extra process of coloring and capping. Or, if material must be added, at least one extra final processing will be necessary. This method is not recommended.

4. The modified impression method allows for as little or as much time as the ocularist wishes to give. If little time is given, the first cosmetic effect may be poor, but the comfort level should be excellent. If adequate time is spent, the method gives the greatest degree of control to all features of the prosthesis. A brief outline of this method is as follows: An impression of the socket is taken using a multiperfor-

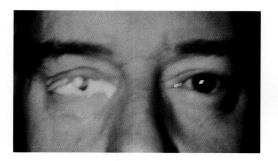

Figure 33-4 *Patient having impression taken.*

ated plastic shield or tray that approximates the shape of the socket. A highly refined alginate impression powder is mixed with the appropriate amount of cold water. In 1 to 2 minutes, the impression material sets to a firm consistency, and the impression material and tray are removed from the socket (Figure 33-4).[7,8] A two-piece dental stone mold is made around the impression. A hard wax, such as dental ivory inlay wax or a paraffin that has a high melting point, is melted into a small crucible and poured into the opening of the mold resulting from removal of the stem of the impression tray. A prepared iris–cornea piece is positioned in the front surface of the wax pattern (Figure 33-5). The wax pattern is inserted into the patient's socket, and the results are evaluated for symmetry with the companion eye. The patient is asked to glance in the extreme directions of gaze to determine whether any edges show and to make sure that the pattern will stay behind the lower eyelid on upward gaze. Any defects are noted, the pattern is removed from the eye socket, and the necessary changes are made. It is seldom ad-

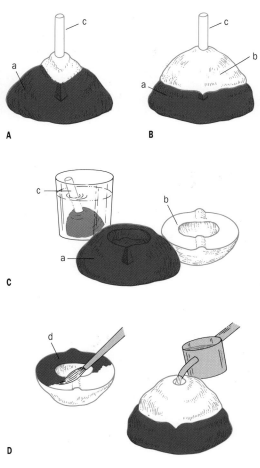

Figure 33-5 *Two-piece dental stone mold. (A) First half of mold of impression (a). Stem of impression shell (c). (B) Second half of mold (b). (C) Mold opened and impression on shell stored in water. (D) Microfilm coating applied (d). Mold with microfilm coating closed and being filled with melted wax for wax pattern.*

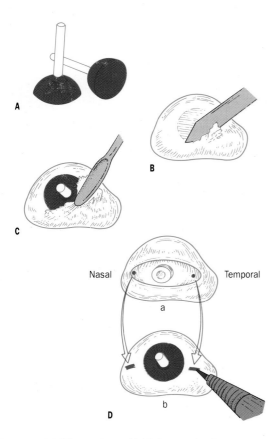

Nasal   Temporal

Figure 33-6 *Wax pattern. (A) Iris–cornea piece with stem. (a) Side view. (b) Rear view. (B) Wax duplicate of impression, space being prepared for iris–cornea piece. (C) Iris piece being waxed in place on pattern. (D) Impression (a) compared with wax duplicate made into pattern (b), nasal and temporal canthal areas being marked with red wax pencil for check on maintaining position of pattern when tried in socket.*

visable to make all of the changes at one time, because some changes in the form of the pattern, while attempting to correct one defect, will introduce other defects. It is necessary to know which of the changes might have caused a new defect (Figure 33-6). After the wax pattern has been modified properly, a two-piece mold of dental stone is made and filled with acrylic, beginning the fabrication of a custom-fit plastic prosthesis, which is then cured, polished, and painted.[7,8]

33-6

PAINTING OCULAR PROSTHESES

The features of a prosthetic eye do not need to be an exact mirror image of the living, companion eye, but they should be near enough so that the differences do not attract attention. There is a method to control the position, size, value, and color of the iris, the size of the pupil, and the coloring of the scleral portions of the eye. The painted colored layer of the prosthetic eye lies underneath a clear protective plastic surface. To obtain the correct positions and colors in painting, a temporary plastic covering is made to be exactly as the final layer in shape and thickness. This is made by using the original mold in which the final shape of the eye has been impressed.

A large drop of contact lens wetting solution is placed between the two layers to create optical continuity, and the piece may be placed in the eye socket for evaluation. If the iris or other details are not in the correct position, the prosthesis may be removed from the socket, the two pieces separated and rinsed, and repainting done as necessary. When all features are judged correct, the painting shell may be discarded and the final layer applied permanently to the eye.

Whether the starting point is an empirically fitted eye, an eye to which an impression has been added on the posterior surface, or a wax pattern copied from an impression, certain well-defined and proven principles of modification may be applied for the sake of comfort, cosmesis, and retention in the socket.

33-7

ANOPHTHALMIC DEFECTS AND THEIR CORRECTION

Some of the more common defects of eyelids and sockets related to the anophthalmic state are discussed in this section, together with recommended methods of prosthesis modification.*

33-7-1 Deep Superior Eyelid Sulcus

This problem is almost commonplace in prosthetic cases because the normal volume of the globe being removed is 7.5 cc, the volume of a 16-mm ball implant placed at the time of surgery is 2 cc, and the average volume of a prosthesis is 3 cc. This leaves a volume deficit after enucleation of 2.5 cc. Often, this amount can be

reduced by adding volume above the superior posterior rim of the prosthesis. Surgical volume augmentation to orbital soft tissue can further reduce this problem.[8]

Globe	7.5 cc
Implant	−2.0 cc
Prosthesis	−3.0 cc
Deficit	2.5 cc

33-7-2 Sagging Lower Eyelid

Prosthetic corrections are attempted by adding material below the nasal and temporal edges and removing material from the front surface and lower edge below the inferior limbus. Many times this situation can be greatly improved prosthetically, so it is best to have the ocularist evaluate the case prior to making a surgical correction.[8]

33-7-3 Exophthalmos

This problem can be corrected by removing material from the anterior or posterior surface of the prosthetic eye or wax pattern.[8]

33-7-4 Horizontally Decreased Palpebral Fissure

Correction may be attempted by adding prominence to the surfaces of the sclera exposed within the nasal and temporal canthal areas and blending these areas with the rest of the scleral surfaces.[8]

---

*See also Chapter 30, "Enucleation and Evisceration," and Chapter 32, "Deformities of the Anophthalmic Socket," in this volume.—ED.

33-7-5 Horizontally Increased Palpebral Fissure

Correction may be attempted by shortening the prosthetic eye or wax pattern horizontally.[8]

33-7-6 Vertically Decreased Palpebral Fissure

This defect may result from lack of adequate prominence of the anterior surface of the prosthesis, causing correctable pseudoptosis. The corneal surface may be moved forward and blended with the surfaces of the surrounding sclera.[8]

33-7-7 Vertically Increased Palpebral Fissure

Correction may be attempted by recessing the cornea. If this is not effective enough, thickness can be added to the upper and lower portion of the prosthetic eye or wax pattern to press behind the distal edges of the tarsal plates, tilting them toward the center of the palpebral fissure.[8]

33-7-8 True Ptosis

Some of the ptosis cases seen after enucleation might be due to stretching or distortion of the tissues during surgery. Damage can be done to vessels and nerves supplying the rectus and levator muscles or directly to the muscles themselves during enucleation surgery. Ptosis can also be a consistent result of the imbrication of the rectus muscles over a simple spherical implant within Tenon's capsule. The ptosis likely evolves in the manner described here.[10-12]

The space within Tenon's capsule is larger than the volume of an 18-mm spherical implant. When the muscles have been imbricated and Tenon's capsule closed over the sphere, there are four rather loose pouches of Tenon's capsule into which the sphere can begin to move between adjacent rectus muscles.* The point of imbrication rests in a very precarious manner in front of the sphere. When the inferior rectus muscle contracts on downward gaze and the medial rectus muscle on adduction, the muscles begin to slip off into an inferonasal direction. The sphere, then, is pressed into the space between the superior and lateral rectus muscles and Tenon's capsule begins to stretch. A rolling movement is imparted to all of the connective tissue around the sphere, and this continues until the rectus muscles are below and nasal to the sphere. Rarely, the sphere will migrate into the superonasal quadrant or another one of the relaxed areas of Tenon's capsule because the presence of the retracted oblique muscles on the nasal side of the orbit and of the ligament of Lockwood below tends to block migration in those directions. Due to the permanent rotation of the connective tissues and because of the forward and downward pull of the sheath of the superior rectus muscle on the sheath of the levator muscle, the entire aponeurosis of the levator is pulled for-

---

*For this reason, many surgeons and ocularists recommend that the rectus muscles not be surgically imbricated over a spherical implant. —ED.

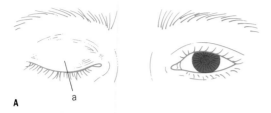

A

ward and downward and is the primary cause of the ptosis. However, the rotation of Tenon's capsule drags the conjunctiva along with it, and the superior fornix moves downward into a position where it can hold an ordinary prosthesis down in an abnormal position. Also, the sphere tends to move very near to the roof of the orbit and somewhat forward, further limiting the space available for a prosthesis. All of these changes have been diagrammed and described by Allen.[10-12]

Traditionally shaped prostheses cannot correct these ptosis cases. Making the eye more prominent to try to prop the upper eyelid upward merely pushes the upper eyelid forward, and the gaze of the prosthetic eye will be toward the floor. Because the ptosis is not the result of a disinsertion of the aponeurosis, the surgery commonly used to reattach it will leave the patient with more prosthetic problems than before.

Schematic prosthetic correction of anophthalmic ptosis is depicted in Figures 33-7, 33-8, and 33-9. Figure 33-7 shows a severe ptosis and the failure to correct it by using a very large prosthesis. Figure 33-8 shows, at A, an impression tray with impression material within the socket; B, a tray with impression removed from the socket; C, a wax pattern with an iris–cornea piece with a stem; and D, the wax

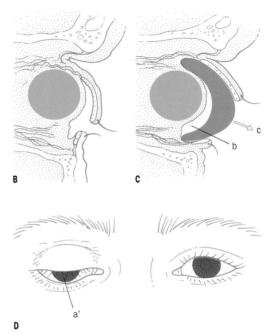

B   **C**

D

Figure 33-7 *Failed correction of ptosis because prosthesis was too large. (A) Ptosis of upper right lid (a). (B) Cross section of same eye showing ball implant in Tenon's capsule. (C) Snellen Reform shaped prosthesis in socket, direction of gaze downward (c), unfilled space (b) behind prosthesis. (D) Front view of unsatisfactory cosmetic result (a') from prosthesis shown in part C.*

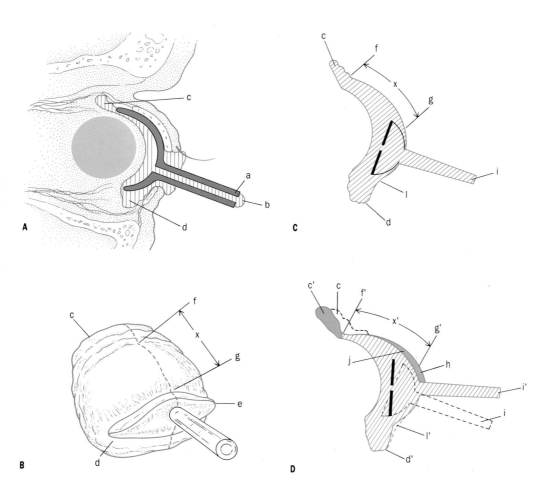

Figure 33-8 *Impression-taking for severe ptosis.*
(A) Taking impression of socket with ptosis of
upper lid. Stem of impression shell (a), impres-
sion material (b), tongue of impression into thin
space in upper fornix (c), fullness of material
from lower fornix (d). (B) Impression removed
from socket. Material from lower fornix (d), rec-
ord of palpebral fissure (e), record of upper
margin of upper tarsus (f), record of lower mar-
gin of upper lid (g), width of upper tarsus (x).
(C) Wax pattern copied from impression. Stem
of iris–cornea piece pointing downward (i),
other features identified as in part B. (D) Modi-
fied wax pattern with stem (i) realigned to
straight ahead (i'); material added to lift upper
lid margin (h) blends off in area of (j). Tongue
at (c) moved to (c') and made larger. Material
removed from lower limbal area (l'). Space for
upper tarsus moved backward (f'-g') with width
of space for upper tarsus (x) maintained as (x').

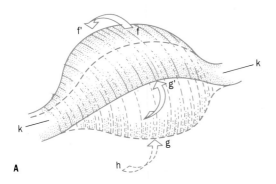

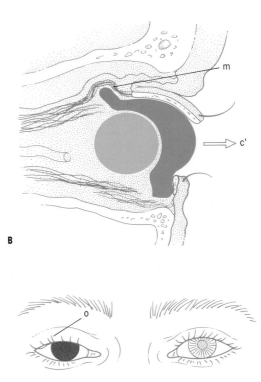

pattern modified in an attempt to correct the ptosis. Figure 33-9A emphasizes the fact that the tarsal plate of the upper eyelid is most important in ptosis correction. The superior tarsal plate, revolving around its axis in the palpebral tendons, must be given room on the upper surface of the prosthesis to drop backward. Added material under Müller's muscle and the levator is shown at *m*, where it places a buckle in the eyelid–levator continuum to help lift the upper eyelid. A final, quite well-corrected appearance of the eyelids over the eye is shown in C.[8,10,11]

33-7-9 Retention Failure

Some prostheses or wax patterns may easily slide over the lower eyelid and out of the socket. Corrections can be attempted by changing the plane of the lower edge of the prosthesis to an exactly vertical plane below the cornea. This form gets behind the lower edge of the tarsal plate of the lower lid, thus rotating it upward and gripping the eye with the entire expanse of the lower tarsal plate. The entire mass of the prosthesis below the limbal area, in the vertical portion of the prosthe-

Figure 33-9 *Importance of tarsal plate in ptosis correction. (A) Principle by which upper tarsus is rotated upward and backward around axis, palpebral tendons (k-k). Prominence added to upper corneoscleral limbus of pattern applies lift (h) to elevate lower margin (g) to level (g'), upper margin (f) moves back to (f'). (B) Cross section showing prosthetic eye of modified impression in same socket as seen in Figures 33-3 and 33-5, upper lid being lifted, prosthesis pointing ahead (c'). Müller's muscle buckled at (m). (C) Front view of cosmetic result, lid opening satisfactory, expanse of upper lid remains slightly greater than in companion eye (o).*

sis, must be very thin. In this form, the prosthesis can make a space for itself behind the tarsal plate and in front of any herniated fat or other tissues lying behind the lower fornix. Sometimes it is necessary to tape the eyelids shut and have the patient wear the prosthesis for 2 or 3 hours before the tissues will adjust and assure retention of the prosthesis. This gives a similar result to sutures placed into the fornices. Fornix sutures should be brought out to deepen the fornix low on the eyelid or evert the eyelid near the ciliary margin.

33-7-10 Entropion

There may be marked entropion to the extent of virtual trichiasis. This may be due to chemical burns of the conjunctiva, conjunctival disease, or a contracted socket. Although correction may be attempted, the modified form will not do more than rotate the lashes 4° or 5° toward their normal positions. Correction is attempted by creating a reverse curve, that is, removing material between the upper limbus and the upper edge and between the lower limbus and the lower edge of the eye to recurve the tarsal plates.[13]

Entropion can be caused by placing an oversized ocular prosthesis. Due to the eyelid's inability to close over the prosthesis, the eyelid margin rolls inward in an attempt to provide more lining to the eye

socket. Eventually, the eyelid will scar in the rolled-down position, causing a gradually increasing entropion, many times to the point of trichiasis.

33-7-11 Ectropion

The rolling outward of the margins of the eyelid, ectropion, can cause several problems, some of which are the inability to retain the prosthesis, inadequate tear distribution, discomfort, and poor cosmesis. Ectropion can result from scarring of the inferior cul-de-sac and lower eyelid or lack of lower eyelid tone in combination with a downward pressure from a malfitting prosthesis. Usually, mild to moderate involutional ectropion can be managed successfully by use of a properly fitted prosthesis. Cicatricial ectropion often requires surgery. Prosthetic contouring for ectropion is similar to correction of retention failure.[8,13]

33-7-12 Pseudoptosis

Pseudoptosis occurs over poorly fitted prostheses, microphthalmos, anophthalmos, and phthisic globes. It most commonly is associated with a lack of support to the upper eyelid and may disappear with a properly fitted prosthetic eye. When the globe is removed and replaced with an implant that is smaller than the globe, the pivot point marked with an arrow is not only lower but more posterior in the orbit. The net effect, assuming levator tone and function remain unchanged, is a lengthening of the levator mechanism, translated as a drop in eyelid level. The laxity of the supporting structures of the levator mechanism, lateral and medial horns and Whitnall's ligament, plays an important role as does tone of the levator muscle itself. To restore normal functioning length to the levator mechanism, a prosthesis must move the pivot point both anteriorly and superiorly (Figure 33-10).[14] Preventive medicine dictates that before correcting surgically, it is prudent to let the ocularist–ophthalmologist team evaluate ptosis jointly. Surgical correction of pseudoptosis may create a too wide palpebral fissure and lagophthalmos, causing mucosal discharge from dryness and poor cosmesis.*

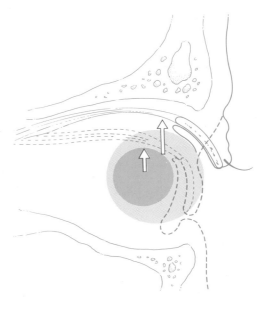

Figure 33-10 *Pivot points marked by arrows before enucleation and after enucleation with implant.*

33-8

TYPES OF SOCKETS FOR PROSTHESIS FITTING

33-8-1 Blind Eye or Phthisis Bulbi

Retaining the globe if at all possible is by far the most preferred situation. The surgery of either partial or complete eye removal will almost certainly have some damaging effects on the tissues of the eyelid or orbit and affect cosmesis and motility. A scarred, full-size globe can be covered with a very thin shell. If the palpebral fissure is enlarged by its presence, the iris–cornea can be enlarged and a minus lens worn over the prosthetic eye in spectacle frames. Motility is usually excellent in such cases. Phthisic globes nearly always allow adequate room for a shell or thicker prostheses. When a phthisic globe

---

*See also Chapter 14, "Management of Entropion and Trichiasis," Chapter 15, "Classification and Correction of Entropion," and Chapter 16, "Classification and Correction of Ptosis," in Volume 2 of Ophthalmology Monograph 8, published in 1994.—ED.

is fitted from an impression, the motility of the prosthetic eye is almost always excellent.

A trial shell is fabricated prior to the fitting of the ocular shell prosthesis. The purpose of making a flush-fitting clear trial shell is threefold:

1. A trial shell can establish whether the patient can wear a lens before the time-consuming fabrication of a final scleral shell is undertaken. If a lens cannot be tolerated by the patient as in the case of crystalline deposits on the cornea, then consideration can be given to a conjunctival flap from the superior fornix to cover the cornea. It is not advisable to use the other quadrants as donor sites because motility can be limited, causing discomfort on movement or creating a retention problem in the lower cul-de-sac.*

2. The patient is instructed to condition the cornea by building up the wearing time until the accumulated wearing time justifies fabrication of the final scleral shell.

3. When the globe and socket shrink, the tissues lining the socket also constrict. Wearing a trial lens will help stretch this contracted tissue. This could save refitting

_____

*If enucleation is ultimately required in a patient who has had a conjunctival flap, the surgeon must be attentive to the possibility of inadequate conjunctiva being available for closure and consider implant options (eg, dermis–fat graft) accordingly.—ED.

the prosthesis as the space is regained. Care for the scleral shell should be the same as for a hard contact lens unless a conjunctival flap is placed. Then longer wearing times are expected as the cornea is protected and has a vascular covering.

33-8-2 Evisceration With Retained Cornea

The next most satisfactory eye socket to fit is following evisceration with a retained cornea and an 18-mm spherical implant. The fact that most of the conjunctiva, Tenon's capsule, and muscles are unaffected by the surgery leaves most of the tissues of the orbit in nearly their original positions and conditions. Most such sockets are relatively easy to fit and the comfort, motility, and general cosmesis are excellent. This should be the first type of surgery to be considered where there is a limited possibility of sympathetic ophthalmia or intraocular malignancy. Care should be given to avoid placing an oversized implant, as exposure can occur or the ocularist may not be able to make a prosthetic eye with enough anteroposterior thickness to create a realistic anterior chamber.

33-8-3 Evisceration With Excised Cornea

Evisceration with the cornea excised and a 16-mm spherical implant is not as satisfactory as with a retained cornea, because there will be a slight tendency toward enophthalmos and less leverage for motility transference to the prosthesis. Otherwise, this operation has the same advantages as the foregoing because there is so little surgical disruption outside the globe. This procedure usually allows enough anteroposterior thickness in the prosthesis for a normal anterior chamber.

33-8-4 Enucleation With Implant

An orbital implant is placed during surgery into the socket or within an eviscerated globe. The purpose is to replace volume, support surrounding tissue, support a prosthetic eye, and impart motility to the ocular prosthesis. In 1884, when Mules placed a glass sphere into an eviscerated globe, the practice of using orbital implants began. Since then, a myriad of materials have been used: glass, gold, Vitallium, silicone, stainless steel, plastic, silk, catgut, ivory, paraffin, petroleum jelly, celluloid, cartilage, fat, charred bone, fascia lata, silicone rubber, and hydroxyapatite.[15] Various sizes and shapes have also been used: small glass or plastic beads, larger spheres, basket, cone, and acorn shapes; some were solid, others hollow or perforated.[16]

The classifications most often used to describe the types of orbital implants are buried nonintegrated, exposed integrated, and buried (quasi) integrated:

1. Buried nonintegrated implants are simple spheres that are completely covered by orbital tissue (conjunctiva and Tenon's capsule). The extraocular muscles are not attached and are allowed to retract into the orbit (Ball implant).[17,18]

2. Exposed integrated implants are attached to the extraocular muscles and then directly linked to the prosthesis through an opening in the conjunctiva. These already exposed implants led to extrusion, secondary to chronic infection.[17,18] Commonly used exposed integrated implants were the Cutler, Stone, Whitney, Johnson, Arruga, and Linn.

3. Buried (quasi) integrated implants are attached to the extraocular muscles and are buried within or behind Tenon's capsule and conjunctiva. The prosthesis is indirectly linked to the implant by matching irregular surfaces between the implant and the prosthesis. The extraocular muscles are sewn to the implants enwrapped with sclera, collagen, fascia, wire mesh, or Dacron mesh. In the case of the Allen implant,[19] they are attached by tunneling between the implant body and imbricating over the implant. With the Iowa[20] and Universal[21] implants, the extraocular muscles are brought up over the implant and sewn between the four mounds. The hydroxyapatite implant[17] also falls into this category because the hole drilled to accommodate its peg is epithelium-lined. In this way, the implant is still buried but coupled with the prosthetic eye by use of the peg.[17,18]

The ideal enucleation technique provides a socket with a centrally located implant of good motility. The conjunctival cul-de-sac should be well defined and not narrowed by the implant. It should provide the patient with comfort and the availability of a natural-appearing prosthesis with few socket complications.

The size of the implant should be determined on an individual case-by-case basis. Usually, it is recommended that a sphere not over 16 to 18 mm[17] be placed into Tenon's capsule because closure of conjunctiva and Tenon's capsule is easier. This size often yields a slightly to moderately enophthalmic appearance and a sunken superior eyelid sulcus. Larger implants of 20 to 22 mm can be used if a patient has undergone several surgical procedures before the enucleation, resulting in retraction or fibrosis of the orbital soft tissue or fat atrophy.

Soll recommended placing the implant within the muscle cone posterior to the deep layer of Tenon's capsule.[22] This permits placement of a larger implant in the orbit and closure of Tenon's and conjunctiva without tension (20 to 22 mm). Less enophthalmos and sunken superior eyelid sulcus is noted with this preferred procedure.

With enucleation, there are a multitude of different implants designed to replace volume and impart motility. Some are designed to be placed in Tenon's fascia and others posterior to Tenon's capsule. Those placed posteriorly can usually be of a larger diameter and still allow easy closure of Tenon's fascia.

33-8-5 Evisceration Without Implant

Eviscerations with no implants are not very satisfactory. Eventually, the sclera shrinks to a nubbin, usually appearing to have four small lobes. The shriveling of the sclera pulls all of the connective tissue in the orbit toward the center, putting it on tension across the fornices. As a result, there can be very little motility and there can be a marked degree of enophthalmos.

Even though the muscles have remained attached to the globe, they have been pulled into the center, where they have very little leverage to more than rock the nubbin of sclera that remains.

33-8-6 Enucleation Without Implant

Although sometimes medically necessary, the least satisfactory operation is simple enucleation without placement of an implant. The rectus muscles fall into the center of the orbit and slightly downward by gravity, tugging against all of the connective tissues from the periphery of the orbit. Because there has been no partial replacement of the volume lost by removal of the globe, the support for the fat in the upper portion of the orbit has been removed and the fat drops downward and backward toward the center of the orbit. The result is a sucking backward of all of the tissue below and in front of the rim of the orbit so that, inevitably, there is enophthalmos as well as deepening and broadening of the superior sulcus.

33-9

TYPES OF IMPLANTS

33-9-1 Hydroxyapatite

Hydroxyapatite, approved as an orbital[15] implant in 1989 by the FDA, is comprised of calcium phosphate in which vascularization occurs. In placement it is often sclera-enwrapped with the rectus muscles attached. Wrapping is not mandatory and actually avoided by some surgeons concerned with residual infection potential of donor sclera. Several surgeons noted initial exposure rates of hydroxyapatite implants as high as 10% to 12%.[18] The high exposure rate was primarily attributed to the roughness of the implant material, with contributing factors of poor surgical technique or improper implant size. The author's data suggest that the rate of exposure is 6% to 8% and that the exposures usually self-correct spontaneously.

With time, the implant becomes vascularized and if it becomes exposed, the blood supply will support tissue growth over the implant. This is probably one of the finest attributes of hydroxyapatite: acrylic, glass, and silicone implants will not re-epithelialize over an exposure. The material also offers good motility in most cases. In approximately 75% to 80% of all cases, the drilling of the implant and peg placement are not necessary for improved motility. However, if additional motility is needed, the drilling and placement of a peg will allow for a direct coupling of the implant and the prosthesis. Refitting of the prosthesis is necessary to accommodate the peg, which prevents any slippage of the prosthesis over the implant. Caution should be exercised in drilling and pegging an implant that already gives excellent motility because the further excursions of movement received from the pegging can cause the medial and lateral edges of the prosthesis to show. Other cases have produced a retention problem on superior gaze. If this occurs, the peg can be removed and the hole will close by granulation. Once tissue ingrowth occurs, the implant is not likely to migrate. With the pegged implant, the weight of the prosthesis is supported on the peg, not on the inferior fornices, and is less likely to create a sagging lower lid.

Although hydroxyapatite makes a good implant, the cost is high compared to other materials. The implant requires one surgery to accomplish placement and a second for subsequent pegging. Added to that are the costs of ocular prosthesis fabrication and refitting to accommodate a peg. Moreover, a bone scan may be needed, to assure complete vascularization before drilling.[15,17] Figure 33-11 shows the implant in position.*

33-9-2 Universal

The Universal is the next-generation Iowa implant.[21] In the Universal implant, the mounds are significantly reduced in height and more smoothly rounded than in the Iowa implant. The implantation technique has also been simplified, to meet a major criticism of the Iowa implant: that the placement procedure required too much time and involved a technique that many ophthalmologists had not performed during their training (Figure 33-12).

The volume of the Universal was also increased posteriorly over the Iowa implant. The Universal, therefore, decreases the possibility of a deep superior sulcus and allows for a smaller prosthesis. Motil-

---

*For a diagram of the implant, see Figure 30-1 in this volume.—ED.

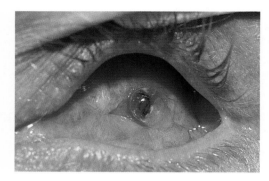

Figure 33-11 *Socket with Biomatrix implant with peg in place.*

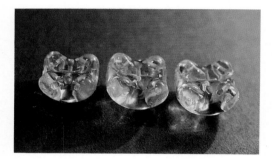

Figure 33-12 *New Universal implant (three sizes).*

ity is still excellent and cost is not a problem. Fitting is accomplished with impression-molding techniques to ensure a proper fit and to prevent points of pressure that can cause discomfort and extrusion.[21]

33-9-3 Iowa

The Iowa remains a well-regarded quasi-integrated implant. In two comparative reviews of orbital implants undertaken at two different facilities,[16,23] the Iowa averaged the lowest exposure rate: 5.4% in one study and 4.2% in the other. This rate was statistically lower than any implant, including spheres. In the larger study, the average exposure rate of all implants was 13%. The Iowa excelled over other implants particularly in trauma cases. At the time these surveys were undertaken, the Universal and the hydroxyapatite implants were not available and therefore not included (Figure 33-13).

The diameter of the Iowa implant in a plane comparable to that of the equator of the living eye is 21 mm—3 mm greater than the largest allowable spherical implant placed in Tenon's capsule. Thus, the mass behind the equator is much greater than that of spherical implants so the fat is supported upward and forward in a more normal position than is done by the spherical implants in Tenon's capsule. The anteroposterior dimension is only 17 mm, leaving adequate room for a well-shaped prosthetic eye. Motility from this implant is nearly as good as that from an eviscerated globe with an 18-mm spherical implant. Fitting this implant must be with impression-molding techniques to prevent pressure points over the implant.[21]

33-9-4 Allen

The Allen, a quasi-integrated implant devised in 1948, can be considered almost as satisfactory as the Iowa.[5] The Allen implant is 21 mm in diameter at the equator and 15 mm in the anteroposterior dimension. Some of the Allen implants give better motility to the prosthesis than does the average Iowa implant. However, the fact that the rim of the implant is exactly circular offers the possibility that the fornices can become almost circular as well, so that some of the prostheses can rather easily make clockwise or counterclockwise rotations, which are noticeable on changes in the direction of gaze.[19] This problem is seldom seen with the Iowa implant, which was designed to avoid this problem.

The Allen implant is also capable of giving such extreme motility that show of the medial and lateral edges of the prosthesis is possible. There also exists the possibility on rare occasions of a retention problem, again due to motility. The fitting of the prosthetic eye usually could alleviate these occurrences. The newest Allen design has been revised to reduce the chances of these fitting difficulties (Figure 33-14).

33-9-5 Spherical

Spherical implants within Tenon's capsule are not as satisfactory as the implants described above. The spherical implant should not exceed 18 mm in diameter. Placing an implant larger than 18 mm within Tenon's capsule creates difficulty in closing Tenon's at the time of enucleation, crowds the cul-de-sac, impedes motility, and complicates prosthesis fitting.

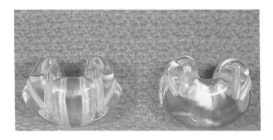

Figure 33-13 *Iowa implants. (Left) Old. (Right) New.*

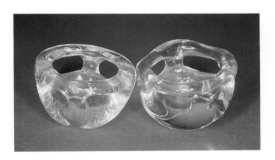

Figure 33-14 *Allen implants. (Left) Old. (Right) New.*

Placing larger spheres (eg, 20 to 24 mm) posterior to Tenon's, rather than *in* the capsule, reduced the difficulty of producing a good cosmetic and therapeutic result.[15]

If an 18-mm or smaller diameter sphere is used, it is preferred that the rectus muscles not be imbricated across its front. Imbrication will almost always result in migration of the sphere, severe ptosis, and lack of motility. If spherical implants are used, the rectus muscles can be left free after removal from the globe. Dissecting the muscles extensively and letting them retract results in little or no movement in the socket. If enucleation is associated with nystagmus or blind wandering eyes, the absence of motility is preferred. When muscles are removed from the globe with minimal disruption of adjacent tissue and/or attached approximately to their former position on Tenon's, a nicely moving soft-tissue socket is usually the result. Without some definite irregularities on the anterior socket surface to which the prosthesis can be anchored, there will be slippage between the implant and the prosthetic eye. This results in a discrepancy between apparent socket movement and the motility of the prosthesis, which can also be seen with the Universal, Iowa, and Allen implants but to a lesser degree than with the spherical implants. PMMA is the material of choice.

33-10

OCULOFACIAL PROSTHESES

Oculofacial prostheses are used after orbital exenteration, when not only the eye, but the eyelids, deep orbital tissues, and perhaps periorbital structures have been excised. Not all ocularists make oculofacial prostheses, for they are very difficult and time-consuming, but the final effects are nearly always gratifying to both the patient and the ocularist.

An oculofacial prosthesis requires about 5 to 7 days to create. An impression of the exenterated orbit and surrounding areas is taken with dental alginate. Some ocularists extend the impression to include the other eye for reference. A mixture of dental stone is poured into the impression to create a positive model of that portion of the face.

A custom prosthetic eye is created to match the companion eye and is incorporated into the prosthesis during the modeling of the eyelid portions. Some ocularists use modeling clay; others use hard dental inlay wax. The prosthesis in progress is lifted from the stone model at an early stage and placed in position on the patient's face. The vertical and horizontal positions and the prominence of the prosthetic eye must be established before the modeling of the eyelids can be finished. Whenever possible, the diameters of the eyelid portion should be relatively small. If the edges can fall directly behind the rim of spectacles, they are less noticeable than if they extend well beyond. They can be further hidden by placing the edges in skin folds or in the eyebrows.

When all of the modeling is finished, a two-piece dental stone mold is made around it in a large denture flask. The eyelid portion of the prosthesis can then be cast in a flexible material such as silicone rubber. Dry powder pigments and flocking materials to represent capillaries can be mixed with the silicone to give a base color. Most ocularists try to avoid a great deal of surface coloring, although a little is needed in every case to match and blend with the patient's skin tone. With the new materials, the edges can be quite thin and therefore easier to hide. With the addition of eyelashes and eyebrow hair, the final prosthesis can look quite realistic. The silicone rubber will flex passively with facial expressions.

A facial prosthesis may be clipped onto a pair of spectacles, or it may be held in place by double-surfaced adhesive tape or a colostomy type of medical adhesive. Adhesives or double-sided tapes can create a skin reaction, prosthetic discoloration, and possible but infrequent retention problems. Other facial prostheses have been anchored by placing a balloon into the socket and anchoring to it. Another choice of affixing the prosthesis to the orbit is by use of bone-anchored orbital implants placed by means of osseointegration.[24] This is accomplished by implanting titanium fixtures into the bony orbital rim. Once osseointegration occurs, an abutment is screwed into the fixture and a framework holding magnets is connected. A facial prosthesis is made with corresponding magnets and held in place by magnetic attraction.[24] If facial prostheses are realistically done, to the point of careful duplication of skin texture and tinting

and the addition of artificial eyelashes, the patients will wear them. Some will remove the prostheses when they are at home but always wear them when they go out. Others will insist on wearing them to bed at night as well as during the day. The use of an antiperspirant where the prosthesis contacts the flesh helps in extended wear, especially in extreme warmth. The limitations of these appliances are obvious: they do not enable blinking or motility, nor will they change color with the skin color variance throughout the year.

33-11

COSMETIC OPTICS

Few people have exact symmetry between the two sides of their faces. However, this fact should not be used as an excuse for stopping short of the best balance and match that can be achieved between the prosthetic and the real eye.

After the ocularist has done everything possible to obtain symmetry, there may still be one or more defects that call attention to the prosthetic eye. Spectacles can be used in an attempt to improve the appearance still further. Spectacle frames, especially plastic ones, will immediately distract from any residual abnormalities. For example, if the remaining problem is a deep and wide superior sulcus, the upper rim of the spectacles may cover it.

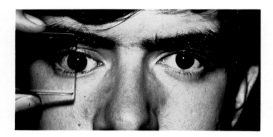

Figure 33-15 *Base-down prism to raise palpebral fissure.*

The upper rim of the frames should not be too high or it will be possible to see the sulcus under the rim.

Any person with only one sighted eye should wear spectacles as a protection. The lenses, then, can be made with optics that will partly or completely correct some of the asymmetries. If the palpebral fissure is vertically increased, a minus cylinder of correct power can be used at axis 180°. If the palpebral fissure is horizontally increased, a minus cylinder may be used at axis 90°. If one of the canthi on the prosthetic eye is too high, crossed cylinders will bring the palpebral fissure to a level position optically. If the palpebral fissure is too small in all dimensions, a plus sphere can be used over the prosthetic eye. In that case, the iris of the prosthetic eye should be painted small in proportion to the palpebral fissure so that it will be enlarged at the same time as the fissure. The opposite is true if the palpebral fissure is too large in all dimensions, in which case the iris should be painted to fill the space and a minus sphere used in the spectacles. If the palpebral fissure is too high or too low or too far from the nose, simple prismatic addition to the spectacle lens can move the image into the proper position (Figure 33-15).

Trial lenses in trial frames can help determine what combination of powers of lenses might be used over the prosthetic eye. Better yet, uncut lens blanks 65 mm in diameter will allow the entire prosthesis, eyelid, and surrounding area to be seen in one glance. An overall tint in the lenses is helpful, or a gradient tint from medium dark at the top to clear at the bottom is especially good to hide deep superior sulcus defects. Cosmetics including eyeliner, artificial eyelashes, eye shadow, and makeup are also useful when properly applied in enhancing symmetry and creating a natural look.

REFERENCES

1. Anson BJ: The ear and the eye in the collected works of Ambroise Paré, renaissance surgeon to five kings of France. *Trans Am Acad Ophthalmol Otolaryngol* 1970;74:249–277.

2. Trester W: The history of artificial eyes and the evolution of the ocularistic profession. *J Am Soc Ocularists* 1982;12:5–13.

3. Scott R, Lodenheim J: *Prostheses: Problems and Treatment of Contracted Sockets, Exenterated Orbits, Alkali Burns*. New York: Intercontinental Medical Book Corp; 1973:99–117.

4. Kelly JJ: History of ocular prosthetics. In: Shannon GM, Connelly FJ, eds: *Oculoplastic Surgery and Prosthetics*. Boston: Little, Brown and Co; 1970;10:713–719.

5. Vistnes L: *Surgical Reconstruction in the Anophthalmic Orbit*. Birmingham, AL: Aesculapius Publishing Co; 1987:14–15.

6. Kelly K: A discussion of custom pressure conformers. *J Am Soc Ocularists* 1991;22:19–24.

7. Allen L, Braley AE, Webster H: Problems in ocular prosthetics. *J Iowa State Med Soc* 1953; 43:329.

8. Allen L, Webster HE: Modified impression method of artificial eye fitting. *Am J Ophthalmol* 1969;67:189–218.

9. Allen L: Modified impression fitting. In: Shannon GM, Connelly FJ, eds: *Oculoplastic Surgery and Prosthetics*. Boston: Little, Brown and Co; 1970;10:747–762.

10. Allen L: Reduction of upper eyelid ptosis with the prosthesis, with special attention to a recently devised, more effective method. In: Guibor P, Guibor M, eds: *Techniques of Anophthalmic Cosmesis*. New York: Stratton; 1976:3–25.

11. Allen L: *One Iatrogenic Ptosis and Its Reduction by a Specially Contoured Artificial Eye*. Third International Symposium, Plastic Reconstructive Surgery of the Eye and Adnexa. Baltimore: Williams & Wilkins; 1981.

12. Allen L: The argument against imbricating the rectus muscles over spherical orbital implants after enucleation. *Ophthalmology* 1983; 90:1116–1120.

13. Erickson M: *A Comprehensive View of Enucleation: Problems and Treatment of Enucleation, Evisceration, Exposure*. New York: Intercontinental Medical Book Corp; 1974:3–9.

14. Vistnes L: *Surgical Reconstruction in the Anophthalmic Orbit*. Birmingham, AL: Aesculapius Publishing Co; 1987:46–51.

15. Bosniak S: The anophthalmic socket. In: Smith B, ed: *Advances in Ophthalmic Plastic and Reconstructive Surgery*. Elmsford, NY: Pergamon Press; 1972;8.

16. Young C: *An Eight-Year Review of Enucleations and Extrusions at the University of Iowa*. March 26, 1975.

17. Perry AC: Advances in enucleation. In: Nunery W, ed: *Ophthalmic Plastic and Reconstructive Surgery*. Philadelphia: WB Saunders Co; 1991:173–182.

18. Nerad JA, Carter KD: The anophthalmic socket. *Focal Points.* Vol X, Module 4. San Francisco: Academy of Ophthalmology; 1992.

19. Allen JH, Allen L: A buried muscle cone implant, 1: development of a tunneled hemispherical type. *Arch Ophthalmol* 1950;43: 879–890.

20. Spivey BE, Allen L, Burns CA: The Iowa enucleation implant: a ten-year evaluation of techniques and results. *Am J Ophthalmol* 1969;67:171–188.

21. Jordan D, Anderson R, Nerad J, Allen L: A preliminary report on the Universal Implant. *Arch Ophthalmol* 1987;105:1726–1731.

22. Soll DB: Enucleation surgery: a new technique. *Arch Ophthalmol* 1972;87:196–197.

23. Jahrling R: Statistical study of extruded implants. *Today's Ocularist* 1979;9:25–27.

24. Nerad, JA, Carter KD, LaVelle WE, et al: The osseointegration technique for the rehabilitation of the exenterated orbit. *Arch Ophthalmol* 1991;109:1032–1038.

Management and Care of Ocular Prostheses

William A. Danz, BCO

A patient with an ocular prosthesis who has complaints regarding comfort, fit, motility, or cosmesis that are not related to infection or other medical problems can be referred to the ocularist for evaluation and correction of the problem.

In addition to providing initial and replacement ocular prostheses and scleral shells, the ocularist affords maintenance of the prosthesis by way of cleaning, polishing, enlarging, reducing, and other modifications. The ocularist also educates patients on the proper care of the prosthesis and is available for preoperative consultation prior to enucleation or secondary procedures.

Surgical procedures planned for an anophthalmic socket to correct superior sulcus recession, blepharoptosis, inferior eyelid sag, socket contraction, conjunctival adhesions, implant migration, exposure, extrusion, entropion, ectropion, or other abnormalities can benefit significantly from participation by the ocularist preoperatively and in the early postoperative management with properly fitting prosthetic devices.

Chronic irritation from an old, rough, improperly fitting ocular prosthesis or the long-term absence of a prosthetic device can result in cicatricial conjunctival contracture of the anophthalmic socket and must be corrected early by referral to an ocularist to prevent permanent loss in size. Additionally, a socket with a history of radiation treatment, caustic injury, congenital anophthalmia, or reconstruction within which the forces of contraction are actively present is in need of immediate care whenever a prosthesis or conformer has been lost or cannot be retained.

A final prosthetic result that does not fulfill the expectations of the ophthalmologist or patient should be discussed with the ocularist to clarify the limitations of the result and to determine the best possible solution. Modification of one aspect of an ocular prosthesis can sometimes have an adverse effect on another aspect. For example, modifications to improve a superior sulcus recession by increasing the superior anterior volume of the prosthesis can create an inferior eyelid sag due to the increased weight and downward displacement.

34-1

ANOPHTHALMIC VS SCLERAL SHELL PROSTHESES

Ocular prostheses are basically of two designs: anophthalmic and scleral shell. The most common type of anophthalmic socket is created by enucleation, with the remainder being congenital. Scleral shells are usually thinner and require a more precise design because they fit over a globe with intact corneal sensation. These globes include phthisis bulbi, evisceration, congenital microphthalmia, and the normal-sized, blind, disfigured globe.

Scleral shell prostheses fit over an intact globe often have greater motility and less enophthalmos than anophthalmic prostheses, making them the prosthesis of choice cosmetically, but they may have shorter wearing times depending on the underlying corneal sensitivity and tolerance. This distinction may be less true today with the current success of the hy-

droxyapatite implant, which allows for retention of larger implants and improved motility from the peg integration of the implant to the prosthesis. However, removal of a quiet, painless, blind, shrunken, and disfigured globe for a purely cosmetic reason is usually unnecessary due to improved fitting techniques for scleral shells.

34-2

GENERAL EVALUATION OF THE PROSTHESIS

In evaluating an ocular prosthesis, the ocularist begins by establishing a thorough history of the conditions and treatments that led up to the need for the prosthesis. In addition, the ocularist examines the type of socket and its contents, the quality of fit and the age of the prosthesis, the amount of eyelid function, the status of the lacrimal system, and the patient's wearing and hygiene habits. Removal of the ocular prosthesis to inspect it and the socket cavity is essential.

Anophthalmic sockets vary greatly in size, configuration, and functioning of the remaining orbital contents due in large part to the fact that enucleation implants vary in design, size, material, placement, and function. The ocular prosthesis, when held in the hand, should closely approximate the contour and size of the socket or globe to provide maximal comfort, fit, and motility. Any space between the posterior aspect of the ocular prosthesis and the socket can be a site for accumulation of mucus and tears, leading to chronic irritation, excessive mucous discharge, and possible infection. The impression fitting technique minimizes this problem and distributes the contact more evenly over the posterior surface of the prosthesis.

Increasing age of the ocular prosthesis decreases the quality of fit, as changes occur within the soft tissues of the socket. Orbital fat atrophy, often associated with a history of trauma, and the changes in orbital anatomy that follow enucleation are often involved. The prosthesis will recede posteriorly, causing a narrowing of the palpebral fissure and misalignment of the prosthetic iris. Problems with rotation or retention of the prosthesis may also be present. This problem can be corrected by enlargement or replacement of the prosthesis, but full correction is difficult because the anophthalmic socket is always going to be volume-deficient compared to a normal orbit and result in some degree of enophthalmos with superior palpebral sulcus recession.

The average life of an ocular prosthesis is 4 to 6 years, depending on the quality of fit, comfort, and cosmesis. Children will require enlargements and replacements more frequently due to growth and to help stimulate bony orbital growth. Replacement of a prosthesis will be indicated when delamination occurs. Delamination is the separation of the pigmentary layer within the middle structure of the prosthesis and often extends to the anterior surface, presenting as a hairline crack near the limbal border. A silvery reflection in the prosthetic pupil and iris is often present.

Indications for prescribing a new ocular prosthesis should be based on medical necessity. Symptoms can include chronic irritation and excessive mucous discharge due to poor fit. There may be problems with rotation or retention of the prosthesis due to laxity of the conjunctiva and eyelids. The conjunctiva may contract, making the prosthesis too large, or the prosthesis may become too small due to orbital fat atrophy. Increasingly larger prostheses for congenital anophthalmia will help minimize socket hypoplasia.

34-3

EVALUATION OF THE SURFACE OF THE PROSTHESIS

The surface condition of a properly fitting prosthesis will often give clues to the cause of excessive mucous discharge and irritation, once an infectious process has been ruled out. Deposits of protein on the surface of the prosthesis are normal, being the socket's method of dealing with a foreign object by providing a protective layer between living tissue and the acrylic plastic. This is evidenced clinically by excessive mucous discharge lasting a few days following removal and cleaning of the ocular prosthesis. During this period, a protein layer is established on the surface of the prosthesis to encapsulate the freshly exposed plastic material. Once established, the amount of discharge decreases to normal levels for continuous prosthetic wear. With time, these protein deposits build up, thicken, and become a rough, irritating surface requiring removal and cleaning of the prosthesis. This is normally done by the patient.

Abrasive scratches in the plastic surface of the ocular prosthesis will require referral to an ocularist for proper polishing. This service is normally recommended once a year. The scratches are often the result of normal wear and handling by the patient but can also be due to improper polishing initially by the ocularist and should be looked for with a minimum of 5-power magnification. Sharp edges on the prosthesis should be properly repolished to improve comfort. Other surface defects can include cracks, crazing, chips, tool marks, and exposed debris such as dental stone.

34-4

PROPER HYGIENE FOR THE PROSTHESIS

Recommendations to patients on proper care of the prosthesis vary with the type of socket or globe and the quality of fit. A patient with an anophthalmic socket and a properly fitting ocular prosthesis with good eyelid function and normal lacrimal production can often wear the prosthesis for many months without problems. Each patient needs to establish individualized intervals for removal and cleaning. Symptoms indicating the need for cleaning are

an increase in the amount of noninfectious mucous discharge that is not related to a cold, allergy, or sinus condition and a gradual decrease in the level of comfort.

Often, the most troublesome time is in the morning upon awakening. Crusting and mucous discharge that accumulates overnight should be cleaned with the ocular prosthesis in place. Periodic irrigation of the prosthesis with balanced salt solution and hard contact lens solution or artificial tears will aid in daily hygiene and comfort. However, these water-based drops may give only limited relief due to evaporation and absorption, especially in cases of dry eye symptoms or lagophthalmos. The use of ophthalmic ointments and oil-based drops such as silicone, vitamin E, and mineral oil can be helpful. Because the surface of the polymethylmethacrylate prosthesis is hydrophobic and drier than a normal globe, a hydrophilic polymer coating on the plastic surface can be effective in some cases by improved wetting of the surface.

The period of time that a scleral shell prosthesis can be comfortably tolerated by the globe (and cornea if present) varies from daytime-only wear to continuous wear lasting many months. The length of successful wear will be determined by the degree of corneal sensitivity, the quality of fit and polish of the scleral shell, and the willingness of the patient to wear the scleral shell. Any unusual discomfort or redness of the globe or eyelids indicates the need to remove the scleral shell until the symptoms are eliminated. In severe cases, an ophthalmologic examination is indicated. The causative factor is usually excessive wear, foreign debris under the shell, or improper hygiene by the patient. When not worn, the scleral shell should be kept hydrated in a sterile saline or hard-contact-lens soaking solution.

If corneal sensitivity prevents acceptance of a scleral shell, a superficial keratectomy and the creation of a conjunctival (Gunderson) flap to cover the cornea may allow the preservation of the globe and successful wear of the scleral shell prosthesis.

34-4-1 Cleaning the Prosthesis

The best method for cleaning the ocular prosthesis depends on the thickness of the surface deposits and how adherent they are on the plastic surface. After the prosthesis has been removed, the surface should be dried gently with a tissue to permit better visualization of the protein layer that has accumulated on the surface. The use of 5-power magnification is helpful because it is strong enough to reveal the surface condition and weak enough to allow covering the entire surface quickly. Careful inspection of both the anterior and the posterior surface is required.

After inspection, soaking the prosthesis in water, saline, or contact lens solution helps to loosen the deposits. For light surface buildup, a hard contact lens cleaning solution, mild hand soap, or baby shampoo will suffice. For more stubborn deposits, a wet white paper towel to vigorously rub the entire surface removes the deposit without scratching the plastic material. Deposits that appear white in color, often located horizontally on the prosthetic cornea, may be difficult for the patient to remove by cleaning, so that polishing by an ocularist is indicated. An ocular prosthesis that has been treated with a hydrophilic polymer coating requires additional care to ensure that the polymer is not removed by the cleaning process.

Dry cloth should not be used because abrasive particles may be present. Any solvents, such as alcohol, should never come in contact with the ocular prosthesis as they will attack the plastic and craze the surface. Hand-washing prior to handling the prosthesis is obligatory to minimize contamination of the eye socket. Washing the hands is also recommended before wiping the prosthesis while it is worn.

34-5

INSERTION AND REMOVAL OF THE PROSTHESIS

The two methods usually employed for inserting and removing an ocular prosthesis are the use of a suction cup and the use of the fingers. Suction cups may be preferable for patients with manual dexterity problems or unusual sockets or eyelids. A viscous solution such as a hard-contact-lens wetting solution to moisten the suction cup improves adherence of the cup to the surface of the prosthesis. The lubricating agent also improves comfort and ease of insertion, but may make handling a slippery prosthesis with the fingers more difficult for some patients. In that case, the patient may find a suction cup helpful.

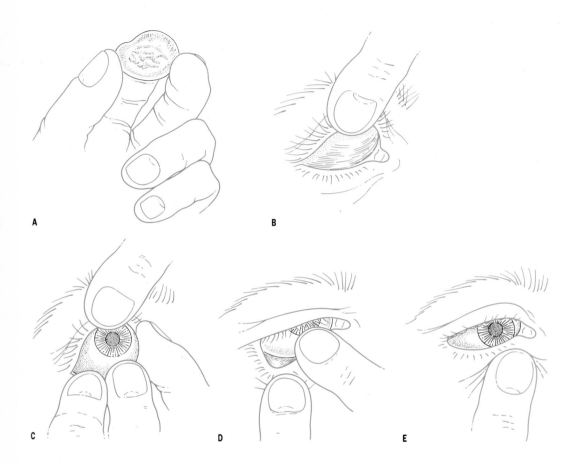

Figure 34-1 *Insertion of ocular prosthesis. (A) Identifying superior aspect of prosthesis. (B) Raising upper lid. (C) Sliding prosthesis up, under, and behind upper lid margin. (D) Pulling lower lid down. (E) Correct positioning of lower lid.*

Both insertion and removal start with thorough hand washing. Care should also be taken to drape a towel over the sink, to prevent breakage or loss in the event the prosthesis is accidentally dropped. As an additional precaution, the drain should be closed or covered.

34-5-1 Inserting the Prosthesis

Insertion begins with identifying the superior aspect of the prosthesis (Figure 34-1A). Some ocularists place an identifying mark or dot at the 12-o'clock position to indicate the superior scleral portion of the prosthesis; occasionally, two dots may be placed at the 6-o'clock position to indicate the inferior portion. The presence of a trochlear notch along the edge of the prosthesis often indicates the superior nasal aspect. The horizontal pattern of the prosthetic blood vessels indicates the canthi, with the nasal scleral portion often shorter and narrower than the lateral scleral portion.

The next step is to raise the upper eyelid high enough to create a space behind the upper eyelid margin (Figure 34-1B). Then the prosthesis is slid up, underneath, and behind the upper eyelid margin (Figure 34-1C). The prosthesis is gradually worked superiorly until its inferior edge falls back behind the lower eyelid margin. This maneuver is aided by pulling down the lower eyelid (Figure 34-1D). The lower eyelid should be checked that it is in the correct position (Figure 34-1E).

34-5-2 Removing the Prosthesis

Removal of the prosthesis is aided by looking upward, as this position of gaze brings the inferior edge of the prosthesis up nearer the inferior eyelid margin. One hand should be cupped on the cheek to catch the prosthesis as it slides out of the socket (Figure 34-2A). The forefinger of the other hand is placed against the lower eyelid at the medial aspect (Figure 34-2B). The finger pushes inward and downward (*a*) and is then pulled laterally (*b*) to invert the lower eyelid margin underneath and behind the inferior edge of the prosthesis. As the prosthesis slides out, the forefinger and thumb of the other hand may be used to grasp it (Figure 34-2C).

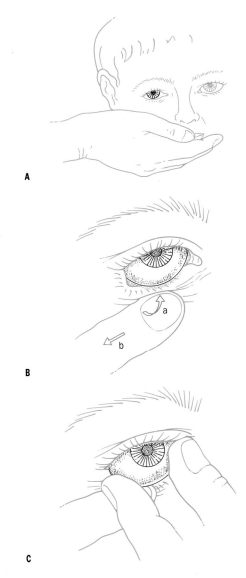

Figure 34-2 *Removal of ocular prosthesis. (A) Positioning one hand on cheek. (B) Placing finger of other hand against lower lid. (C) Grasping prosthesis with forefinger and thumb.*

34-6

SUGGESTED WEARING HABITS

The two most common problems encountered by patients when improperly wiping or rubbing the prosthesis are rotation of the prosthesis out of proper position and expulsion. A prosthesis rotated out of position can be turned in place with a clean finger, a cotton-tipped applicator, or a suction cup. Proper wiping of the prosthesis is suggested as a temporal-to-nasal motion to minimize these problems. Caution should always be exercised whenever the lower eyelid or the adjacent area is pulled down or stretched, as when washing the face.

Loss of the prosthesis can occur during water sports. Whenever water strikes the face, as in diving, water skiing, or swimming underwater with the eyes open, the water can enter behind the prosthesis and expel it. Wearing swim goggles, tightly closing the eyelids, patching, or not wearing the prosthesis at all during these activities is recommended.

Minimizing some of the more obvious differences between a prosthetic eye and the normal eye requires the development of good wearing habits. The best attitude for the patient to cultivate is to try to forget that the prosthesis exists, as self-consciousness often draws more attention than do the cosmetic discrepancies.

All ocular prostheses entail some form of limited motility, and the patient should learn to turn the head, shoulders, and body when looking up, down, or to the side. Maintaining the primary gaze with both eyes will maximize the cosmetic effect. Facial expressions, such as smiling, add animation to the muscles surrounding the ocular prosthesis and distract attention from the prosthetic eye.

Eyeglasses with a light tint help minimize the obviousness of any ocular prosthesis. Gradient tints in large frames can draw attention away from a deepened superior eyelid sulcus. Cosmetic optics, involving minus or plus cylinder or prism lenses can bring dissimilar palpebral fissures into more symmetric alignment. The most important reason for a monocular patient who wears an ocular prosthesis to wear glasses, other than to improve vision, is to protect the other eye from injury.

With proper care from both ophthalmologist and ocularist, plus good wearing and hygiene habits, most patients can enjoy successful wear of an ocular prosthesis or scleral shell.

SUGGESTED READING

Bethke EG: Criteria and guide for evaluation of ocular prostheses. *Am J Ophthalmol* 1952;35: 527–536.

PART IX

Orbital Trauma

CHAPTER 35

Orbital and Periorbital Fractures

David B. Soll, MD
Stephen M. Soll, MD

The amount of damage to the globe, surrounding soft tissue, and bony orbit depends on the amount of force applied, its direction, and its duration, as well as the type of object that strikes the orbital area. The freedom of motion of the head at the time of injury is also pertinent, because the amount of damage is greater if the head is immobile. If the head moves with the force, damage to the orbit may be less but damage to the neck may be greater because of the sudden motion of the head.

35-1

ANATOMY OF THE ORBIT IN BRIEF

The orbit is roughly pyramidal or conical in shape (Figure 35-1).* It consists of an apex, a base, and four sides: roof, floor, medial wall, and lateral wall. The orbital entrance (the base of the pyramid) is cir-

---

*See also Chapter 6, "Anatomy of the Eyelid, Orbit, and Lacrimal System," in Volume 1 of Ophthalmology Monograph 8, published in 1993.—ED.

cumscribed by the orbital margin. The bony rim provides anterior support for the thinner bones located behind it. The walls are slightly rounded so that no sharp line of demarcation is present between the superior, medial, inferior, and lateral walls. Because of the slight curvature of the walls, the widest portion of the orbit lies about 1 cm behind the orbital margin. The volume of the orbit is approximately 30 cc.

The floor of the orbit serves as the roof of the maxillary sinus. The floor is thinnest medial to the infraorbital groove and canal. The posterior portions of the orbital floor are thinner than the anterior portions. The main area of weakness of the floor is the medial posterior aspect and its continuation into the medial orbital wall, especially in the area where the medial wall is not yet supported by the bony portions of the ethmoidal labyrinth (Figure 35-2). The inferior orbital foramen, located near the midpoint of the inferior orbital rim, is also a weak area where fractures frequently occur.

The infraorbital canal extends from the infraorbital fissure anteriorly and medially toward the center of the inferior orbital rim. Anteriorly, the fissure is roofed over to form the infraorbital canal. This canal

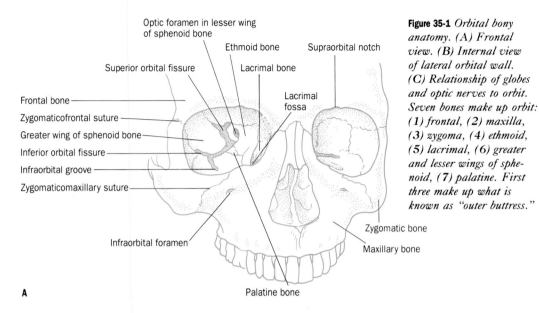

Optic foramen in lesser wing of sphenoid bone

Ethmoid bone

Supraorbital notch

Superior orbital fissure

Lacrimal bone

Lacrimal fossa

Frontal bone

Zygomaticofrontal suture

Greater wing of sphenoid bone

Inferior orbital fissure

Infraorbital groove

Zygomaticomaxillary suture

Infraorbital foramen

Zygomatic bone

Maxillary bone

Palatine bone

A

Figure 35-1 *Orbital bony anatomy. (A) Frontal view. (B) Internal view of lateral orbital wall. (C) Relationship of globes and optic nerves to orbit. Seven bones make up orbit: (1) frontal, (2) maxilla, (3) zygoma, (4) ethmoid, (5) lacrimal, (6) greater and lesser wings of sphenoid, (7) palatine. First three make up what is known as "outer buttress."*

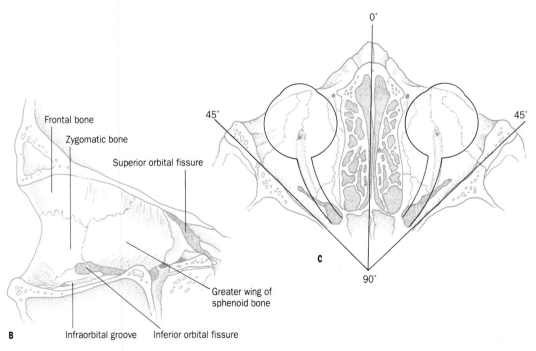

Frontal bone

Zygomatic bone

Superior orbital fissure

Greater wing of sphenoid bone

Infraorbital groove

Inferior orbital fissure

B

0°

45°

45°

90°

C

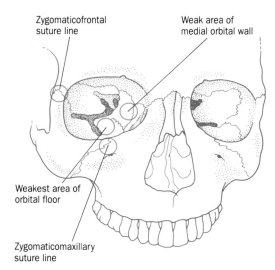

Zygomaticofrontal
suture line

Weak area of
medial orbital wall

Weakest area of
orbital floor

Zygomaticomaxillary
suture line

Figure 35-2 *Areas of weakness of orbit (circles) where fractures are most likely to occur.*

opens below the rim in the canine fossa and is seen as the infraorbital foramen. Occasionally, it is a sulcus or groove at the infraorbital rim.

The medial wall, called the *lamina papyracea*, is thin with natural dehiscences. It is thinner than the floor; however, the dividing thin bony walls of the ethmoidal air cells are perpendicular to the lamina papyracea and act as supports.

The periosteal lining of the orbit is known as the *periorbita* and is easily dissected from the underlying bone except at suture lines, fissures and canal openings, and the trochlear fossa. At the optic canal, it fuses with the dura mater.

35-2

CLINICAL EXAMINATION

35-2-1 Inspection

The initial examination of the orbital area should take place after the patient's general medical situation has been evaluated and stabilized. This is especially true for accidents when high-velocity injuries, such as occur with automobile accidents, have taken place. Cranial, spinal, thoracic, and abdominal injuries can all be life-threatening.

The main function of the bony orbit is to protect the eye. The ophthalmologist's primary concern is evaluation of the globe; visual acuity should be assessed if possible. Meticulous observation of the face from all directions is important. When possible, photographic documentation should be obtained. The change of facial contours caused by displaced fractures can be appreciated easily soon after the injury. However, these signs will be masked by varying degrees of edema and hemorrhage that inevitably occur. Thus, the patient should be examined as soon after the injury as possible.

A fracture dislocation of the zygoma may cause a depression of the malar prominence, which is best evaluated when viewing the patient's face from above and behind. There is usually flattening on the side of the fracture with facial asymmetry that is easily recognized unless masked by edema. A nasoethmoidal orbital fracture, with flattening of the bridge of the nose, is best viewed from the side. This type of fracture is usually accompanied by widening of the intercanthal distance (telecanthus), which should be measured.

The size, type, and location of lacerations should be accurately documented. Underlying fractures should always be suspected when a deep laceration is caused by the force of blunt trauma. Hemorrhage may be caused by soft-tissue injury to the eyelid or to an underlying fracture. Hemorrhage in the orbital area is an early associated sign of orbital fracture. The following types of hemorrhages can be differentiated:

1. Hemorrhage in the eyelid anterior to the orbital septum

2. Hemorrhage posterior to the orbital septum, including subconjunctival hemorrhage

3. Hemorrhage within the muscle cone

4. Subperiosteal hematoma

5. Intracranial hemorrhage, which spreads to the orbit via the medial portion of the supraorbital fissure or via the space between the dura mater and the optic nerve in the optic canal (Figure 35-3)

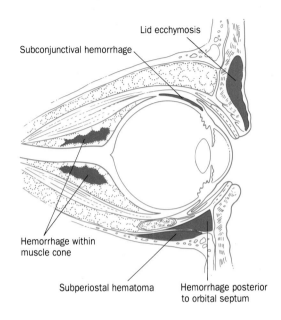

Figure 35-3 *Possible locations of hemorrhage in orbital area occurring after fracture or contusion injury.*

Ecchymosis of the eyelids is usually caused by soft-tissue injury. Extravasation of blood located anterior to the orbital septum spreads easily and may not be confined by the orbital septum. It may cause considerable swelling of the eyelids, extending anteriorly to the tarsal plate up to the eyelid margin. It may also spread under the loose skin of the bridge of the nose to the opposite side. Fractures of the orbital walls may be accompanied by subperiosteal hematomas, especially if the periorbita remains intact. A hematoma of this type usually is of limited size but occasionally may cause a mild exophthalmos. These hematomas are limited by the bony suture lines because the periorbita is firmly adherent to bone at these areas. A subperiosteal hematoma sometimes may be visible as a crescent-shaped discoloration just within the orbital margin. Computed tomography (CT) demonstrates a localized convexity emanating from the bony surface. If the periorbita is damaged, as is usually the case, extravasation of blood spreads forward until it reaches the orbital septum and conjunctiva. Deep orbital hemorrhages are sharply limited by the orbital septum and tarsal plate. Externally, the blood may be visible as a bulge and vague discoloration extending from the orbital margin up to the tarsal plate.

Subconjunctival hemorrhage is usually present.

Occasionally, damage to one of the branches of the ophthalmic vessels causes hemorrhage within the muscle cone. Exophthalmos may result, along with mobility disturbances. The differentiation of this condition from an orbital fracture with muscle entrapment is necessary. The possibility of a fracture of the optic canal should also be considered when a retrobulbar hemorrhage is present. A retrobulbar hemorrhage usually spreads through the openings between the muscles into the peripheral orbital space.

If the hemorrhage is extensive, orbital pressure may increase and compromise the retinal vascular circulation. If visual loss occurs, immediate lateral canthotomy and cantholysis with division of the tendon's attachment to the lateral orbital rim is indicated to decompress the orbital hematoma. This maneuver is usually effective in decreasing the intraorbital pressure. If it is not, more extensive surgery such as an orbital exploration with bony wall decompression may be necessary.

Careful inspection of the position of the eyeball and eyelids should be performed. The eyeball should be evaluated in relation to its position in the orbit, and a comparison of both sides made. Exophthalmos, enophthalmos, and horizontal or vertical displacement of the globe should be noted. Traumatic exophthalmos may be caused by hemorrhage, orbital emphysema, or a complete third nerve palsy (due to loss of muscle tone). Initially, enophthalmos secondary to displacement of orbital soft tissue through fracture sites into adjacent sinuses may be masked by orbital edema, hemorrhage, and transient exophthalmos. The amount of axial displacement should be measured with an exophthalmometer.

35-2-2 Palpation

Palpation of the orbital margin should be gentle and systematic. Rough manipulation causes discomfort and may further displace a dislocated fragment. Because of the superficial location of the orbital margin, palpation is of great value in diagnosing the presence of a displaced fracture.

Special attention should be given to define the point of maximal tenderness. Usually, the fracture is located under this area. A displaced fracture may be palpated as a step-like deformity or discontinuity of the orbital margin. When in doubt, it is useful to palpate both orbital margins simultaneously for comparison.

Palpation may reveal a small chip fracture of the orbital rim even in the presence of negative roentgenographic views. This seems to occur more frequently when the superior orbital rim is involved. These small chip fractures, however, may be demonstrated by computed tomography.

Orbital emphysema can be palpated as crepitus and is diagnostic of orbital fractures involving the paranasal sinuses. Fractures of the medial wall are the most common cause of orbital emphysema. Most cases of orbital emphysema are caused by air being forced through the fracture site and periosteal defect during nose blowing or sneezing, and air thus accumulating in the peripheral orbital space behind the orbital septum.

35-2-3 Sensorimotor Examination

The peripheral branches of the trigeminal nerve lie in close contact with the bony plates. The infraorbital nerve passes along the floor of the orbit, the frontal nerve passes along the roof of the orbit, and the zygomaticotemporal and zygomaticofacial nerves pass through the lateral wall. Thus, the peripheral sensory nerves are easily damaged by orbital fractures. Careful examination of the area for facial anesthesia or hypesthesia often reveals the involved nerve or branch and may be a clue to the possible fracture site.

The infraorbital nerve is most frequently involved in an orbital floor fracture and an inferior rim fracture. This nerve gives off various branches before it enters the infraorbital groove (Figure 35-4). It also gives rise to branches in the groove, in the infraorbital canal, and at the infraorbital foramen. The posterior and anterior superior alveolar nerves are branches of the infraorbital nerve, and injury to them often gives a clue regarding the fracture site and level of injury. The posterior alveolar nerve supplies the upper molar and bicuspid teeth; the anterior alveolar nerve supplies the upper canine and incisor teeth. Numbness in these teeth is indicative of injury to one or both of these branches. In the presence of a

Figure 35-4 *Distribution of infraorbital nerve. Location of orbital floor fracture may often be determined clinically by associated area of numbness.*

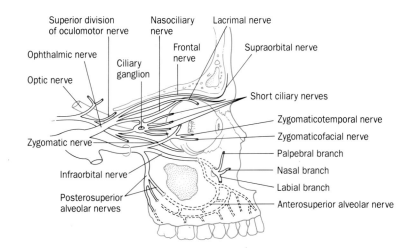

fracture of the inferior orbital rim in which only the nerve in the canal is involved, loss of sensation and/or numbness of the lower eyelid and cheek can be expected. However, if more sensory loss is encountered, such as numbness of the teeth and the mucous membrane of the upper lip and cheek, a fracture of the posterior floor of the orbit involving the orbital groove should be strongly suspected.

When a fracture of the roof of the orbit occurs, the supraorbital nerve may be damaged, producing an area of numbness around the upper eyelid and eyebrow.

Although the zygomaticotemporal and zygomaticofacial nerves are usually damaged when the zygomatic bone is fractured, numbness caused by discontinuity of these nerves is rare because of considerable overlap of nerve distribution.

Loss of sensation along the course of any of the sensory orbital nerves, when caused by an orbital fracture, is usually secondary to a contusion injury to these nerves, and sensation frequently returns after several months.

Evaluation of the action of the orbicularis, frontalis, and other facial muscles may reveal unexpected nerve injury. Pain and limitation of movement of the mandible may indicate a fracture of the zygomatic arch impinging on the coronoid process of the mandible or the temporalis muscle.

35-2-4 Ophthalmic Examination

The severity of an orbital fracture does not necessarily correlate with the degree of injury to the globe. Conversely, any blow to the midfacial area may cause damage to the globe even if there is no associated fracture. Therefore, before any fracture repair is attempted, a thorough examination of each eye should be made. Whenever possible, slit-lamp and indirect ophthalmoscopic examinations should be included. Visual acuity of each eye, even if only a rough estimate, should be assessed. This measurement is important, not only to reveal damage to the optic pathways, but also from a medicolegal point of view. Visual field testing should be performed as soon as possible. The shape, size, and reactions of the pupils should be noted carefully. In general, the pupils should not be dilated if there is any possibility of intracranial injury.

The globe should be examined carefully for laceration, perforation, foreign bodies, lens dislocation, angle recession, hemorrhage, choroidal rupture, retinal edema, tears, and detachment.

Examination of the levator muscle and the extraocular muscles is of paramount importance in orbital trauma. Traumatic ptosis may be the only sign of a roof fracture. Such ptosis usually improves with time unless there is permanent nerve injury. Ptosis, particularly if secondary to a third nerve injury, may mask an extraocular movement disorder and diplopia.

Diplopia is one of the most frequent and distressing sequelae of orbital fractures. Determining the cause of the diplopia is critical. Most often, it is caused by entrapment of one of the extraocular muscles or the fascial tissue attached to an extraocular muscle. Usually, the inferior rectus, inferior oblique, or less frequently the medial rectus muscle is involved. It may also result from nerve damage or hematoma formation.

Forced-duction testing is an important aid for the preoperative diagnosis of entrapment of an extraocular muscle. If positive and if there is imaging evidence of a fracture, the test is highly indicative of entrapment. However, on occasion, a forced-duction test may be positive, secondary only to orbital hemorrhage and not muscle entrapment. If the test is negative, there may still be entrapment of some tissue attached to an extraocular muscle, especially if the patient complains of diplopia. A negative forced-duction test in the absence of imaging evidence of fracture is an indication for conservative management. If there is clinical evidence of limitation of extraocular motion during the forced-duction test and if there is no imaging evidence of fracture, the possibility of an intraorbital hemorrhage should be considered, especially if exophthalmos exists.

A forced-duction test is performed to determine whether there is mechanical restriction of rotation of the globe. The test is performed by injecting a small amount of anesthetic at the inferior limbus, grasping the conjunctiva with forceps, and asking the patient to look in the direction opposite to that of the involved muscle. If the involved muscle or attached tissue is incarcerated in a fracture site, resistance is felt on ocular excursion when pulling with the forceps. This test is also positive if the involved muscle is fibrotic. Both sides should be compared. An example of a positive forced-duction test when the inferior rectus muscle is incarcerated in an orbital floor fracture site is the examiner feeling resistance to elevation of the eye as the eye is rotated up when the patient looks up. It is advisable to coordinate the forced-duction test with the active force-generation test. This test is used to make a qualitative judgment of muscle force. For example, if the inferior rectus muscle is paralyzed, the patient is unable to look down, the eye is freely movable, and the examiner does not feel any tug on the muscle when the patient is asked to look down.

If the fracture is large, there may be little entrapment of tissue and diplopia may be minimal or nonexistent. Prolapse of tissue into a large fracture defect is the primary cause of enophthalmos and globe displacement. Delayed onset of diplopia may occur as scar tissue contracts. This is especially true of an orbital fracture associated with a rim fracture. To avoid the development of enophthalmos and diplopia in these situations, early repair is indicated.

Involvement of the lacrimal drainage system should be suspected when a fracture involves the medial portion of the orbit, as in a naso-orbital fracture. The intraosseous portion of the lacrimal duct is vulnerable. The patency of the lacrimal drainage system should be determined before and after surgical intervention.

35-2-5 Nasal Examination

The nasal bones often are the first to fracture after frontal trauma has been sustained. Following external inspection and palpation of the nose, the interior should be examined. The presence of cerebrospinal rhinorrhea indicates a communication between the nasal cavity and the intracranial cavity through a fracture of the cribriform plate or inner table of the frontal sinus. Nasal bone fractures are often associated with orbital fractures.

35-3

IMAGING STUDIES

Imaging studies of the orbit should be performed in all instances of orbital contusion injury where the possibility of a fracture is suspected. When severe general body trauma has occurred, it may not be possible to initially obtain computed tomography (CT) or magnetic resonance imaging (MRI) scans of the orbits, but standard skull x-ray views can usually be obtained. Therefore, the ophthalmologist should be familiar with the various standard x-ray views of the skull and orbits, especially the Waters view, which is most useful to the ophthalmologist (Figures 35-5 and 35-6). Whenever possible, axial and coronal CT views and also MRI views should be obtained. CT scans demonstrate bony pathology best, whereas MRI

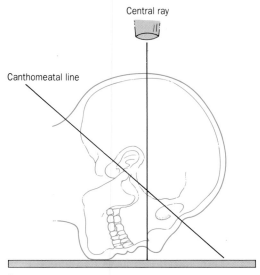

Canthomeatal line

Central ray

A

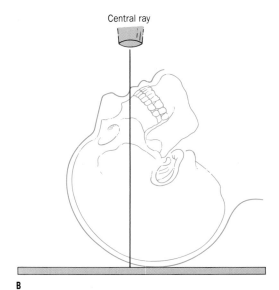

Central ray

B

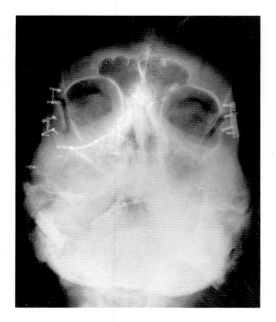

Figure 35-5 *Head positions for Waters x-ray views. (A) Waters view. (B) Reverse Waters view.*

Figure 35-6 *Postoperative Waters view showing intraosseous screw and plate fixation of patient with bilateral orbital fractures.*

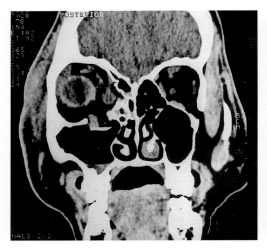

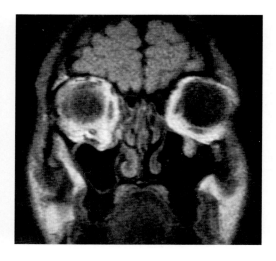

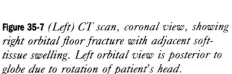

Figure 35-7 *(Left) CT scan, coronal view, showing right orbital floor fracture with adjacent soft-tissue swelling. Left orbital view is posterior to globe due to rotation of patient's head.*

Figure 35-8 *(Right) MRI scan, coronal view, showing herniation of orbital contents into maxillary sinus. Bony structures are better visualized by CT scans. MRI scans are most useful for soft-tissue definition.*

scans show soft-tissue pathology best (Figures 35-7 and 35-8). Often, the combination of the two is invaluable in determining the best treatment approach. In most instances, however, axial and coronal CT scans yield sufficient information. Both CT and MRI scans have largely supplanted plain x-rays in the diagnosis and evaluation of orbital trauma and disease.

Special attention should be given to the presence of foreign bodies, especially metallic foreign bodies in the orbital area. If the foreign body is suspected to be magnetic, MRI scans are contraindicated. Conditions associated with various types of orbital fractures that may be demonstrated by imaging include fragmentation and displacement of the orbital rim and floor, hairline fractures, prolapse of orbital contents into the adjacent paranasal sinuses, hemorrhage into a paranasal sinus, and orbital emphysema. Diagnosis and evaluation of optic canal fractures and associated optic nerve pathology are best achieved with a combination of CT and MRI studies. Although these fractures are not as common as other orbital fractures, the physician should be aware of them. Decompression of the optic nerve in the optic canal may occasionally be required to relieve pressure caused by edema and/or displaced fracture fragments.

CT scans give coronal and axial views. When coronal views cannot be obtained, axial views can be rearranged to demonstrate coronal views by a process called *re-formation*. Additionally, three-dimensional imaging reconstruction of the orbit can be achieved. Magnified views of any given area can also be produced, thus demonstrating even subtle changes. Actual incarceration of tissue in fracture sites, difficult to visualize with ordinary x-ray films, can often easily be seen on a CT scan.

35-4

GENERAL MANAGEMENT OF ORBITAL FRACTURES

Patients with an orbital fracture often have associated facial injuries. Immediate management should consist of maintenance of an adequate airway, control of hemorrhage, and treatment of shock. Consultation with other specialists often is necessary. Soft-tissue injuries frequently accompany orbital fractures. As a rule, any laceration around the face and orbit should be cleansed and properly sutured as early as possible to minimize the possibility of infection and scarring.

The most common indications for surgical intervention are as follows:

1. Displacement of bone fragments disfiguring the normal facial contours

2. Interference with normal binocular single vision caused by extraocular muscle entrapment

3. Interference with mastication in the presence of a zygomatic fracture

4. Obstruction of the nasolacrimal duct

There is no immediate urgency concerning repair of an orbital fracture when the fracture involves the inferior orbital rim, the naso-orbital structures, or the orbital floor. The bones usually can be easily moved into correct position for as long as 10 to 14 days after injury. This gives the surgeon time to evaluate the patient's ocular status and the function of the extraocular muscles and nasolacrimal system. It also allows enough time for the patient's general medical condition to be stabilized. After 3 weeks, union between the fractured bony fragments becomes fairly firm, especially between thicker bony edges, so that these fragments are hard to move and an osteotomy is necessary for realignment. It is desirable to repair orbital fractures while the bone fragments are still fairly easy to move, because an osteotomy, especially in the orbital region, may be accompanied by severe orbital hemorrhage, which in turn threatens vision.

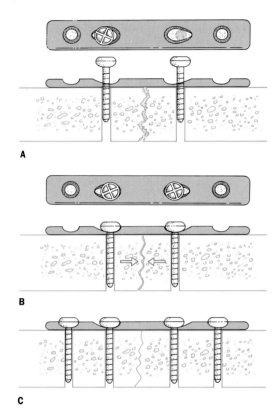

Figure 35-9 *Compression plating achieves three-dimensional rigid fixation and compression of fractured edges. Oval configuration of plate holes forces edges together as screws are tightened. (A) Central screws are partly inserted through oval holes. Linear fracture edges are still apart. (B) Central screws are fully inserted. Fracture edges are compressed. (C) Lateral screws are inserted for additional fixation.*

Because of the thickness of the zygomatic bone, the reduction preferably should be performed within the first week, when the displaced fragment is easily moved and may snap into position. When a zygomatic fracture is not reduced during the first week, reactive tissue and callus form so that the fracture reduction is more difficult. A reduction of any facial fracture, especially a fracture involving the zygomatic bone, requires some additional means of stabilization such as wiring or the use of bone fixation plates.

General anesthesia is preferred when repairing orbital fractures; however, fracture surgery may be satisfactorily performed with local anesthesia, especially with the use of nerve blocks.

With the advent of craniofacial techniques, the use of plating systems for fracture immobilization has been developed, the most popular being made of Vitallium and titanium. To decrease the thickness of a plating system in the orbital and midfacial area where cutaneous tissue closely approximates bone, microplating systems have evolved. Vitallium is generally favored for use in the orbital area because it is stronger than either stainless steel or titanium and it can be used as a thinner plate.

Some plating systems use the principle of compression to bring edges of fractured bone together so that firm bony union rather than fibrous union occurs during healing. As screws are tightened in the compression plates, the fractured ends of bone are moved closer together. The principle is achieved by oval holes in the compression plates with the narrow portion outward so that when the screws are securely in place, the adjacent fracture ends of bone are in tight apposition (Figure 35-9). Compression plates are most useful in the repair of fractures of thicker bone such as in the zygoma and orbital rims.

The general principle of immobilizing a fracture must be adhered to whether wires or compression plates are used. In most instances, a displaced fracture must be secured in at least two positions to prevent rotation. This is especially true of a zygomatic fracture because of significant pull of muscle groups on the fracture fragments.

Lag screws can occasionally be used for repair of a zygomatic fracture if the fracture is oblique. The principle underlying the lag screw is that the bone adjacent to the screw bed is overdrilled so that the screw head pushes the fragment against the opposite fragment of bone where the threads are engaged (Figure 35-10).

It is perfectly acceptable to combine compression plates, lag screws, and wires in any given operation. The surgeon should use the modality that works best and most efficiently for the specific site and problem. For example, compression plates may not be easily applied to thin bones, while wiring may accomplish the intended goal (Figure 35-11).

Some problems that may be encountered in patients with delayed diagnosis or inadequate early treatment are the following:

1. Deformity of the facial contours and palpebral fissure caused by displacement of the medial or lateral canthal tendon

2. Obstruction and subsequent suppuration of the lacrimal passages

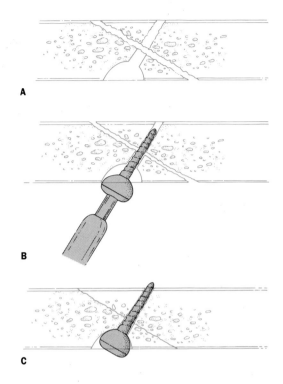

Figure 35-10 *Principle of lag screws in oblique fractures. (A) Initial hole is drilled larger than screw shaft, to depth of size of screw head, to allow for recession of screw head when screw is tightened. (B) Screw threads engage distal bone fragment. (C) Bone fragments are compressed against each other, and screw head is recessed.*

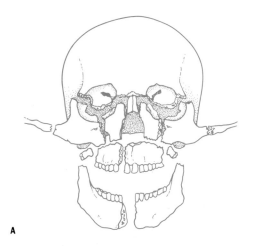

A

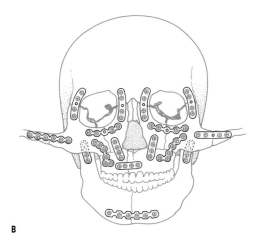

B

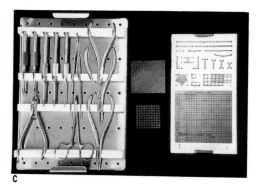

C

Figure 35-11 *Fixation plates. (A) Multiple facial and orbital fractures. (B) Reduction of fractures using fixation plates. (C) Different configurations of plates and screws, with cutting and bending instruments.*
Part C courtesy of Leibinger LP.

3. Paranasal sinus obstruction and deformity

4. Sinusitis

5. Disturbances of mastication caused by fracture of the zygomatic arch

6. Late traumatic enophthalmos

7. Late diplopia

8. Ptosis

The early diagnosis and treatment of fractures will reduce or avoid these problems.

35-5

MIDFACIAL FRACTURES

A working knowledge of the Le Fort classification of facial fractures is indispensable because these fracture lines follow weak areas in the facial skeleton and involve the orbit in Le Fort types II and III.

A Le Fort I fracture is a transverse fracture that involves the lower portion of the maxilla (Figure 35-12A). The maxil-

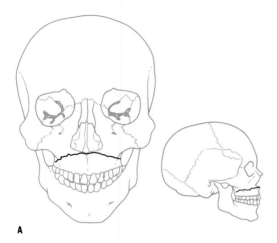

A

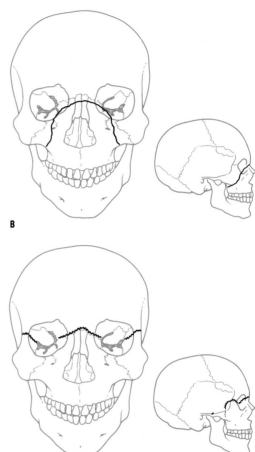

B

C

lary fragment that contains the teeth is dislocated from the remainder of the facial bones, and if the bones are not impacted, a free-floating fragment may result.

A Le Fort II fracture is also called a *pyramidal fracture* (Figure 35-12B). The fracture lines go through the thick portion of the frontal processes, extend laterally to involve the lacrimal bones and the floor of the orbits, and then traverse the area of the zygomaticomaxillary suture lines along the lateral walls of the maxillae and through the pterygoid plates into the pterygomaxillary fossae. This configuration of the fracture gives it a pyramidal shape. When the fragments are markedly displaced, as can occur with a dashboard injury, the ethmoidal, nasoseptal, and lacrimal areas are significantly involved and result in flattening of the orbitonasal complex and splaying of the interorbital distances.

The level at which this type of fracture crosses the nose is highly variable. The distal nasal bones on one side may be in-

Figure 35-12 *Le Fort classification. (A) Le Fort I or transverse fracture: fracture line does not involve orbits. (B) Le Fort II or pyramidal fracture: orbital floors and nasal bones are involved. (C) Le Fort III fracture, or craniofacial dysjunction: both orbits are involved.*

volved and the cartilage on the opposite side, or the nasal bones may actually become separated from the glabella at the junction of the nasal bones and frontal bone. Damage to the ethmoidal area always occurs in a pyramidal fracture, and the lacrimal drainage system may also be involved. Extraocular muscle imbalance is not uncommon following Le Fort II fractures.

In a Le Fort III fracture, the fracture line follows the approximate areas of attachment between the facial skeleton and the cranium (Figure 35-12C). The fracture line involves the area near the upper part of the nasal bones, crosses the orbital margin near the frontomaxillary suture, and continues through the ethmoids and lamina papyracea in a downward and backward direction, passing below the optic canal to the infraorbital fissure. Here the fracture line divides. One line continues forward and upward, following the zygomaticosphenoid suture between the roof of the orbit and the lateral orbital wall, and crosses the orbital margin near the frontozygomatic sutures. The second or inferior fracture line runs downward and backward and crosses the upper part of the pterygoid process near its base. The zygomatic arch is also fractured. In a Le Fort III fracture, there is a complete craniofacial dysjunction and the entire facial skeleton floats freely, being held together only by soft tissue. When this occurs, the facial bones are usually dislocated posteriorly and inferiorly. Le Fort II and III fractures roughly outline the strong zygomatic buttress and involve the orbit.

Pure Le Fort fractures are rarely seen in clinical practice. More often, a variation or an incomplete type is observed. Nasoorbital fractures, which the ophthalmologist most frequently encounters, result from automobile accidents in which the face hits the dashboard of a car. These fractures resemble Le Fort II fractures in that the orbital rims and floors are often involved and there is posterior telescoping of the nasal structures. A midfacial fracture may also occur unilaterally, involving only one orbit and the nasal bones. In facial fractures, the sense of smell may be destroyed if the cribriform plates and olfactory nerves are involved.

35-6

LATERAL ORBITAL FRACTURES

A lateral orbital fracture requiring repair is usually associated with dislocation of the zygomatic bone, classically resulting from a lateral blow on the cheek. This type of zygomatic fracture is also known as a *tripartite fracture* if the zygoma is fractured in three places: in the region of its junction with the zygomatic process of the frontal bone; near the zygomaticomaxillary suture line and infraorbital foramen; and at the arch. The zygomatic bone fragment may be entirely depressed and the rim rotated internally. If the fragment is not reduced, a flattening of the involved side of the face persists, the lateral canthal tendon becomes inferiorly displaced, and the globe and socket demonstrate a depressed

as well as an enophthalmic appearance
(Figure 35-13A). The orbital floor is usually involved; however, a blowout fracture
of the floor with prolapsed orbital soft tissue is not often present in this type of
fracture. Later, as scarring and healing occur, if the extraocular muscles or attached
tissues are involved, diplopia may ensue.

The globe is usually intact, but there
may be subluxation or dislocation of the
lens, angle recession, herniation of vitreous into the anterior chamber, and retinal
and vitreous hemorrhage in the temporal
periphery with retinal edema. There is
usually no intracranial damage other than
a concussion-type injury.

The signs and symptoms of a zygomatic
fracture depend on the amount and direction of the displacement. Flattening of the
cheek is present, but it may be masked
once edema of the surrounding tissue occurs. Gaps, step deformities, and points
of tenderness can be palpated along the
orbital margin, especially at the fracture
site. Subconjunctival, palpebral, and retroseptal or subperiosteal hemorrhage may be
present. Hemorrhage into the antrum, as
demonstrated by roentgenographic studies, is not unusual. Eyelid emphysema is
rare, as is epistaxis.

Not all zygomatic fractures conform
to the previous description, and various
types may be subclassified. In some instances, displacement is minimal, especially when the displaced fragment in a
tripartite fracture is hinged at one of the
fracture sites. If displacement is minimal
and there is no appreciable alteration of
the level of the eye or the lower eyelid,
the fracture does not require reduction
(Figure 35-13B). If the fracture fragment

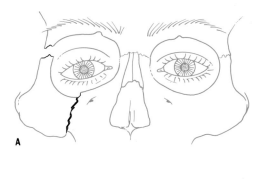

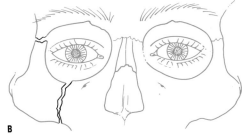

Figure 35-13 *Zygomatic fractures. (A) Downward displacement of lateral canthal tendon secondary to rotation of fragment. Globe is also displaced. (B) Minimal displacement of fragments and no appreciable alteration of level of eye. This type requires no treatment.*

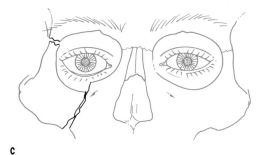

C

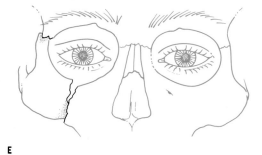

E

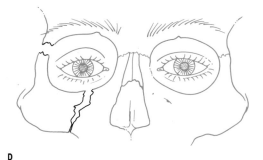

D

Figure 35-13 *(C) Hinged at frontal bone. Lower lid appears dragged downward because of attachment of orbital septum to displaced bone fragment. (D) Hinged at maxillary bone. Lateral orbital tubercle is displaced downward with resultant downward pull of lateral canthus. Displacement of globe depends on rotation of fragment. (E) Upward and backward displacement causes malar flattening associated with lateral orbital bulge. Direction of force is from below and moves upward.*

hinges at the frontal bone and displacement is significant, it takes place mainly along the inferolateral margin. In this instance, the level of the globe remains undisturbed but the lower eyelid appears to be dragged downward (Figure 35-13C).

If the hinge is at the maxillary bone and the main displacement is at the zygomaticofrontal process, the lateral orbital tubercle will be displaced downward with the fragment pulling the lateral canthus downward (Figure 35-13D). Occasionally, the zygoma can be displaced upward and backward, causing malar flattening associated with a lateral orbital bulge (Figure 35-13E).

As mentioned earlier, sensory disturbance of the zygomaticofacial and zygomaticotemporal nerves is difficult to demonstrate because of the overlapping nerve distribution. The infraorbital nerve is frequently involved in a tripartite fracture of the zygoma; thus, hypesthesia or anesthesia of the lower eyelid and cheek may be present. The auriculotemporal nerve is sometimes damaged by a fracture of the zygomatic arch. A depressed zygomatic arch occasionally impinges on the coronoid process of the mandible and temporalis muscle, causing limitation of movement and pain on opening and closing the mouth. Usually, opening the mouth is more difficult than closing, especially when the arch is severely involved or depressed.

35-6-1 Management

As with any fracture, if a lateral orbital fracture is minimal or if there is no displacement of the fragment, no associated displaced floor fracture with entrapment of muscle or attached tissue, and no symptoms, no operative treatment is necessary. The patient is reminded not to sleep on the involved side. Although uncommon, visual loss has been reported following reduction of orbital fractures.

If surgery is deemed to be necessary, several different surgical approaches are available. The one selected depends on the type of fracture and the amount of displacement. Oral surgeons and otolaryngologists prefer the intraoral or antral approach; plastic surgeons often prefer the coronal approach. Most ophthalmologists prefer a direct approach through an area that produces minimal scarring.

In a tripartite fracture, if the fragment is impacted on adjacent bone and the breaks are fairly regular, the Gillies temporal approach for reduction is preferred. The hair is shaved for approximately 5 cm posterior to the hairline in the temporal region. The operative area is prepared, and a 4-cm incision is made parallel and 2 to 3 cm posterior to the hairline and carried down to the temporalis fascia (Figure 35-14). An attempt is made to avoid the temporal vessels. If they are inadvertently cut, they should be ligated. After the temporalis fascia is exposed and identified, it

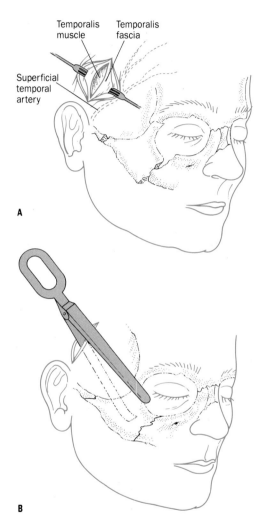

Figure 35-14 *Gillies temporal approach for reduction of tripartite fracture of zygoma. (A) Incision is made to level of temporalis fascia. (B) Kilner elevator or similar instrument, such as a curved urethral sound, is used for reduction in order to manipulate zygoma into position.*

is incised to expose the temporalis muscle within its sheath. The temporalis fascia is attached inferiorly to the zygomatic arch and anteriorly to the lateral border of the zygomatic bone. A space is dissected bluntly with the surgeon's finger or a blunt instrument placed between the temporalis fascia and the temporalis muscle.

A Kilner elevator or similar instrument is preferred for use in the reduction. This instrument has two handles and, once inserted in position, the elevating blade may be lifted without using the temporal bone and overlying tissue as a fulcrum. The blade of the instrument is inserted under the temporalis fascia, guided under the zygoma, and the zygoma is manipulated into position. If this type of instrument is not available, a Bristow elevator or a small urethral sound works well. It is preferable not to exert excessive pressure on the temporal bone and adjacent tissue to avoid tissue injury. By an upward and outward movement, assisted externally by the surgeon's opposite hand, the bone fragment is guided into position and the fracture is reduced. A click is often heard after the fracture has been reduced, indicating that the fracture fragment has snapped into position. The zygomatic bone usually maintains its position once it is reduced, especially if the fracture is new. If the arch is depressed and there is interference with mastication, the fragments should be elevated into position. Because muscle forces on the fracture fragments can produce misalignment with subsequent functional and cosmetic problems, the fracture should be stabilized with miniplate or wire immobilization.

The temporalis fascia is closed with absorbable suture material, after which subcutaneous and skin closure procedures are performed. Antibiotics are prescribed routinely whenever an open reduction is performed, a compound fracture is present, or a fracture communicates with a sinus cavity.

If the displacement is considerable or the fragments are comminuted and free-floating, the direct approach with compression plating or wiring of at least two fracture sites is preferred (usually the zygomaticofrontal and zygomaticomaxillary areas). The incision for the zygomaticofrontal suture should be in the lateral one third of the brow or through an upper eyelid blepharoplasty incision. For plating or wiring of the fracture site in the zygomaticomaxillary suture area, a lower eyelid blepharoplasty type of incision or an incision made in one of the lower eyelid folds is made (Figure 35-15). Alternatively, an inferior conjunctival fornix approach can be used. Once these two incisions are made, the fragment can usually be rotated into position with the aid of an elevator inserted through the lateral incision. A bone hook may also be used. A towel clip occasionally helps in manipulating the fragment; however, this instrument must be handled with extreme care when used for this purpose so as not to cause additional fractures. Once in position, the fragments are secured by compression plates or interosseous wiring. If wires

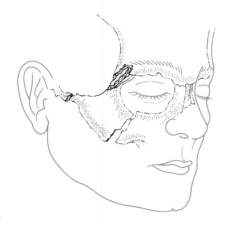

A

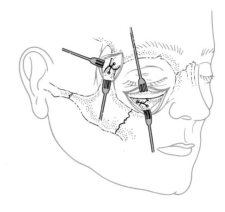

B

are used, an air or electric drill with a 1- to 2-mm burr is used to make the bony holes.

If drilling a hole in the direction of the orbital cavity is necessary, a malleable retractor or other protective instrument should be placed on the internal surface of the bone after the periosteum has been elevated to prevent damage to the orbital tissue or globe. The drill holes are made 5 to 6 mm on either side of the fracture line.

When drilling is performed in the area of the zygomaticotemporal suture, the burr is angulated from the anterior surface of the orbital margin toward the temporal fossa. With this angulation, perforation of the drill into the orbital cavity is avoided. The soft tissue of the temporal fossa is retracted, and the drilling area is copiously irrigated while the hole is being made. When a plating system is not available, wiring is used; a No. 3-0 (30-gauge) stainless-steel wire is threaded through the holes and twisted externally until perfect apposition of the fragments is obtained.

Figure 35-15 *Direct approach for repair of zygomatic fracture when fragments are comminuted and free-floating or fracture has been present for more than 10 to 14 days so that callus and healing between fragments have occurred. Wiring or plating of at least two fracture sites is usually necessary. (A) Incision is made directly over fracture sites. (B) Bone fragments are held together by wires or plates.*

Excessive tightening of the wire should be avoided; else, the wire will break or additional fragmentation of bone will be produced. Once the proper tightness of wire has been achieved, the wire is cut 5 mm long and bent so that the exposed end can be pushed into a drill hole. Alternatively, the wire may be pressed flat on the bone.

The fracture at the zygomaticomaxillary separation is held together by wire extending from the anterior surface of the orbital margin toward the antrum. When drilling or working in the area of the inferior orbital rim, the surgeon must take special care to preserve the integrity of the infraorbital vessels and nerve—plates are often more easily used in this area than wires. Usually, the fragments of the zygomatic arch do not need to be wired if the other two fracture sites are mobilized. The periosteum is closed, and skin and subcutaneous tissue are approximated at the end of the procedure.

The Gillies approach has the advantage of a concealed scar. However, the fragments may not be perfectly aligned and no fixation is used. With the direct approach, visible incisions are necessary although they are not conspicuous. A better reduction can usually be obtained when fragments are held securely in position by plate or wire immobilization. This approach also affords the surgeon the opportunity to inspect the orbital floor and to insert an implant when necessary. The ophthalmologist doing fracture repair must be familiar with both approaches.

A headlight is helpful when performing orbital surgery, especially when looking at the orbital floor or other areas to determine if herniation of contents or entrapment of muscle or attached tissue is present.

The patient should not lie on the involved side for about 3 weeks, longer if much comminution was present. Various devices such as large fluff bandages, boxes, and metal bars have been devised to remind the patient to lie on the uninvolved side.

35-7

SUPRAORBITAL FRACTURES

Following severe supraorbital fracture, the patient is usually admitted to the neurosurgical service because of accompanying intracranial injury. Lacerations of the brow and upper eyelid often accompany fractures of the superior orbital margin, which anatomically protects the eye superiorly. Depression of the supraorbital ridge may be present. A step-like irregularity and a point of tenderness may be elicited on palpation. Eyelid ecchymosis and retroseptal hemorrhage are located mainly around the upper eyelid. Ptosis may be caused by damage to the third nerve, mechanical entrapment, or injury to the levator muscle. In fractures involving the trochlea, diplopia may result. The supraorbital nerve runs adjacent to the periorbita, exiting at the supraorbital notch or foramen at the margin. Its anatomic position makes the nerve vulnerable to injury in supraorbital fractures.

Orbital emphysema and epistaxis may be present because of involvement of the frontal sinus and nose. Cerebrospinal rhinorrhea occurs if the fracture involves the posterior wall of the frontal sinus or cribriform plate. Because of this intracranial communication, the patient may have other neurologic complications. In severe injury, the fracture may extend posteriorly to involve the superior orbital fissure and optic canal. Damage to the optic, oculomotor, trochlear, or abducens nerve may result.

In all supraorbital injuries, the brain sustains a concussion injury. If a comminuted fracture exists, the brain may be lacerated. The patient must be observed closely. The thin orbital roof may be perforated by any long and sharp object passing through the upper eyelid without any injury to the globe (Figure 35-16). This possibility should always be kept in mind when examining the patient, especially a child with a small laceration wound of the upper eyelid.

Supraorbital fractures may be arbitrarily subdivided into two types. The first type, a chip fracture of the supraorbital rim, may occur without involving the inner table (Figure 35-17A). This type of fracture most often occurs when a blunt or sharp instrument, such as a hammer or a prong, hits the rim from above in a downward direction. When a prong is the causative instrument, the fracture is compound and repair involves replacement of the fragments. Because the blow usually comes from above, passing downward and posteriorly, the possibility of a perforating

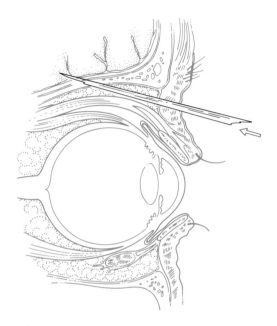

Figure 35-16 *Perforation of orbital roof through upper lid by long, sharp object. Possibility of intracranial injury must always be considered.*

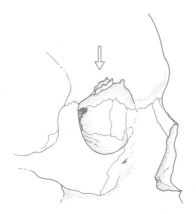

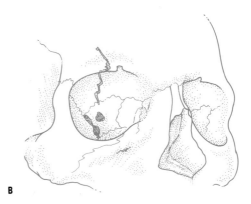

A

B

Figure 35-17 *Supraorbital fractures. (A) Chip fracture of supraorbital rim without involvement of inner table, usually occurring from force directed downward from above. (B) Supraorbital fracture involving orbital rim and roof. Both are associated with hematoma formation of upper lid and ptosis.*

injury to the globe should always be strongly suspected. The levator muscle is involved if the globe is perforated and may be damaged even in the absence of perforation. There is usually a large hematoma of the upper eyelid, and initial assessment of levator muscle function is, at best, difficult. Plain roentgenographic studies may be misleading because chip fractures are not always well visualized in standard views and CT scans are preferred because they allow visualization of eye and brain as well as bone.

The second type of supraorbital fracture involves the orbital rim and roof (Figure 35-17B). The blow producing this type of fracture is usually more direct than the blow that causes a chip fracture. If there is comminution of fragments, herniation of cranial contents into the orbit may occur. If the injury was primarily orbital, orbital contents may herniate into the cranial cavity. This type of fracture is usually associated with a large eyelid hematoma and a traumatic ptosis. Traumatic optic neuropathy may occur with supraorbital trauma and should be suspected if clinical findings are suggestive.

35-7-1 Management

No operative treatment is required for a supraorbital fracture if there is no or minimal displacement of fragments. With a simple rim fracture dislocation, closed reduction may be all that is indicated. If associated with a laceration, the fracture fragment may be reduced through the laceration and sutured or wired in place before the wound is closed.

Open reduction may be necessary in fractures involving the superior oblique trochlea. Accurate reduction under direct observation is required. The trochlea should be sutured back into the periosteum if necessary.

Open reduction of an orbital roof fracture that communicates with the cranial cavity should be performed with a neurosurgeon. The surgical approach is through an existing laceration or a brow or coronal incision with repositioning of fragments into proper position and plating or wiring when indicated. The decision as to the ideal time to repair a roof fracture that communicates with the cranial cavity is a neurosurgical one.

A traumatic ptosis following a roof fracture should not be repaired for at least 6 months after the injury because recovery of function may occur spontaneously. Certainly at the time of initial repair, any lacerations of the levator muscle should be repaired.

If the patient complains of loss of vision, ophthalmoscopic examination suggests reduced circulation to the central retinal artery, and a fracture line or bony chip impingement on the optic nerve is demonstrated through the optic canal, surgical decompression may be indicated. A rapid deterioration of vision or a failure of the pupillary reflex after a period of normal findings may indicate the need for optic canal decompression. Occasionally, some vision can be restored if the patient's condition is stable enough to allow surgical intervention, which can be intracranial, transethmoidal, or transorbital in approach.

When there is evidence of optic nerve injury, with or without a documented optic canal fracture, megadosages of systemic corticosteroids have been recommended to minimize inflammation and swelling.

An afferent pupillary defect in an anatomically normal eye with decreased vision that previously had useful vision is indicative of traumatic optic neuropathy. This condition is usually unilateral but can be bilateral. Traumatic optic neuropathy can occur indirectly, without radiographic evidence of a fracture in the optic canal. The disease process can include hemorrhage, severance of optic nerve fibers, and secondary optic nerve edema with subsequent infarction of tissue. Approximately 20% to 30% of patients improve spontaneously; however, the current trend is to treat these patients with high-dose intravenous corticosteroids. Clinical and research studies of the National Acute Spinal Cord Injury Study Group have shown that patients with spinal cord injuries who were given high doses of intravenous methylprednisolone early, within 8 hours of injury, had significant improvement in both motor and sensory function as compared with those given a placebo. These findings have been shown to be statistically significant. The average dose advised is 30 mg/kg of body weight as an initial bolus followed by an infusion at 5.4 mg/kg of body weight per hour for 23 hours. The intravenous methylprednisolone is thought to have a neuroprotective effect and because of the similarity of structure of the optic nerve and spinal cord tracts, this treatment is advised for patients with severe optic nerve injuries.

This high dose of methylprednisolone is given only for the single day period described because death rates from infection are significantly higher in patients with multiple injuries (head, spinal cord, etc) when corticosteroids are continued. Also, head injury studies have shown that prolonged use of corticosteroids can actually be detrimental. In addition to infection, patients may develop an aseptic necrosis of bone that can occur even after several weeks of corticosteroid use.

If a CT or MRI scan demonstrates an intrasheath hemorrhage compressing the optic nerve, decompression by fenestration of the optic nerve sheath should be performed. The approach for optic nerve fenestration can be either medial, with removal and reattachment of the medial rectus muscle, or lateral, with or without bone removal.*

Additional CT and MRI studies should be performed on patients whose vision does not improve or actually worsens. Hemorrhage within the canal and/or optic nerve sheath should be suspected in patients who had good vision when initially seen after injury but whose vision subsequently deteriorated. However, to date, reliable statistics are lacking to evaluate the best medical or surgical treatment for the management of traumatic optic neuropathy.

35-8

INFERIOR ORBITAL RIM FRACTURES

The inferior orbital rim is located between the thin bony plates of the floor of the orbit and the anterior wall of the maxillary sinus. A fracture of the inferior orbital rim is likely to involve these two anatomic boundaries (Figure 35-18). An inferior orbital rim fracture often is associated with a zygomatic fracture.

Often, infraorbital rim fractures are comminuted and the fragments displaced downward and inward. A step-like irregularity and a point of maximal tenderness can be palpated. Isolated fragments of bone may be displaced into the sinus cavity or may be missing. Palpebral and orbital hemorrhage is present adjacent to the lower eyelid. Orbital emphysema may be

---

*See Chapter 28, "Optic Nerve Sheath Decompression," in this volume.—Ed.

present. Diplopia, which is common, may be caused either by incarceration of the inferior rectus or inferior oblique muscle and/or attached tissue in the orbital floor fracture or by involvement of the origin of the inferior oblique muscle.

A fracture involving the inferior medial orbital rim is likely to damage the intra-osseous portion of the lacrimal duct. Patency of the lacrimal passage should always be checked at the time of repair and after the swelling subsides.

Fractures of the inferior orbital rim may be associated with fractures of the medial or lateral wall. When they occur as isolated entities, there is usually a V-shaped depressed fragment with cracks at the apex and both sides of the V. Because of the mechanics of this type of fracture, a floor fracture is always present. The area of the infraorbital foramen is almost always involved. Diagnosis from roentgenographic studies is not difficult, and the fracture can be demonstrated on Waters and CT views. Antral clouding from hemorrhage is usually present. The amount of associated herniation of orbital contents into the antrum can be demonstrated with coronal CT scans. Occasionally, only a crack with no or minimal displacement of the anterior orbital rim is present. In this case, no treatment other than conservative management is necessary. Numbness along the course of the infraorbital nerve indicates contusion or injury of the nerve.

35-8-1 Management

In the reduction of a depressed fragment, exposure is obtained through an infralash incision or through one of the folds of the lower eyelid skin in the region of the frac-

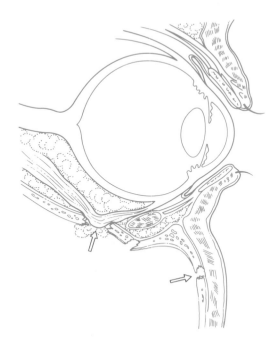

Figure 35-18 *Orbital rim fracture and associated floor fracture with entrapment of inferior rectus muscle and attached tissue. In all inferior orbital rim fractures, floor involvement with entrapment of tissue should be ruled out.*

ture. A skin–muscle flap is retracted to expose the orbital rim. A periosteal incision is made over the fracture site, preferably several millimeters inferior to the rim on the anterior wall of the maxilla, and the periosteum is elevated. An alternative incision utilizes the concept of the swinging lower eyelid flap. A lateral canthotomy is performed and the inferior aspect of the lateral canthal tendon is severed, allowing the lower eyelid to be fully retracted. An inferior fornix incision through conjunctiva and underlying structures is made, dissecting anteriorly and inferiorly to the septum, to the periosteum. This approach does not seem to affect the retractors of the lower eyelid, and scarring and disability are minimal. The rim fragments are elevated with bone hooks and wired or plated into position as previously described.

A headlight is useful when repairing these fractures because an associated fracture of the floor may be present. When this occurs, the orbital contents should be reposited by a hand-over-hand maneuver, using malleable retractors, until all orbital contents have been repositioned. An inferior rectus muscle traction suture is important to determine that no muscle or its fascia remains herniated into the antrum. When the inferior rectus muscle suture is pulled, no movement of the bone fragments or of the retractor should be seen after all of the contents have been reposited into the orbit.

Once all of the orbital contents have been repositioned, a floor implant is inserted and the inferior rectus muscle moved again. There should not be any movement of the floor implant. Plating systems alone or in conjunction with other synthetic implants such as Supramid, Medpor, Teflon, or silicone may be used in the repair. Bone grafts and hydroxyapatite have also been employed. The usual thickness of a synthetic implant is approximately 0.4 to 0.6 mm. When not used with a plating system, the implant is wedged or wired into position. Wedging works well when an anterior shelf is present, even if the anterior fragments have been wired into place. When a floor implant is used, it is essential to keep the anterior edge posterior to the inferior orbital rim to prevent loss of the inferior fornix. It is important not to use too large an implant because damage to the posterior orbital contents, including the optic nerve, may occur. Also, an oversized implant may eventually extrude. After the fracture is reduced, closure consists of a nonabsorbable suture reuniting the cut inferior lateral canthal tendon, several absorbable conjunctival sutures, and one or two skin sutures in the canthotomy site.

Postoperatively, the patient's vision should be checked. If the patient develops acute sudden pain and loss of vision, then the possibility of an intraorbital hemorrhage and/or impingement of the implant on the optic nerve must be considered and the implant removed.*

---

*See also Chapter 36, "Blowout Fractures of the Orbital Floor," in this volume.—ED.

If the fracture is comminuted and a portion of the orbital rim bone is missing, it is desirable to cover the missing area on the rim with a piece of Supramid sheet to avoid a sucked-in appearance of the skin after scar tissue has formed (Figure 35-19). Other material (such as methylmethacrylate, porous polyethylene, metal mesh, or autogenous bone) may be used to close the defect; however, synthetic grafts should not be used in any potentially infected wound such as may occur in compound fractures. Later removal may be extremely difficult. Cranioplastic material, once inserted, sometimes has to be drilled out. Special shapes of hydroxyapatite implants have been used in bony reconstruction. These implants become invaded by blood vessels, resemble bone, and are well tolerated.

It is usually not necessary to close the periosteum at the orbital rim when repairing floor fractures. Care should be taken to avoid incorporating the orbital septum during wound closure to avoid retraction of the lower eyelid due to vertical shortening of the orbital septum. Orbicularis muscle closure is not necessary. Skin closure should be meticulously performed. In any patient in whom a synthetic material is used in contact with an open sinus cavity, prophylactic broad-spectrum intravenous antibiotics should be prescribed preoperatively and in the immediate postoperative period. Some surgeons prefer to use intravenous antibiotics intraoperatively. In general, the antibiotic regimen is started orally immediately following the injury and continued orally for 5 to 7 days postoperatively. Many surgeons also soak the implant in an antibiotic solution prior to insertion.

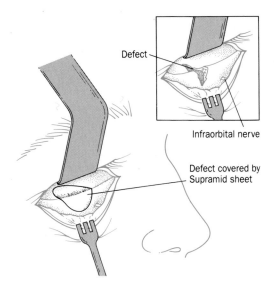

Figure 35-19 *Supramid sheet is draped over orbital rim to substitute for missing bone in inferior orbital rim fractures.*

35-9

MEDIAL WALL FRACTURES

Medial wall fractures are not uncommon. They are associated with other orbital fractures. Frequently, subcutaneous emphysema occurs but because of the thinness of the lamina papyracea, the fracture may not be demonstrable on roentgenograms. Orbital hemorrhage can be present and enophthalmos ensue if the fracture site is large. CT scans are more effective in demonstrating medial wall fractures than are standard x-rays.

The medial rectus muscle or attached tissue may become entrapped in the fracture, thus limiting abduction. The clinical appearance of a patient who has a healed medial wall fracture with entrapment of the medial rectus muscle may mimic Duane's syndrome or abducens nerve paralysis.

35-9-1 Management

Surgery should be performed when there is clinical or radiographic evidence of a medial wall fracture together with the clinical findings of a positive forced-duction test of the medial rectus muscle or when herniation of orbital contents into the ethmoidal sinus is significant.

Good exposure of the medial wall may be obtained through a medial eyelid incision in one of the skin folds of the lower eyelid or by a Lynch type of ethmoidectomy incision (Figure 35-20). Once the medial orbital rim is identified, the periosteum is incised along its anterior surface 2 to 3 mm inferior to the margin, and the superior edge is elevated using a Freer periosteal elevator directed toward the medial wall.

The dissection is carried upward and backward, avoiding injury to the lacrimal apparatus and medial canthal tendon. Once the medial rectus muscle is freed, the defect in the medial orbital wall may be covered with a Supramid or other synthetic sheet of appropriate thickness, or an absorbable gelatin film (Gelfilm or Gelfoam) may be inserted between the bone and the orbital tissue.

The periosteum is closed with interrupted absorbable sutures, and the skin is closed with nonabsorbable sutures. Orbicularis muscle closure is not necessary. The prophylactic use of antibiotics, as described, is indicated because sinus exposure has occurred. If a medial wall blowout fracture is large and not fully reduced, persistent enophthalmos and extraocular muscle imbalance may ensue.

35-10

NASOETHMOIDAL FRACTURES

A nasoethmoidal orbital fracture results from a force delivered across the bridge of the nose. This type of fracture most commonly occurs during an automobile accident in which the face strikes the dashboard. The nasal bones are fractured and depressed; the lacrimal and ethmoidal bones are crushed. Because the bridge of

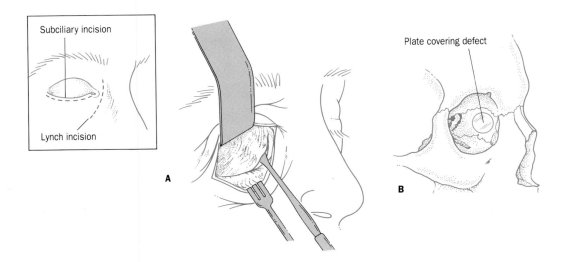

Figure 35-20 *Medial wall fracture. Exposure is obtained by medial lid incision in one of skin folds or by Lynch type of incision. Gelfilm, Gelfoam, or thin sheet of nonabsorbable material is inserted between bone and orbital tissue to prevent herniation and adhesions from forming. (A) Exposure of medial wall through incision in lower lid. Medial wall periorbita is being reflected. (B) Representation of plate covering medial wall defect.*

the nose is flattened, one or both medial canthi are displaced laterally and deformed. Usually, there are associated orbital floor fractures and comminuted fractures of the inferior orbital rim bilaterally. If the force is severe, the zygomatic bones may be fractured at the junction with the frontal bones. All combinations are possible, and frequently injury to the eyeball is also present. Most of these are compound fractures, often with pieces of bone missing. The nasolacrimal apparatus may be irreparably damaged by this type of fracture, and a subsequent dacryocystorhinostomy may become necessary. Therefore, patency of the lacrimal passages should be checked.

35-10-1 Management

In naso-orbital and medial wall fractures, damage to the lacrimal passages commonly occurs. If not detected and corrected early, dacryocystitis can result and necessitate secondary surgical correction via a dacryocystorhinostomy. It is important when repairing a naso-orbital fracture in which telescoping of the fragments has occurred to reduce the fracture as early as possible, while the fragments are still mobile. Reversal of the telescoping fragments may be accomplished by inserting the blades of an Asch or comparable nasal forceps in each nostril and pulling the fragments forward. Internal compression plates, wires, and external medial canthal plates and transnasal wiring can be used to secure the fragments until healing has occurred.

As mentioned, an integral step in the correction of a naso-orbital fracture is the evaluation of the lacrimal drainage system. If at the conclusion of the reduction, there is free irrigation of the system, nothing further need be done. However, if there is some resistance to irrigation, then gentle probing and silicone intubation of the system are indicated. This is performed by passing silicone tubing attached to malleable probes (Quickert type or a modification) through the upper and lower canaliculi, then through the nasolacrimal duct with both ends of the silicone tubing secured under the inferior turbinate. This maneuver may prevent posttraumatic naso-

lacrimal duct occlusion and secondary dacryocystitis. The tubing should be left in place for at least 3 to 6 months.

35-11

LATE COMPLICATIONS OF ORBITAL FRACTURES

Early treatment of nasoethmoidal orbital fractures is important to prevent late cosmetic and functional deformities that can be extremely difficult to manage. If there is lateral displacement of the medial canthus, an osteotomy, contouring by burring, and intercanthal transnasal wiring can be performed at the same time. If there is marked depression of the bridge of the nose, a bone graft can be inserted during the same procedure or later, or a synthetic implant may be inserted secondarily. With the use of systemic antibiotics before and after surgery, infection of the graft is not a common problem.

In neglected displaced fractures of the inferior orbital rim and orbital floor, deformities of the facial contour, sagging of the lower eyelid, and enophthalmos often result. A new orbital rim can be created by using a bone graft or one of the synthetic implants. Both Medpor and hydroxyapatite implants are used for bony reconstruction. These implants become invaded by fibrous tissue and heal securely in place.

Late traumatic enophthalmos in a patient with a useful eye is extremely difficult to correct, and surgical correction poses a further threat to vision. When late enophthalmos secondary to orbital fracture occurs, the globe usually is displaced inferiorly as well as posteriorly. The late insertion of an orbital floor implant elevates the globe but may not displace it anteriorly, resulting in persistent enophthalmos. It is not advisable to insert a large implant behind a seeing eye to push the eye forward, because circulation may be compromised. The treatment of late enophthalmos may require craniofacial techniques involving osteotomy and bone grafting. Prevention by proper early treatment of a naso-orbital fracture is the best treatment.

A flat Medpor implant, several millimeters thick, placed on the orbital floor, is often useful to eliminate hypo-ophthalmos and make an enophthalmic appearance less noticeable. An additional camouflage procedure consisting of a contralateral upper eyelid blepharoplasty further reduces the appearance of a unilateral enophthalmos. If there is residual ptosis on the involved side, a minimal ptosis procedure further camouflages the enophthalmic appearance. If there is no levator function, a frontalis suspension operation may be needed.*

In the management of all orbital fractures, ample time should be allowed for spontaneous recovery of levator and extraocular muscle function. In late repair of extraocular muscle problems, it is often preferable to operate on the uninvolved eye because results may be more predictable.†

---

*For information on this operation, see Chapter 16, "Classification and Correction of Ptosis," in Volume 2 of Ophthalmology Monograph 8, published in 1994.—ED.

†See also Chapter 37, "Late Repair of Posttraumatic Deformities," in this volume.—ED.

35-12

FRACTURES IN THE PEDIATRIC AGE GROUP

The management of facial and orbital fractures in infants and children is significantly different from the management of adult orbital fractures. The bones of infants and children are more pliable, and many of the fractures are incomplete and comparable to a greenstick fracture of the long bones of the extremities.

The brittleness of facial bones increases significantly after the age of 3 years. Furthermore, the sinuses are not well developed in young children. Injury to permanent tooth buds can occur following maxillary or mandibular fractures and repair. Because of the unique characteristics of pediatric bones, remolding occurs during the growth phase. The surgeon who treats pediatric patients must be aware that not only the injury but also the treatment, unless properly planned, may interfere with normal growth. While plates may be left permanently in adults, they often have to be removed in children because of bony overgrowth. Paying particular attention to the basic principles of restoration of function and adopting a plan that gives the most satisfactory long-term cosmesis are particularly pertinent when treating the pediatric age group.

SUGGESTED READINGS

Aguilar EA: The reevaluation of the indications for orbital rim fixation and orbital floor exploration in zygomatic complex fractures. *Arch Otolaryngol Head Neck Surg* 1989;115:1025.

Anderson DK, Demediuk P, Saunders RD, et al: Spinal cord injury and protection. *Ann Emerg Med* 1985;14:816–821.

Anderson RL, Panje WR, Gross CE: Optic nerve blindness following blunt forehead trauma. *Ophthalmology* 1982;89:445–455.

Arthurs B, Silverstone P, Della Rocca RC: Medial wall fractures. *Adv Ophthalmic Plast Reconstr Surg* 1987;6:393–401.

Bracken MB, Collins WF, Freeman DF, et al: Efficacy of methylprednisolone in acute spinal cord injury. *J Am Med Assoc* 1984;251:45–52.

Bracken MB, Shepard MJ, Collins WF, et al: A randomized, controlled trial of methylprednisolone or naloxone in the treatment of acute spinal-cord injury: results of the Second National Acute Spinal Cord Injury Study. *N Engl J Med* 1990;322:1405–1411.

Crockett DM, Funk GF: Management of complicated fractures involving the orbits and nasoethmoid complex in young children. *Otolaryngol Clin North Am* 1991;24:119–137.

Dufresne CR, Manson PN, Iliff NT: Early and late complications of orbital fractures. *Clin Plast Surg* 1988;15:239–253.

Freeman JN, Seiff SR, Aguilar GL, et al: Self-compression plates for orbital rim fractures. *Ophthalmic Plast Reconstr Surg* 1991;7:198–207.

Glassman RD, Manson PN, Vanderkolk CA, et al: Rigid fixation of internal orbital fractures. *Plast Reconstr Surg* 1990;86:1103–1109.

Gruss JS, Van Wyck L, Phillips JH, Antonyshyn O: The importance of the zygomatic arch in complex midfacial fracture repair and correction of posttraumatic orbitozygomatic deformities. *Plast Reconstr Surg* 1990;85:878–890.

Hes J, de Man K: Use of blocks of hydroxylapatite for secondary reconstruction of the orbital floor. *Int J Oral Maxillofac Surg* 1990;19:275–278.

Hornblass A: Dacryocystitis: a late complication of orbital floor fracture repair with implant. *Ophthalmology* 1987;94:1360.

Joseph MP, Lessell S, Rizzo J, Momose KJ: Extracranial optic nerve decompression for traumatic optic neuropathy. *Arch Ophthalmol* 1990;108:1091–1093.

Koornneef L: Eyelid and orbital fascial attachments and their clinical significance. *Eye* 1988;2:130–134.

Lam BL, Weingeist TA: Corticosteroid-responsive traumatic optic neuropathy. *Am J Ophthalmol* 1990;109:99–101.

McLachlan DL, Flanagan JC, Shannon GM: Complications of orbital roof fractures. *Ophthalmology* 1982;89:1274–1278.

Mahapatra AK: Does optic nerve injury require decompression? *J Indian Med Assoc* 1990;88:82–84.

Marcucci L, Vellucci A, Miani P, et al: Antibiotic prophylaxis in ear, nose and throat surgery: a comparison of a single preoperative dose with three peri-operative doses of ceftazidime. *J Hosp Infection* 1990;15(suppl A):81–85.

Messinger A, Radkowski MA, Greenwald MJ, Pensler JM: Orbital roof fractures in the pediatric population. *Plast Reconstr Surg* 1989;84: 213–216.

Nockels R, Young W: Pharmacologic strategies in the treatment of experimental spinal cord injury. *J Neurotrauma* 1992;9(suppl 1): S211–S217.

Nunery WR: Lateral canthal approach to repair of trimalar fractures of the zygoma. *Ophthalmic Plast Reconstr Surg* 1985;1:175–183.

Paskert JP, Manson PN, Iliff NT: Naso-ethmoidal and orbital fractures. *Clin Plast Surg* 1988;15:209–223.

Pospisil OA, Fernando TD: Review of the lower blepharoplasty incision as a surgical approach to zygomatic-orbital fractures. *Br J Oral Maxillofac Surg* 1984;22:261–268.

Raflo GT: Blow-in and blow-out fractures of the orbit: clinical correlations and proposed mechanisms. *Ophthalmic Surg* 1984;15:114–119.

Rohrich RS, ed: *Advances in Craniomaxillofacial Fracture Management.* Philadelphia: WB Saunders Co; 1992.

Segrest DR, Dortzbach RK: Medial orbital wall fractures: complications and management. *Ophthalmic Plast Reconstr Surg* 1989;5:75–80.

Spoor TC, Hartel WC, Lensink DB, Wilkinson MJ: Treatment of traumatic optic neuropathy with corticosteroids. *Am J Ophthalmol* 1991;111:526.

Stanley RB, Mathog RH: Evaluation and correction of combined orbital trauma syndrome. *Laryngoscope* 1983;93:856–865.

Sullivan WG: Displaced orbital roof fractures: presentation and treatment. *Plast Reconstr Surg* 1991;87:657–661.

Waite PD, Carr DD: The transconjunctival approach for treating orbital trauma. *J Oral Maxillofac Surg* 1991;49:499–503.

Wildfeuer A, Luckhaupt H, Springsklee M: Concentrations of ampicillin and sulbactam in serum and tissues of patients undergoing ENT surgery. *Infection* 1991;19:58–60.

Young W, Bracken MB: The Second National Acute Spinal Cord Injury Study. *J Neurotrauma* 1992;9(suppl 1):S397–S405.

CHAPTER 36

Blowout Fractures of the Orbital Floor

Richard K. Dortzbach, MD
Don O. Kikkawa, MD

The term *blowout fracture* refers to a specific type of fracture of the orbital floor. A true blowout fracture is related to increased intraorbital pressure at the time of trauma and is associated with an intact orbital rim. Fractures of the orbital floor often occur with fractures of the orbital rim and adjacent facial bones. The most common site for a blowout fracture of the orbital floor is the thin portion of the maxillary bone in the posterior medial aspect of the floor. Because the ethmoid bones along the medial orbital wall are also quite thin, there may be significant associated fracture into the ethmoid sinuses. Although the bony septa in the ethmoid sinuses afford some support, sometimes very large fractures into these sinuses can be present.

36-1

STRUCTURES CLINICALLY RELEVANT TO BLOWOUT FRACTURES

A complex system of connective-tissue septa is present throughout the orbit, serving as a means of support and linkage among the various orbital structures.[1] Each extraocular muscle has its own connective-tissue system. The inferior rectus muscle, with its long course along the floor, is the extraocular muscle most likely to be involved. The muscle or its connective-tissue system may be involved through entrapment of the muscle itself or its connective-tissue system or by damage to its innervation. The branch of the oculomotor nerve to the inferior oblique passes along the lateral border of the inferior rectus, and trauma to the nerve along this route will cause paresis of the inferior oblique. If a medial orbital wall fracture is associated with a fracture of the floor, the medial rectus muscle or its connective-tissue system may be involved and tether the globe, limiting horizontal movement.

The inferior orbital fissure lies between the sphenoid and maxillary bones in the posterior part of the orbit. The infraorbital groove and canal extend anteriorly along the middle of the orbital floor, ending at the infraorbital foramen. The infraorbital groove and canal contain the infraorbital neurovascular bundle, which may be compromised in an orbital floor fracture. Damage to the infraorbital artery leads to hemorrhage, and trauma to the infraorbital nerve causes sensory dysfunction within its distribution on the face. The infraorbital groove may be quite long and can be mistaken for the fracture itself at the time of surgery. The neurovascular bundle also may be mistaken for an entrapped inferior rectus muscle.

36-2

CAUSES OF BLOWOUT FRACTURES

Currently, two theories account for blowout fractures. The predominant theory is that a blowout fracture results from a sudden increase in intraorbital pressure due to the application of force by a nonpenetrating object greater in diameter than the orbital entrance (Figure 36-1).[2] Most often, the orbital area is hit by a ball or fist or is struck by the dashboard in an automobile accident. The contents of the orbit are compressed posteriorly toward the apex of the orbit. Because the posterior orbit cannot accommodate this increased volume of tissue, the orbital bones break at their weakest point, which is the posteromedial part of the floor in the maxillary bone. This weak area in the orbital floor provides some measure of protection to the globe and orbital contents, allowing them to expand into the area of the maxillary antrum rather than be compressed against the more rigid bones of the orbit. Although concomitant rupture of the globe may occur, it is rare in these cases. An associated blowout fracture of the thin medial orbital wall may occur at the same time and by the same mechanism.

A more recent theory concerning the production of isolated orbital floor fractures suggests that the striking object causes a compressive force on the inferior orbital rim and leads directly to buckling of the orbital floor.[3,4] The bony orbital floor, therefore, is fractured directly by this buckling force. This theory also explains why it is possible for a "blow-in" fracture to occur, in which the orbital floor is fractured into the orbit and not into the maxillary sinus.[5] The degree of increased intraorbital pressure then determines whether or not orbital tissues are pushed down through the fracture into the maxillary antrum.

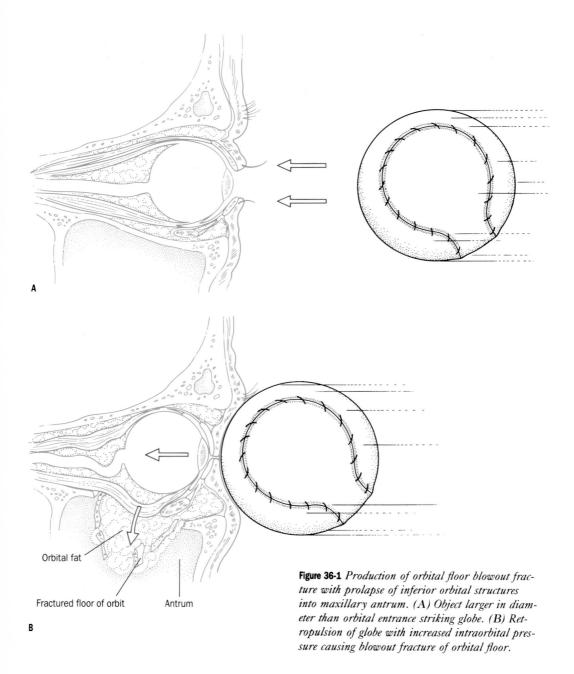

A

B

Orbital fat

Fractured floor of orbit

Antrum

Figure 36-1 *Production of orbital floor blowout fracture with prolapse of inferior orbital structures into maxillary antrum. (A) Object larger in diameter than orbital entrance striking globe. (B) Retropulsion of globe with increased intraorbital pressure causing blowout fracture of orbital floor.*

36-3

DIAGNOSIS OF BLOWOUT FRACTURES

36-3-1 Eyelid Signs

Ecchymosis and edema of the eyelids usually are present.

36-3-2 Diplopia With Upgaze–Downgaze Limitation

The patient complains of double vision, and examination shows limitation of the globe on upgaze and/or downgaze. Seldom is there limitation on horizontal gaze unless a medial wall fracture is also present. The restriction of vertical movement of the eye commonly is caused by entrapment of the inferior rectus or its associated connective tissues (orbital septa). The inferior oblique muscle is infrequently involved. Pain may be present on attempted vertical movement of the globe because of traction on the incarcerated muscle. Entrapment of the inferior rectus is most likely to occur with small fractures in which the muscle or its associated orbital septa are wedged into the fracture. With larger fractures, on the other hand, marked limitation of the globe is less likely to occur initially. Although some vertical diplopia in these cases may be present in the primary position, it is more likely to be noted in extreme upgaze and downgaze. However, in large fractures of longer standing in which fibrosis of the prolapsed tissues has had time to develop, vertical movement of the globe may be significantly limited.

Evaluation of the extraocular muscle limitation can be done with prism measurements in the cardinal fields of gaze, a red glass test for diplopia, a forced-duction test, an active force-generation test, and diplopia fields. With a forced-duction test, anesthetic drops are instilled in the eye and toothed forceps are used to grasp the conjunctiva and Tenon's capsule just inferior to the limbus at the 6-o'clock position (Figure 36-2). If the patient is limited on upgaze and the examiner cannot elevate the globe with forceps, it is likely that entrapped inferior orbital structures are tethering the globe. There are, however, other causes of limited globe movements, such as hematoma and edema of the orbit or damage to the extraocular muscles or their innervation. A strongly positive forced-duction test is of some help in distinguishing entrapped inferior orbital tissues from these latter causes, particularly in association with radiographic evidence of an orbital floor fracture. In an active force-generation test, the relative strength of the inferior rectus muscle may be evaluated by asking the patient to look down while fixating the eye with toothed forceps. This test is useful for differentiating paralysis from entrapment. Diplopia fields are obtained binocularly by having the patient follow a small test object with either a Goldmann perimeter or a tangent screen

Figure 36-2 *Forced-duction test with forceps grasping Tenon's capsule and conjunctiva.*

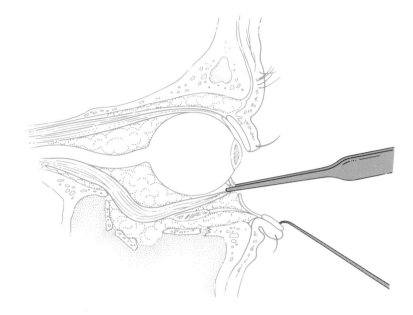

(Figure 36-3). When the patient states that the test object appears double, the point is plotted. This procedure is continued until the entire field is plotted, noting the area in which there was single vision and that in which there was double vision. The diplopia field can be repeated to determine if improvement has occurred during the early period of observation.

36-3-3 Exophthalmos

Proptosis may be seen if marked edema and/or an early orbital hemorrhage accompanies the floor fracture. This situation may confuse orbital evaluation and mask factors leading to enophthalmos.

36-3-4 Enophthalmos and Globe Ptosis

Enophthalmos may occur by any of four mechanisms:

1. A large fracture of the orbital floor may allow orbital fat and other posterior and inferior orbital tissues to prolapse into the maxillary antrum, thereby removing support behind and below the globe.

2. Bone fragments in the area of the orbital floor can sag into the maxillary antrum, thus enlarging total orbital volume. The orbital structures, particularly the orbital fat, expand into this larger volume, removing support behind the eye.

3. The inferior rectus muscle can be caught in the fracture at the time of the trauma, when the orbital contents are compressed into the posterior orbit. The

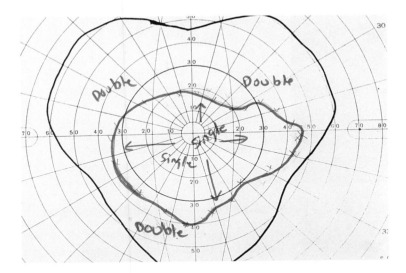

Figure 36-3 *Diplopia fields plotted by Goldmann perimetry.*

trapped inferior rectus muscle can then tether the globe in this posterior location.

4. Atrophy of the orbital fat following trauma can contribute further to poor support behind the globe, allowing the eye to sink farther back into the orbit.

Medial wall fractures, particularly if they are very large, may significantly contribute to enophthalmos when the orbital fat and other orbital soft tissues bulge into the ethmoid sinuses. If a large medial wall fracture is present, it should be repaired at the same time as the floor fracture; otherwise, significant enophthalmos could persist even though the orbital floor has been reconstructed.

Enophthalmos is measured with an exophthalmometer. Immediately following injury, enophthalmos may be masked by orbital edema, but exophthalmometer readings repeated every few days will disclose the enophthalmos as the orbital

edema subsides. Enophthalmos of 2 mm or less may be within the range of normal; enophthalmos greater than 5 mm can be quite noticeable.

Enophthalmos decreases the support of the upper eyelid, resulting in ptosis and a deepening of the superior sulcus. In large orbital floor fractures with associated damage to Lockwood's ligament and other suspensory structures, ptosis of the globe results from migration of the eye, not only posteriorly in the orbit, but also inferiorly into the maxillary sinus. In rare instances, the globe may be displaced entirely into the maxillary sinus.[6]

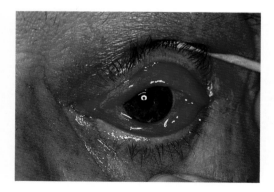

Figure 36-4 *Emphysema of orbit with conjunctival prolapse.*

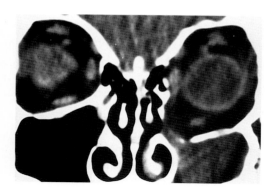

Figure 36-5 *Coronal view of orbital CT scan showing blowout fracture in right orbital floor.*

36-3-5 Infraorbital Nerve Dysfunction

The infraorbital nerve carries sensation from the area of the face extending from the lower eyelid margin down to the upper lip on the ipsilateral side. Alveolar branches from the infraorbital nerve transmit sensation from the ipsilateral upper teeth. Fractures involving the central part of the orbital floor usually affect this nerve, resulting in hypesthesia or paresthesia in the cheek and upper teeth.

36-3-6 Emphysema of the Orbit and Eyelids

Any fracture that extends into a sinus may cause air to escape into the tissues of the orbit and eyelids (Figure 36-4). The air causes crepitus in the tissues, a problem that can be exacerbated if the patient blows the nose or sneezes. Thus, a patient should be urged not to blow the nose. Emphysema of this nature is more likely to occur with fractures of the medial wall than the orbital floor. In rare instances, the orbit can be so filled with air that severe proptosis, markedly elevated intraocular pressure, decreased blood supply to the eye, and loss of vision can occur.

36-3-7 Imaging Studies

Orbital computed tomography (CT) with coronal views is invaluable in the diagnosis and management of orbital floor fractures (Figure 36-5).[7] The size of the fracture, as well as the extent of incarceration of extraocular muscle and soft tissue, can be directly estimated by this technique. If direct coronal images are not possible, coronal views should be obtained by refor-

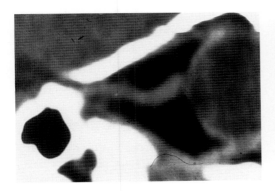

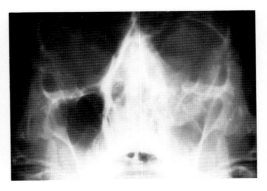

matting axial views. Sagittal views also can depict the extent of floor fractures (Figure 36-6). Axial cuts are parallel with the floor and, therefore, are not helpful in delineating fractures there. However, axial views are important in evaluating fractures of the medial orbital wall.

When CT is not available, a Waters view of the skull is the best radiologic means for screening patients suspected of having a blowout fracture of the orbital floor (Figure 36-7). This view may show fragmentation of the bone of the floor, prolapse of orbital soft tissues into the maxillary antrum, fluid due to blood in the maxillary antrum, and sometimes air in the orbit or eyelids. Soft-tissue densities visualized within the maxillary sinus may be hematoma, fat, or muscle, and do not prove muscle entrapment. A Caldwell view is helpful in screening the ethmoid sinuses for medial orbital wall fractures.

Magnetic resonance imaging (MRI) shows soft-tissue details particularly well. However, because MRI does not image cortical bone, it is not very useful in evaluating orbital fractures.

Figure 36-6 *(Left) Sagittal view of orbital CT scan showing blowout fracture.*

Figure 36-7 *(Right) Waters view showing blowout fracture in left orbital floor with maxillary sinus opacification.*

36-4

ASSOCIATED INJURIES

Blowout fractures commonly are associated with injuries to the globe and ocular adnexa. The most serious (but rare) injury is blindness due to damage to the optic nerve. Injury may be related to the initial trauma, with immediate or delayed loss of sight due to contusion, avulsion, or infarction of the nerve. Improper placement of an orbital floor implant at the time of surgery also may cause damage to the nerve.

Intraocular injuries such as hyphema, traumatic cataract, retinal tears, and commotio retinae can occur. Ptosis of the upper eyelid, damage to the lacrimal drainage system, and avulsion of the medial canthal ligament are some of the extraocular injuries that may be present. As with any other type of head trauma and as noted in the preceding section, neurologic symptoms and signs should be sought and may take precedence over repair of the fracture.

36-5

INDICATIONS FOR SURGERY

Historically, the indications for blowout fracture repair have been controversial. Initially, surgery was recommended for virtually all patients with the clinical and radiographic features of a blowout fracture.[1,8,9] Subsequent studies recommended the nonsurgical management of blowout fractures because relatively few patients who were managed without surgery developed significant enophthalmos and/or diplopia.[10] Currently, surgery is recommended for selected patients.[11-13]

Certain guidelines are helpful in determining whether surgery is advisable:

1. Limitation of upgaze and/or downgaze within 30° of the primary position with a positive traction test and with radiologic confirmation of a blowout fracture of the orbital floor is an indication for surgery (Figure 36-8). These findings indicate extraocular muscle entrapment. Diplopia may improve significantly over the course of the first 2 weeks as edema or hemorrhage in the orbit resolves and as some of the entrapped tissues stretch. However, if there is no significant improvement over the course of 2 weeks after the initial injury and if the above findings are present, surgery is advisable to prevent sequelae. If the entrapped tissues are not freed, vertical diplopia is likely to persist. Furthermore, globe limitation may become worse if significant fibrosis and contracture of the entrapped tissues occur.

2. Enophthalmos greater than 2 mm that is cosmetically unacceptable to the patient is a reasonable indication for surgery (Figure 36-9). Enophthalmos commonly is masked by orbital edema immediately after the trauma, and several weeks or months may pass before the extent of this problem is fully appreciated. If significant enophthalmos is present within the first 2 weeks and is associated with a large orbital floor fracture, greater enophthalmos can be anticipated in the future, and in most cases surgical repair is advisable.

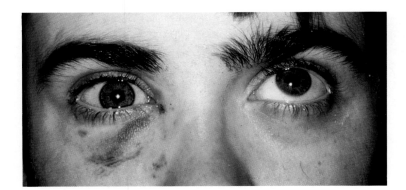

Figure 36-8 *Patient with blowout fracture of right orbital floor and marked restriction of upgaze.*

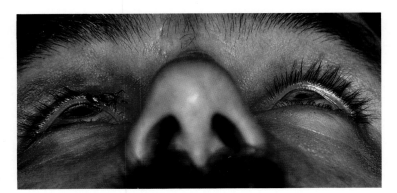

Figure 36-9 *Patient with enophthalmos following blowout fracture of right orbital floor.*

3. A large fracture involving one half the orbital floor or more, as determined by CT, particularly when associated with a large medial wall fracture, is an indication for surgery (Figure 36-10). These extensive floor fractures have a high incidence of subsequent significant enophthalmos and limitation of globe movement. Restriction of the globe may result from progressive fibrosis and contracture of the prolapsed tissues. Cosmetically unacceptable enophthalmos is even more likely to occur when such large orbital floor fractures are associated with a large fracture into the ethmoid sinuses.

4. A patient with an entrapped inferior rectus muscle shown on CT should be considered a candidate for surgical intervention.[14] Such a patient will most likely have clinically significant diplopia if untreated. A patient with a hooked inferior rectus, in which only one side of the muscle abuts a bony fragment, generally has spontaneous resolution of the diplopia and does not require surgery.

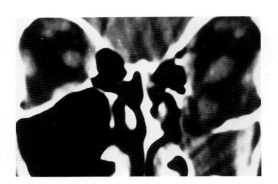

Figure 36-10 *Large blowout fracture (more than half of orbital floor) of right orbital floor as determined by CT scan.*

If significant ocular damage is present, surgery may be contraindicated or at least should be delayed. The surgeon should know what the patient is willing to accept as an adequate final result—a most important factor that also alters the above indications for surgery. If surgery is to be undertaken, it generally is preferable to proceed with the blowout fracture repair within 2 weeks of the trauma. Scar-tissue formation, with contracture of the prolapsed orbital tissues, makes later correction more difficult. Edema of the orbit and eyelids immediately after the injury should be allowed to resolve before an operation is performed. Systemic corticosteroids have been shown to speed resolution of orbital edema and may delineate earlier those surgical cases with unresolving motility deficit and/or enophthalmos.

36-6

TREATMENT OF BLOWOUT FRACTURES

A headlight may be helpful for better visualization within the orbit. If a significant fracture of the medial orbital wall is present, it may be repaired at the same time through the same lower eyelid incision.

Treatment of blowout fractures may be divided into early treatment and delayed treatment. Early treatment may be defined as repair of the fracture up to 1 month after injury but usually within 2 weeks. The three principal operations comprising early treatment are (1) the transconjunctival approach with lateral cantholysis, (2) the infraciliary transcutaneous approach through the lower eyelid, and (3) the combined approach with the Caldwell-Luc technique.

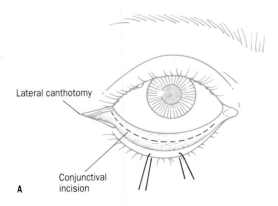

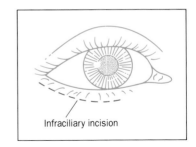

Delayed treatment refers to management of the sequelae of an untreated fracture or the residual enophthalmos or motility disturbance of a fracture that has been previously operated on, usually 2 months or more after the injury.* Some fractures may undergo late repair because they were not recognized at the time of injury, or treatment was delayed purposely because the patient may not have been medically stable to undergo surgery.

36-6-1 Transconjunctival Approach Combined With Lateral Cantholysis

The transconjunctival approach provides good exposure and has the advantages of a largely hidden incision (with only a small skin incision at the lateral canthus) and of minimizing the possibility of postoperative lower eyelid retraction.[15,16]

This approach involves incising the conjunctiva of the inferior fornix combined with a lateral canthotomy and an inferior cantholysis (Figure 36-11). The

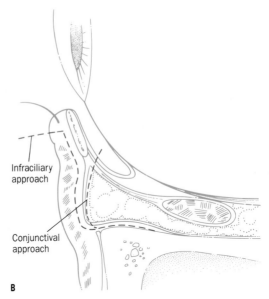

Figure 36-11 *Conjunctival approach with lateral cantholysis. (A) Inferior fornix approach, front view. (B) Inferior fornix approach, side view.*

---

*See also Chapter 37, "Late Repair of Posttraumatic Deformities," in this volume. —ED.

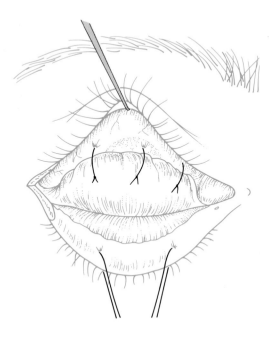

Figure 36-12 *Suturing of conjunctiva and lower lid retractors to superior bulbar conjunctiva to provide corneal protection during surgery.*

inferior cantholysis detaches the lower eyelid from the lateral orbital rim. The conjunctiva and lower eyelid retractors are then incised across the width of the inferior fornix about 3 mm below the inferior tarsal border. The conjunctiva and lower eyelid retractors inferior to the incision can be sutured to the superior bulbar conjunctiva to provide corneal protection throughout the operation (Figure 36-12). The dissection proceeds to identify the orbital fat and inferior orbital rim. Careful attention is paid to avoid dissection through the orbital septum, which can lead to lower eyelid retraction postoperatively.

The periosteum is incised at the inferior orbital rim, and a periosteal elevator is used to detach the periosteum from the rim and floor back to the fracture. Most orbital floor fractures involve the posteromedial aspect of the floor, close to the infraorbital groove. The infraorbital nerve enters the infraorbital canal through the infraorbital groove, and it is important to remember that, posteriorly, the infraorbital nerve is not housed within bone. Safe subperiosteal dissection can be accomplished approximately 25 mm posterior to the inferior orbital rim before risking injury to orbital apex structures. The prolapsing orbital contents are gently lifted out of the fracture, and an implant is placed over the fracture to maintain the orbital structures in proper position. If the orbital tissues are tightly wedged into a linear fracture, it is advisable to enlarge the fracture slightly so that the entrapped contents may be lifted out easily without further trauma to them. The traction test is repeated to ensure that the inferior orbital structures are free. The fracture must be clearly exposed on all sides (360°) so that adequate posterior support of the floor implant can be obtained. It is important to avoid using an unnecessarily large implant or placing the implant too far posteriorly, both of which could result in damage to the optic nerve. Implant stabilization is rarely needed. If the implant moves with forced ductions, orbital soft tissue is still incarcerated in the fracture. If fixation is needed, a suture is preferred because, unlike wire, it is not magnetic and would allow future MRI examination of the orbit if necessary.

Many different materials have been used as implants to cover the defect in the orbital floor, including silicone, Teflon, Supramid extra, Gelfilm, methylmethacrylate, autogenous cartilage, autogenous bone, and Vitallium mesh.[17] Sometimes no implant is necessary, especially when the fracture is small. If an implant is used with small fractures, its main purpose is to cover the defect and provide a nonadherent surface on the floor. Very thin implants of Supramid extra or Gelfilm are suitable for this purpose. In the presence of larger fractures, however, more rigidity in the implant is required to provide satisfactory support for the orbital contents. In such defects, a stronger material, such as Teflon or thicker Supramid extra (0.4 to 0.6 mm), should be used. Autogenous iliac bone grafts and outer-table cranial bone grafts have the advantages of being more physiologic and easily penetrated by systemic antibiotics after vascularization has taken place.[18] These bone grafts, however, have the disadvantage of being more difficult to obtain and sometimes resorbing over time. Vitallium mesh implants have the advantage of being rigid

and yet malleable and can be contoured to reconstruct very large orbital floor defects.

All bleeding in the orbit should cease before closure of the wound. Thrombin-soaked Gelfoam may be helpful in stopping persistent oozing. The periosteum at the inferior orbital rim is closed with absorbable sutures. Care should be taken not to place these sutures through the orbital septum, an error that could lead to postoperative vertical shortening of the lower eyelid and ectropion. After closure of the conjunctiva and lower eyelid retractors to the inferior fornix and reattachment of the lateral canthal ligament, a Frost traction suture is placed in the lower eyelid and taped to the forehead for 1 or 2 days to prevent postoperative contracture of the eyelid.

No pressure dressings are used, and only iced compresses and local antibiotic ointment are applied to the eyelids. Prophylactic broad-spectrum antibiotics may be given intraoperatively and then orally for 3 to 5 days postoperatively. Vision should be monitored closely for the first 24 hours after surgery.

36-6-2 Infraciliary Transcutaneous Approach Through the Lower Eyelid

An alternative approach involves a skin incision and an anterior approach through the lower eyelid. This provides exposure of the involved area with good access to the orbital floor for proper exploration and placement of an implant. It is preferable to make a subciliary skin incision to hide the scar. An alternative is to make the skin incision in the lower eyelid crease. In the case of the subciliary incision, dissection is continued through the pretarsal orbicularis muscle to the tarsus. A skin–muscle flap is then elevated from the tarsus and the orbital septum in an almost bloodless plane down to the inferior orbital rim. Care should be taken to avoid damaging the orbital septum; a torn septum allows protrusion of orbital fat, which interferes with visualization of the orbital rim. The periosteum at the rim is incised and elevated to expose the fracture, which is then reduced as described for the transconjunctival approach. Closure includes suturing of the orbicularis muscle and skin.

A disadvantage of the infraciliary incision approach is the increased possibility of lower eyelid retraction postoperatively. Furthermore, although this incision usually heals well, it still may be more noticeable than that in the transconjunctival approach. The lower eyelid crease incision approach places the postoperative scar in a more obvious, hence undesirable, location.

36-6-3 Combined Approach With the Caldwell-Luc Technique

The Caldwell-Luc technique involves the creation of an opening into the maxillary sinus in the area of the upper gingiva (maxillary bone). The orbital floor is then approached through the maxillary sinus. Petroleum gauze packing or a catheter balloon is placed in the antrum to provide postoperative support of the floor for 1 to 2 weeks. One end of the packing or the catheter attached to the balloon is brought out through an antrostomy in the nose to allow removal at the appropriate time.

The Caldwell-Luc approach should not be used alone to repair blowout fractures because the area of the fracture, where orbital contents may be incarcerated, is poorly visualized. There also is the danger that bone fragments may be pushed into important orbital structures, particularly the optic nerve. Therefore, the Caldwell-Luc technique should be combined with an anterior approach to the floor through the inferior fornix or lower eyelid, in which better visualization can be accomplished.

Two indications for the combined approach are (1) a very large fracture in which the orbital floor implant needs support from below during the immediate postoperative period (if a Vitallium mesh implant is not available), and (2) an associated maxillary sinusitis in which it is inadvisable to place a foreign-body implant on the orbital floor. In the latter instance, the Caldwell-Luc operation allows the flexibility of removing the support for the floor if the infection cannot be controlled.

36-6-4 Delayed Treatment of Diplopia

Diplopia may persist following a blowout fracture. It may also improve over a period of time as orbital hemorrhage and edema clear and entrapped tissues stretch. Furthermore, there may be residual diplopia even after corrective surgery for the fracture has been performed.

Fresnel prisms may relieve diplopia and allow flexibility in adjusting the prism power to changing patterns in extraocular muscle imbalance. An occluder is another alternative. About 4 to 6 months should be allowed for the diplopia to clear or stabilize. If diplopia remains after that time, permanent prisms in spectacles may obviate the need for strabismus surgery. Otherwise, a strabismus procedure may be considered.

When extraocular muscle surgery is performed to correct the diplopia, recession of the involved inferior rectus, commonly on an adjustable suture, can be done. Exploration of the orbital floor with as much freeing of the entrapped, often contracted tissues as possible may be helpful prior to such an operation. Operating on other extraocular muscles, in addition, may be required to enhance the field of single binocular vision.

36-6-5 Delayed Treatment of Enophthalmos

If there is cosmetically unacceptable enophthalmos 4 to 6 months after the trauma, several procedures may be considered to improve the patient's appearance.[19] The orbital floor may be explored and the prolapsed tissues replaced in the orbit. A recessed globe gives less support to the upper and lower eyelids, with consequent narrowing of the palpebral fissure. If the palpebral fissure is widened vertically, the enophthalmos is not so obvious. Minimal blepharoptosis procedures, such as Müller's muscle resection[20] or a tarsoaponeurectomy,[21] can widen the palpebral fissure and thereby decrease the noticeability of the enophthalmos. If a deep superior sulcus is a cosmetic deformity, the patient's appearance may be improved by operating on the contralateral upper eyelid, excising fat from the preaponeurotic and nasal fat pads, and elevating the upper eyelid crease.*

---

*See also Chapter 37, "Late Repair of Posttraumatic Deformities," in this volume.—ED.

POSTOPERATIVE COMPLICATIONS

Numerous complications can occur following orbital blowout fracture repair. For the most part, many of them are correctable.

1. *Blindness* Blindness following surgery for blowout fractures of the orbital floor is fortunately rare.[22] Such loss of vision is usually caused by either orbital hemorrhage compromising the blood supply to the optic nerve or trauma to the optic nerve by the orbital implant or by orbital dissection. The risk of visual loss or injury to a seeing eye must be carefully weighed against the potential benefits of surgery when planning early or late surgical correction of an orbital floor fracture or its associated findings. The surgeon must be particularly judicious with the use of orbital floor implants.

2. *Residual diplopia* An injured inferior rectus muscle that has been trapped in the fracture may have impaired function for several weeks or months after it has been freed. This impairment and paresis result in hypertropia and diplopia postoperatively. Often, the muscle function returns and the hypertropia resolves. If muscle imbalance remains after 6 months, the diplopia may be treated by the use of prisms or surgery. Frequently, surgical therapy consists of resection of the involved inferior rectus muscle and may require operating on the other extraocular muscles as well.

3. *Undercorrection of enophthalmos* Undercorrection of enophthalmos is much more common than overcorrection, and treatment is difficult because of contracture of orbital tissues and atrophy of orbital fat. Attempts to correct this problem usually are made by placing thicker implants, such as silicone or autogenous bone grafts, between the periosteum and the orbital floor. Care should be taken with these thicker implants not to create globe elevation or hyperglobus.

4. *Overcorrection of enophthalmos* Overcorrection of enophthalmos is more likely to occur with thicker implants and may be present in the immediate postoperative period, gradually improving over the course of weeks or months as edema resolves and contracture occurs. Reoperation is rarely necessary.

5. *Lower eyelid retraction* Apparent lower eyelid retraction may be caused by mechanical elevation of the globe because an implant is too thick. In such cases, the implant should be reduced in thickness or removed completely. True lower eyelid retraction also may occur due to adhesions of the orbital septum to the orbital rims (Figure 36-13). Such adhesions are particularly likely to occur if the septum is vertically shortened during wound closure. Correction of this problem may be accomplished by making a horizontal incision along the inferior border of the tarsus and recessing the orbital septum, lower eyelid retractors, and conjunctiva. A spacer is placed between the recessed tissues and the inferior tarsal border. Although donor sclera can be used, autogenous hard palate mucosa or auricular cartilage is commonly used because of rigidity and decreased immunologic reaction. Generally, the spacer measures 2 mm for each 1 mm of vertical elevation desired in the lower eyelid. The development of lower eyelid retraction is less common with the transconjunctival approach than with the infraciliary transcutaneous approach, because the dissection avoids the orbital septum and less scarring results in this plane.

6. *Infection*   Infection is treated with systemic antibiotics, but treatment usually necessitates removal of the orbital floor implant as well.

7. *Extrusion of the implant*   Extrusion of the implant can result from infection, trauma, oversized implant, or inadequate closure of the periosteum along the inferior orbital rim. Frequently, an extruded implant does not need to be replaced, depending on the time of extrusion and the size of the fracture, because scar tissue heals beneath the implant.

8. *Lymphedema*   Lymphedema is more likely to occur with a lower eyelid crease incision that is curved upward in the lateral canthal area, severing the lymphatic vessel drainage, particularly from the upper eyelid. To avoid this complication, the incision should not be extended into the lateral canthal area. The lymphedema may clear slowly over the course of several months (Figure 36-14).

9. *Infraorbital nerve dysfunction*   The infraorbital nerve may be damaged in the initial injury or by the surgeon during explo-

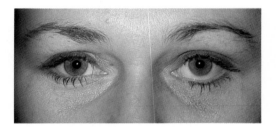

Figure 36-13 *Left lower lid retraction following infraciliary transcutaneous approach to blowout fracture repair.*

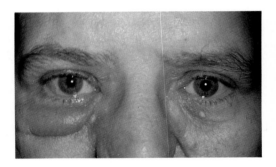

Figure 36-14 *Chronic lymphedema in right lower lid following fracture repair via lower lid crease incision.*

ration of the orbital floor. This damage results in numbness, hypesthesia, or anesthesia in the area of sensory distribution of the nerve. If bone fragments impinge on the nerve, they should be removed. Usually, sensory function of the infraorbital nerve gradually returns over a period of several months to 1 year.

REFERENCES

1. Koornneef L: Orbital septa: anatomy and function. *Ophthalmology* 1979;86:876–880.

2. Smith B, Regan WF: Blow-out fracture of the orbit: mechanism and correction of internal orbital fractures. *Am J Ophthalmol* 1957;44: 733–739.

3. Fujino T: Experimental blowout fracture of the orbit. *Plast Reconstr Surg* 1974;54:81–82.

4. Fujino T, Makino K: Entrapment mechanism and ocular injury in orbital blowout fracture. *Plast Reconstr Surg* 1980;65:571–576.

5. Antonyshyn O, Gruss JS, Kassel EE: Blow-in fractures of the orbit. *Plast Reconstr Surg* 1989;84:10–20.

6. Berkowitz RA, Putterman AM, Patel DB: Prolapse of the globe into the maxillary sinus after orbital floor fracture. *Am J Ophthalmol* 1981;91:253–257.

7. Grove AS Jr, Tadmor R, New PF, Momose KJ: Orbital fracture evaluation by coronal computed tomography. *Am J Ophthalmol* 1978;85: 679–685.

8. Converse JM: On the treatment of blow-out fractures of the orbit. *Plast Reconstr Surg* 1978;62:100–104.

9. Converse JM, Smith B, Wood-Smith D: Orbital and naso-orbital fractures. In: Converse JM, ed: *Reconstructive Plastic Surgery: Principles and Procedures in Correction, Reconstruction, and Transplantation.* 2nd ed. Philadelphia: WB Saunders Co; 1977;2:748–775.

10. Putterman AM, Stevens T, Urist MJ: Nonsurgical management of blow-out fractures of the orbital floor. *Am J Ophthalmol* 1974;77: 232–239.

11. Hawes MJ, Dortzbach RK: Surgery on orbital floor fractures: influence of time of repair and fracture size. *Ophthalmology* 1983;90: 1066–1070.

12. Millman AL, Della Rocca RC, Spector S, et al: Steroids and orbital blowout fractures: a new systematic concept in medical management and surgical decision-making. *Adv Ophthalmic Plast Reconstr Surg* 1987;6:291–300.

13. Putterman AM: Management of orbital floor blowout fractures. *Adv Ophthalmic Plast Reconstr Surg* 1987;6:281–285.

14. Gilbard SM, Mafee MF, Lagouros PA, Langer BG: Orbital blowout fractures: the prognostic significance of computed tomography. *Ophthalmology* 1985;92:1523–1528.

15. Goldberg RA, Lessner AM, Shorr N, Baylis HI: The transconjunctival approach to the orbital floor and orbital fat: a prospective study. *Ophthalmic Plast Reconstr Surg* 1990;6:241–246.

16. McCord CD Jr, Moses JL: Exposure of the inferior orbit with fornix incision and lateral canthotomy. *Ophthalmic Surg* 1979;10:53–63.

17. Sargent LA, Fulks KD: Reconstruction of internal orbital fractures with Vitallium mesh. *Plast Reconstr Surg* 1991;88:31–38.

18. Levin PS, Stewart WB, Toth BA: The technique of cranial bone grafts in the correction of posttraumatic orbital deformities. *Ophthalmic Plast Reconstr Surg* 1987;3:77–82.

19. Putterman AM: Late management of blowout fracture of the orbital floor. *Trans Am Acad Ophthalmol Otolaryngol* 1977;83:650–659.

20. Dortzbach RK: Superior tarsal muscle resection to correct blepharoptosis. *Ophthalmology* 1979;86:1883–1891.

21. McCord CD Jr: An external minimal ptosis procedure: external tarsoaponeurectomy. *Trans Am Acad Ophthalmol Otolaryngol* 1975;79: 683–686.

22. Cullen GC, Luce CM, Shannon GM: Blindness following blowout orbital fractures. *Ophthalmic Surg* 1977;8:60–62.

SUGGESTED READINGS

Hawes MJ, Dortzbach RK: Blow-out fractures of the orbital floor. In: Dortzbach RK, ed: *Ophthalmic Plastic Surgery: Prevention and Management of Complications.* New York: Raven Press; 1994:195–210.

Kikkawa DO, Lemke BN: Orbital and eyelid anatomy. In: Dortzbach RK, ed: *Ophthalmic Plastic Surgery: Prevention and Management of Complications.* New York: Raven Press; 1994: 1–29.

Natvig P, Dortzbach RK: Facial bone fractures. In: Grabb WC, Smith JW, eds: *Plastic Surgery.* 3rd ed. Boston: Little, Brown and Co; 1979:251–259.

Stasior OG: Complications of ophthalmic plastic surgery and their prevention. *Trans Am Acad Ophthalmol Otolaryngol* 1976;81:OP543–552.

Westfall CT, Shore JW: Isolated fractures of the orbital floor: risk of infection and the role of antibiotic prophylaxis. *Ophthalmic Surg* 1991;22:409–411.

CHAPTER 37

Late Repair of Posttraumatic Deformities

Jurij R. Bilyk, MD
John W. Shore, MD

The integrity of the orbital skeleton is often compromised by severe orbital or midfacial trauma, resulting not only in disruption of normal bony anatomy, but also in changes to intraorbital soft-tissue relationships. Although immediate or early repair is preferable, a delay in repair may be necessary because other life-threatening injuries take precedence. Consequently, late complications of orbital fractures and soft-tissue injuries may develop, including globe malposition, diplopia, and traumatic telecanthus.

Delayed correction of orbital deformities presents the surgeon with a formidable task usually requiring multiple and staged procedures. Because of the inherent uniqueness of each case, surgical techniques and materials must be tailored for each patient. However, certain basic clinical and surgical principles should be followed. Adequate preoperative assessment and planning are essential to the success of any procedure. The patient must understand that late reconstruction demands a stepwise approach, with sufficient time between procedures to allow for healing and orbital remodeling. Late orbital reconstruction should never be rushed. If the time and effort are taken to explain to the patient in a realistic manner the goals and expectations of orbital reconstruction, then the surgical results can be most gratifying to both the patient and the surgeon.

37-1

GLOBE MALPOSITION

37-1-1 Enophthalmos

Enophthalmos, defined as a posterior displacement of a normal-sized globe, may result from a variety of mechanisms. Traumatic enlargement of the orbital space with disruption of the orbital ligament support system, causing loss of support for the globe and surrounding soft tissues, may lead to enophthalmos (Figure 37-1).[1] In addition, loss of orbital contents through a fracture site with cicatricial

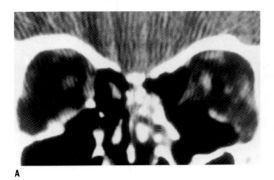

A

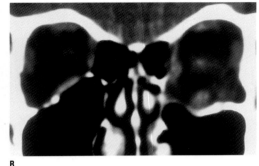

B

changes to the orbital tissue may also cause a posterior shift of orbital contents. Finally, traumatically induced displacement (and to a lesser extent resorption of orbital tissues, usually intraconal fat[2]), as well as posterior soft-tissue fibrosis (scar formation), may result in enophthalmos. In most cases, posttraumatic enophthalmos is postulated to be a combination of these factors, although imaging studies have demonstrated that an increase in bony orbital volume, rather than a decrease in orbital soft tissue, is a consistent finding in patients with traumatic enophthalmos.[2,3] Surgical correction is therefore directed at restoring the natural bony volume of the orbit, as well as freeing any tethered soft tissue.*

37-1-2 Hypo-Ophthalmos

Hypo-ophthalmos, an inferior displacement of the globe, occurs in the setting of marked disruption to the suspensory support of the eye, namely, Lockwood's liga-

Figure 37-1 *Coronal images of orbital floor fracture. (A) Acute. (B) At followup 4 months after injury. Second CT scan shows enlargement of bony orbit, consistent with clinical findings of enophthalmos and hypo-ophthalmos.*

---

*For information on anophthalmic enophthalmos and its management, see Chapter 32, "Deformities of the Anophthalmic Socket," in this volume. —ED.

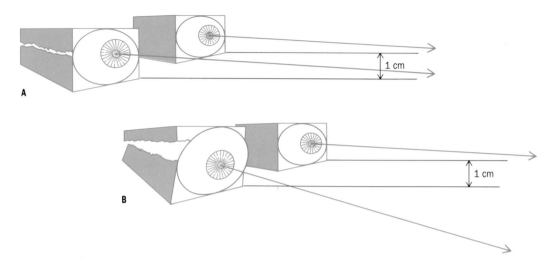

Figure 37-2 *Two types of vertical displacement of globe. (A) Translatory displacement with minimal induced vertical phoria. (B) Angulating displacement frequently induces large hypertropia with diplopia.*

ment and the orbital floor. Depending on the nature of the injury, it may be seen either unilaterally (with extensive orbital rim, orbital floor, or trimalar fractures) or bilaterally (as is seen with Le Fort II or III fractures involving the maxilla). Hypo-ophthalmos may manifest in conjunction with enophthalmos.

Hypo-ophthalmos need not necessarily result in diplopia. The degree of diplopia depends to a great extent on the type of ocular displacement: angulating versus nonangulating. A "translatory displacement," ie, without an angular component, may be well tolerated. A downward displacement of up to 10 mm may produce only a slight hyperphoria that is easily overcome by the patient's vertical fusional vergences. Angular displacement, on the other hand, is poorly tolerated, and a large hypertropia resulting in diplopia may result even if minimal inferior displacement is present (Figure 37-2).

Determination of the degree of enophthalmos or hypo-ophthalmos may be difficult following trauma because of the disruption of bony landmarks. Exophthalmometry is useful in measuring the amount of enophthalmos only if the lateral orbital rims are intact. Photographs, both before and after trauma, as well as full-face and lateral views, help in the preoperative assessment (Figure 37-3). In addition, computed tomography (CT) may be helpful in determining relative bone and globe position as an aid to surgical correction and in detecting any evidence of coincident sinusitis.

Preoperative assessment of visual acuity, ocular motility, the pattern of diplopia, and the condition of the eye is of paramount importance. The patient must also understand that posttraumatic orbital reconstruction may not resolve all problems after only one procedure and that further intervention may be necessary.

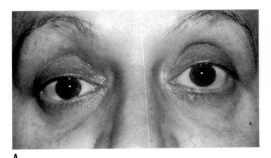

A

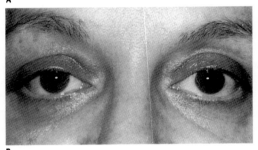

B

Figure 37-3 *Late posttraumatic hypo-ophthalmos and enophthalmos. (A) Preoperative appearance of right eye, with associated malar flattening. Brow recruitment was used to overcome pseudoptosis on right side. Despite asymmetry of globe position, patient did not complain of diplopia. (B) Postoperative appearance after orbital and malar augmentation with porous polyethylene.*

37-2

STRABISMUS–DIPLOPIA

Posttraumatic strabismus may be related to several causes, and it is important to differentiate these possibilities preoperatively. The surgeon must classify strabismus in one of two categories: (1) that due to muscle entrapment or orbital fibrosis with muscle tethering versus (2) that due to contusion injury to the muscle (or to the nerve supplying the muscle), ie, traumatic disinsertion of the muscle, transection of the nerve, or intracerebral injury to a cranial nerve.

Forced-duction testing is a quick and practical method of determining whether a mechanical restriction is present.[4] After topical proparacaine has been applied, two pledgets of either 4% lidocaine or 4% cocaine are placed on the appropriate quadrants of the limbus and kept there for 1 minute. Alternatively, a subconjunctival injection of lidocaine may be administered. Two Bishop-Harmon forceps are used to grasp the episclera at the 12- and 6-o'clock positions. Traction in the horizontal axis is applied to test for any restriction of adduction or abduction of the globe. Vertical movement is likewise tested by placing the forceps at the 3- and 9-o'clock positions. It is important not to apply posterior pressure when testing the rectus muscles, as this may give a false sense of full excursion although tethering is present. The oblique muscles are tested in a similar fashion. If incyclotorsion and excyclotorsion are tested, then gentle posterior pressure on the globe should be applied to accentuate the torsional component of the oblique muscles.

If forced-duction testing is negative for restriction, then the cause of strabismus should be further investigated. This may require additional neuroimaging (computed tomography or magnetic resonance imaging), as well as neuro-ophthalmic and strabismic consultations. The clinician and the patient must also be aware that the presence of restriction does not necessarily rule out the possibility of concomitant neuromuscular injury; orbital exploration may not resolve the strabismus.

Force-generation testing should be performed at the same time as forced-duction testing to rule out damage to the neural supply of the extraocular muscle. The test is performed in a similar manner as forced ductions, except that the examiner stabilizes the globe in primary gaze at the limbus with toothed forceps and then asks the patient to look in the direction of the muscle being tested. If the muscle is functioning properly, the examiner will perceive an active force generation as the globe begins to rotate. For instance, to test the inferior rectus muscle, the patient is asked to look down after the globe is grasped at the limbus. Active force indicates that the neural supply to this muscle is intact. An abnormal test result is more difficult to interpret, because it could indicate either neural or muscular damage. For example, contusion or hematoma within the muscle may cause a decrease in force generation. In most cases, however, such direct, blunt trauma to the extraocular muscle is seen in the acute setting and resolves in 1 to 2 weeks. As more time elapses, abnormal force generation becomes more indicative of neural damage.

At this time, forward traction should also be tested to give some indication of whether significant orbital fibrosis is the cause of enophthalmos (Figure 37-4). The globe is grasped at the horizontal limbus as described, and anterior traction is applied in an effort to displace the globe anteriorly. If the globe is tightly fibrosed, this anterior movement will be minimal

(<3 mm). In cases of significant orbital fibrosis, volume augmentation exclusively for correction of enophthalmos should be avoided, because the volume implant will tend to push the globe superiorly rather than forward.

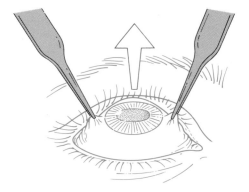

Figure 37-4 *Forward traction. As toothed forceps grasp perilimbal conjunctiva at 3- and 9-o'clock positions, globe is displaced gently out of orbit (arrow), to ascertain degree of enophthalmos-related orbital cicatrix.*

37-3

TELECANTHUS

Telecanthus, defined as an increased distance between the medial canthal angles, is a finding commonly associated with midfacial fractures, resulting from a splaying out of the bony nasoethmoidal complex between the medial orbital walls, the so-called central fragment or frontal process of the maxilla, which provides bony support to the medial canthal tendon.[5] Traumatic telecanthus may occur either unilaterally or bilaterally. Clinically, this condition presents as a rounding of the medial canthal angle. An associated disruption of the lacrimal drainage system is also common and results either from soft-tissue disarray or more frequently from fractures of the lacrimal sac fossa or nasolacrimal canal, compromising the membranous lacrimal sac and duct.

As a general principle, lacrimal drainage should be re-established prior to reconstructive orbital surgery, including telecanthus repair, to eliminate epiphora and possible dacryocystitis. However, if conjunctivodacryocystorhinostomy with Jones tube insertion is planned, then the telecanthus must be repaired initially, because Jones tube placement requires a normally shaped medial canthal angle.

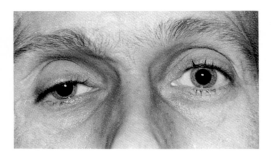

Figure 37-5 *Patient presented 2 years after injury, complaining of facial asymmetry. Clinical examination was consistent with trimalar fracture involving orbital floor. Note lateral canthal dystopia, malar flattening, and deep superior sulcus from enophthalmos on right side.*
Courtesy Francis C. Sutula, MD.

37-4

ORBITAL WALL MALPOSITION

Although orbital and facial fractures are described as following certain patterns, trauma often results in unpredictable fractures that involve more than one wall of the orbit. In addition to orbital floor* and nasoethmoidal complex fractures, deformities of the orbital roof, zygoma, and medial wall must be addressed.

Zygomatic fractures involving the lateral orbital wall often present with lateral canthal dystopia (Figure 37-5).[6] The zygomatic arch and malar eminence may be flattened, and an orbital rim stepoff deformity may be palpable if a trimalar (tripod) fracture is present. If the orbital rim is involved, the orbital floor is also usually fractured to some degree. Entrapment of the lateral retinaculum or lateral check ligaments may be present, resulting in either an abduction or an adduction deficit, or both. Forced-duction and force-generation testing is especially useful in this setting to differentiate restrictive myopathy from an abducens palsy. It is important to document and address this issue with the patient preoperatively. If an abducens nerve palsy is suspected, the patient must understand that surgical repair of the fracture may not improve ocular motility, although spontaneous improvement in abduction may occur in the weeks to months following surgery.

Repair of late zygomatic deformities usually requires osteotomies to separate

---

*See also Chapter 36, "Blowout Fractures of the Orbital Floor," in this volume.—ED.

any bony malunion. If additional bone is needed for augmentation of the zygomatic arch or the malar eminence, a variety of autogenous and alloplastic materials are available. The zygoma is repositioned and secured in place with intraosseous wires or microplates (discussed later in this chapter).

The lateral orbital wall and rim may be exposed beyond the level of the fronto-zygomatic suture by a lateral canthotomy approach (described below). Exposure of the zygomatic arch may necessitate a second incision made through the scalp in the temporalis region (Gillies approach). This is especially useful when a large amount of leverage is needed to reposition the zygoma. Alternatively, an incision may be made through the buccal mucosa (Caldwell-Luc approach), and the bony fragment and zygomatic arch may be elevated from below.

Malar flattening may be present despite adequate bone repositioning. This is often seen with comminuted fractures of the anterior maxillary wall, in which bone is either missing or too fragmented for satisfactory reconstruction (Figure 37-6). Indeed, patients may present with malar flattening as their only complaint following repair of trimalar fractures. The malar eminence may be augmented with either bone grafts or alloplasts placed in a subperiosteal pocket via an inferior cul-de-sac or Caldwell-Luc approach. Porous polyethylene is available as preshaped malar implants (Figure 37-7). Hydroxyapatite and other alloplasts must be contoured to the appropriate shape from premade blocks. The advantages and disadvantages of these materials are described below.

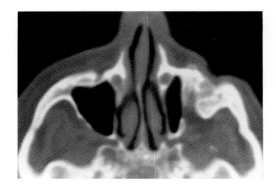

Figure 37-6 *CT axial image of patient with facial trauma incurred two decades before presentation. Note bony deformity of left anterior maxillary wall with overlying soft-tissue deformity from entrapment and cicatrix. Patient underwent release of scar tissue and malar augmentation. Courtesy Francis C. Sutula, MD.*

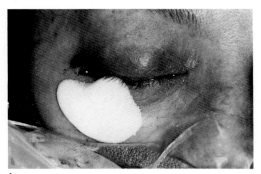

A

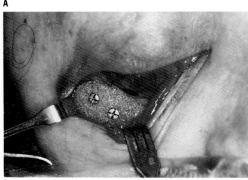

B

Figure 37-7 *Prefashioned porous polyethylene malar implant. (A) Implant in approximate position over malar ridge. (B) Implant was placed in subperiosteal pocket through subconjunctival approach and secured to underlying bone with titanium screws.*

Orbital roof fractures usually result from frontal trauma. The orbital roof is in close proximity to the frontal lobe dura, the cribriform plate, and the frontal sinus. Acutely, the patient may present with ptosis, hypesthesia in the distribution of the frontal nerve, anosmia, and cerebrospinal fluid rhinorrhea. In the late stage, many of these findings may have resolved. Ptosis and hypesthesia may take several months to improve. Evidence of residual traumatic optic neuropathy should be ruled out by careful clinical examination (and visual field testing when indicated), because a frontal blow is the most common cause of traumatic optic neuropathy.[7] A trochlear nerve palsy, which is also caused by a frontal injury, may be present if the patient complains of diplopia. Direct injury to the trochlea is sometimes coexistent.

Neuroimaging can reveal fractures extending through the orbital roof into the intracranial space or limited to frontal sinus involvement. The presence of overlying chronic subdural hematoma should be ruled out. Repair of residual deformities of the orbital roof must be undertaken with caution and may necessitate a team approach involving neurosurgeons and otorhinolaryngologists.

Medial wall fractures may result in entrapment of the medial rectus muscle in the fragments of the lamina papyracea. Traumatic telecanthus and nasolacrimal duct fractures may also be present. If the fracture is small and located inferomedially with a concomitant orbital floor fracture, then an inferior conjunctival cul-de-sac approach may be satisfactory. This is usually true in the acute setting. However, late repair often requires greater exposure to divide scar tissue and free any tethered tissue. A medial orbitotomy (with or without external ethmoidectomy) is often necessary. A traction suture passed beneath the insertion of the medial rectus muscle is helpful for distinguishing muscle fibers from the surrounding cicatrix. Once the tissue is freed, an implant is placed to bridge the bony defect. If stable bone is absent, a microplate cantilevered from the nose is useful in providing a scaffold for the implant.[8]

37-5

PRINCIPLES OF TREATING ORBITAL DEFORMITIES

Depending on the specific circumstances, a displaced globe may be well tolerated and need not be repositioned. However, if globe repositioning is indicated, it should precede any strabismus or secondary eyelid surgery. Some surgeons believe that restoration of the bony orbit is best managed by an osteotomy and open reduction of bone malunion. Other surgeons, recognizing that this approach can be difficult, recommend the use of volume implants with the application of alloplastic or autogenous materials over bone to restore the configuration of the orbit and allow a repositioning of the globe. Returning the eye to a more normal position often yields excellent cosmetic results, but diplopia may persist postoperatively, especially with angular displacement. Fortunately, extraocular muscle surgery can frequently resolve this problem. The adjustable suture technique is ideally suited in these cases.[9] Strabismus surgery should be delayed for

3 to 6 months until any orbital augmentation has had a chance to stabilize and strabismic measurements are constant.

37-6

SURGERY FOR HYPO-OPHTHALMOS AND ENOPHTHALMOS

Downward displacement of the globe may be improved by implanting various substances in the subperiosteal space along the orbital floor to augment this area, thereby raising the globe and moving it anteriorly. Materials used in the past included cancellous bone from the iliac crest, rib cartilage or bone, blocks of silicone rubber, RTV (room temperature vulcanizing) silicone, and cold-curing methylmethacrylate (cranioplastic). The use of split-thickness calvarial bone has increased dramatically in recent years. Newer alloplastic materials such as hydroxyapatite and porous polyethylene are now available for use in orbital volume augmentation and are supplanting the older alloplasts in many centers.

Exposure of the orbital floor can be obtained by either a subciliary incision or a transconjunctival approach through the inferior fornix.* The latter is the preferred

---

*See also Chapter 36, "Blowout Fractures of the Orbital Floor," in this volume.—ED.

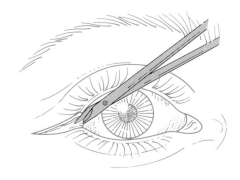

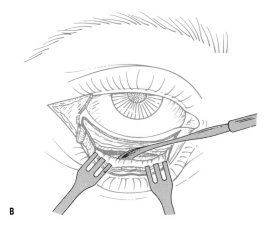

A

B

Figure 37-8 *Exposure of orbital floor through inferior fornix incision with cantholysis: "swinging lower lid flap." (A) Lateral canthotomy and inferior cantholysis. After conjunctival incision at junction of bulbar and palpebral conjunctiva, capsulopalpebral fascia is held under tension and incised directly over inferior orbital rim. (B) Periosteum of inferior orbital rim is incised and periorbita of orbital floor is elevated. Malleable retractor is used to retract periorbita and orbital contents upward, to give excellent exposure of fracture site in orbital floor.*

method, because it provides wide exposure of the inferior orbit and orbital floor, yet avoids a cutaneous scar through the lower eyelid, which may interfere with lower eyelid movement and in some cases lead to cicatricial ectropion and lower eyelid retraction. When used in conjunction with a superomedial orbital, buccalgingival, or bicoronal incision, the entire midface is exposed.

The surgical technique is independent of the material to be implanted (Figure 37-8).[10-12] The lateral canthal angle, the inferior fornix, and the orbital floor are infiltrated using a mixture of lidocaine with epinephrine and hyaluronidase.* A lateral canthal incision is made, and the inferior crux of the canthal tendon is severed with sharp scissors. It is important to cut all lateral canthal attachments of the lower eyelid to the lateral orbital rim, thus allowing the lower eyelid to swing freely over the inferior orbital rim without tethering the canthal angle.[10] Rotation of the lower eye-

---

*Many surgeons employ a large contact lens–like corneoscleral device to protect the eye.—ED.

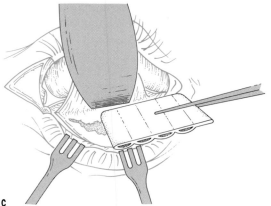

C

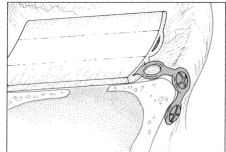

lid is maintained with Blair rake retractors, and the conjunctival fornix is incised with sharp scissors.

Although an incision at the lower border of tarsus theoretically maintains a plane anterior to the orbital septum and prevents the prolapse of orbital fat, this approach is avoided in trauma cases for two reasons. First, periosteal and periorbital planes are usually disrupted by orbital fractures, and prolapsed fat most likely already exists. Second, in the setting of traumatic scarring in the area of the orbit and eyelids, a fornix approach provides the surgeon with easier access, faster closure, and lower incidence of complications.

The Blair retractors are replaced by two larger Senn rake retractors placed in the conjunctival incision. Care must be taken to avoid an "accordion" effect on the skin during retraction, as this may result in an inadvertent skin laceration during further dissection. Inferiorly directed traction reveals the white, glistening capsulopalpebral fascia. A large malleable retractor is placed in front of the globe and pressed

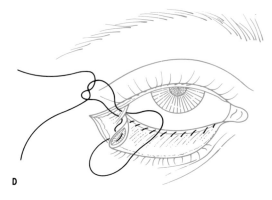

D

Figure 37-8 *(C) Alloplast placement in cases of poor bony support: slotted porous polyethylene is fashioned to cover fracture defect and fixated to inferior orbital rim with microplate (inset). (D) Following implant placement, conjunctiva is closed with running 6-0 plain suture and canthal tendon is refixated.*

firmly against the orbital floor just inside the orbital rim to protect the orbital contents and the inferior oblique muscle. The capsulopalpebral fascia is opened exactly over the inferior orbital rim with a No. 15 blade or cutting cautery. Orbital fat will prolapse and is retracted with a ribbon retractor. The periosteum is incised over the bony rim and elevated with a periosteal elevator posteriorly into the orbit. Any bleeding encountered during incision of the capsulopalpebral fascia and periosteum is controlled with cautery. Traction sutures are then passed transconjunctivally under the tendons of the medial and lateral rectus muscles. As anterior traction on the sutures is maintained, the globe is elevated with the malleable retractor. This maneuver will open a subperiosteal pocket along the floor of the orbit, into which the selected augmentation material is placed. The surgeon can quantitate the volume of material needed by grading the upward movement of the ribbon retractor while placing anterior traction on the rectus muscles until the globe is in proper position and the supratarsal sulcus is equal to the unaffected side. In patients with hypo-ophthalmos, the vertical alignment of the globe is matched to the normal side as volume is added subperiosteally. The implant must remain behind the orbital rim to avoid compromise to the inferior fornix postoperatively. Periosteum is not closed over self-fixating implants.

During placement of the implant, the assistant carefully observes the pupil to ensure that the optic nerve and its vascular supply have not been compromised. Epinephrine in the local block often dilates the pupil on the operative side, and this dilation should not be confused with an amaurotic pupil. One way to rule out vascular compromise to the optic nerve or globe is to check for a relative afferent pupillary defect, although doing so may be difficult if the general anesthetic agents have influenced pupillary reactivity (making the pupil miotic or sluggish, for example). If any question remains, funduscopic examination is indicated. After implant placement, the optic nerve and the central retinal artery should be examined with indirect ophthalmoscopy prior to wound closure. Forced-duction testing should be done to ensure that the implant is not tethering extraocular muscles.

In severe trauma, other areas of the craniofacial skeleton may also require repair by an otorhinolaryngologist or a craniofacial, general plastic, or maxillofacial surgeon at the time of orbital reconstruction. These repairs often necessitate manipulation of the face in the periorbital region, and may dislodge the implant. It is therefore important not to close the wound until all facial manipulation is completed and to then recheck the orbit for correct positioning of the implant.

The conjunctival incision is closed with an absorbable 6-0 suture. The capsulopalpebral fascia need not be closed, as it is well reapproximated during conjunctival closure. The lateral canthal angle is reformed by suturing the lateral edge of tarsus to the periosteum of the inner aspect of the lateral rim. Alternatively, drill holes in the lateral rim may be made to achieve canthal fixation. If the lateral rim is severely deformed or missing, tarsus may be sutured to a properly placed miniplate.

The skin of the canthotomy is closed. A Frost suture is not required, as no lower eyelid skin incision has been made. To protect the cornea from exposure that may occur from eyelid edema, a temporary tarsorrhaphy may be placed. However, the surgeon must be satisfied that the neurovascular supply of the globe is not compromised, because the tarsorrhaphy will limit postoperative examination of the globe. The temporary tarsorrhaphy sutures are removed 5 to 7 days later. In most cases, visual acuity may still be checked postoperatively despite the temporary tarsorrhaphy. Prophylactic antibiotics are used perioperatively.[13]

Correction of hypo-ophthalmos may accentuate a pre-existing ptosis, because the upper eyelid will not be elevated as much as the globe during orbital augmentation. Therefore, patients should be informed before the procedure that subsequent ptosis surgery may be necessary. The surgical technique for ptosis correction is not affected by orbital augmentation. Any damage to the eyelid, levator complex, or oculomotor nerve from the original trauma will, of course, change the surgical management of the eyelid malposition. The use of minimal ptosis surgery to "mask" enophthalmos has also been suggested as an alternative to orbit augmentation.[14] This technique is especially helpful when orbital fibrosis is significant and volume augmentation is of little use.*

37-7

IMPLANTATION MATERIALS AND TECHNIQUES

37-7-1 Autogenous Bone

Cancellous (endochondral) bone was one of the earliest materials to serve as a volume implant for orbital reconstruction. It can be fashioned to fit the orbit and because it is autogenous, infection and migration are less likely and rejection does not occur. However, sequestration and absorption do occur and with time about 60% to 80% of the implanted volume is lost. In addition, the technique requires a procedure at the donor site to obtain bone, and complications at this donor site, including hematoma or seroma formation and infection, must be considered. Potential donor sites for endochondral bone grafts include the iliac crest and the rib.

The iliac crest is prepped and the skin over the crest is stretched superiorly. Stretching allows the scar to lie over the hip and be less conspicuous. Subcutaneous tissue is retracted to expose periosteum over the crest. Periosteum is incised and reflected medially from the inner surface of the iliac bone. Large vessels inside the periosteum are protected by malleable retractors. The bone along the inner crest is cut with a sharp osteotome, removed in one piece, and later fashioned to fill the defect in the orbit. The periosteum is closed and drainage (either Penrose drain

---

*See also Chapter 24, "Late Repair of Soft-Tissue Deformities," in Volume 2 of Ophthalmology Monograph 8, published in 1994.—ED.

or suction) is established as the subcutaneous tissue is closed in layers. The patient should be ambulatory on the first postoperative day. The drain is advanced and then removed as drainage decreases in 2 to 3 days.

Split-thickness calvarial (membranous) bone has distinct advantages over the endochondral bone of the iliac crest. Studies have shown far less resorption of calvarial bone volume over time,[15,16] 15% to 30% as compared to the aforementioned 60% to 80% for endochondral bone.[17,18] In addition, increased graft survival is seen with calvarial bone. Calvarial bone also has specific advantages in orbital reconstruction.[10,19] The donor site is in close proximity and easily accessible to the orbital surgeon.[17] In addition, bone harvest and orbital reconstructive exposure sites may be well exposed by the same bicoronal scalp incision. This can be supplemented by an inferior fornix approach as necessary for wider orbital exposure.[10] The calvarial graft also has a curvature that approximates that of the orbital rim and orbital floor, necessitating less sculpting by the surgeon. Finally, calvarial bone graft harvesting is associated with a lower incidence of morbidity than either iliac crest or rib grafts. Nonetheless, complications of split-thickness calvarial bone grafts do occur and must be emphasized. These include hematoma or seroma at the donor site, infection, dural exposure or tears, subarachnoid bleeding, cerebrospinal fluid leaks,[15] and intracerebral hematoma.[20]

The technique for harvesting a calvarial graft begins with an incision in the parietal region and the creation of a subgaleal flap.[15,19,21] The appropriate curvature of the skull is selected to correspond to the defect at the recipient site. Periosteum over the parietal bone is exposed and incised, and a periosteal flap is dissected. Cranial sutures and the midline cranium should be avoided. Bone cuts should be made at least 1 cm from the suture lines. A cutting burr is then used to create a groove through the outer cortical table to the level of the diploë, with generous irrigation by the assistant to prevent burning of the bone. An osteotome inserted into this groove is used to carefully elevate the brittle outer table in one piece (in 1- to 2-cm strips). If a full-thickness bone graft is inadvertently excised, it is split and the inner table is replaced over the exposed dura. Bone wax is applied to the donor site for hemostasis. Periosteum is closed over the donor site, followed by closure of the galea and skin in layers. The graft is fashioned to the necessary shape and placed over the defect, with the cortical side against the recipient bone if possible.[17] If the fit is not snug, the graft is secured to the recipient bone by a variety of methods. Microplates or miniplates are well suited for this purpose (described below).

37-7-2 Cranioplastic

Historically, cranioplastic was used to correct cranial bone defects. Its use is also readily adaptable to the orbit for volume augmentation. After a subperiosteal pocket is created and adequate hemostasis obtained, the methylmethacrylate polymer and copolymer are mixed according to the manufacturer's instructions. Once the mixture reaches a doughy consistency, the volume required for augmentation is estimated and cut from the mixture with Mayo scissors, trimmed, and placed in the pocket for further molding. The material remains malleable for 3 to 5 minutes as it polymerizes, and can be shaped with moistened cotton-tipped applicators during this time. Excess material is cut free with scissors or scooped out with a periosteal elevator. It is essential that the assistant maintain anterior traction with the bridle sutures on the rectus muscles as the cranioplastic is inserted and molded firmly back in the orbit to correct enophthalmos. As already mentioned, the assistant should also pay close attention to the pupil during this posterior insertion to ensure that the optic nerve is not compromised.

If hypo-ophthalmos is the primary concern, then the bulk of the material should be placed under the globe to promote upward displacement. The cranioplastic must not be allowed to protrude over the inferior orbital rim, as this may compromise the inferior fornix. The material must be trimmed to avoid this complication. If it hardens before all molding has been completed, a pneumatic drill with a rotating burr will allow final sculpting of the implant. This is not usually necessary. The surgeon must realize that as the material hardens, heat is generated. The surgical field should be irrigated to help dissipate this heat. After the implant has been placed and hardens, further hemostasis is obtained and any small pieces of cranioplastic are removed. Forced ductions are performed to ensure that no muscle en-

trapment has occurred, especially with posterior insertion, and the incisions are closed as previously described. Intravenous dexamethasone or methylprednisolone for 24 hours helps reduce postoperative orbital edema. Oral prednisone is tapered over 5 days. Oral antibiotics are continued for 7 days postoperatively.

Cranioplastic is an easy and predictable material to use in volume implantation for the correction of posttraumatic enophthalmos and hypo-ophthalmos but, like silicone, it is an alloplastic substance. Therefore, it carries the same risks as any alloplastic material, including extrusion and infection. To date, the authors have not encountered complications such as systemic toxicity, embolic phenomena, or thermal injury. Several late infections, however, have occurred in patients with a history of sinusitis, and its use in these patients should be avoided.

37-7-3 Silicone

Medical-grade silicone rubber continues to be a popular alloplastic material for orbital augmentation. Its use avoids the additional surgery necessary to obtain bone, and it is easy to fashion into the shape needed to fit the pocket created for it. RTV silicone is also popular because it can be prepared and molded in the operating room and vulcanized at room temperature in contact with the tissue surrounding it; however, it is no longer commercially available in the United

States. Solid silicone is biologically inert and becomes encased in a fibrous capsule with time. Until this occurs, however, migration of the implant can occur. Infection, either immediate or delayed, can also occur, particularly if communication with an exposed sinus cavity exists. Alloplastic materials of any type should be avoided if an anatomic communication of this kind is present. Extrusion of larger blocks of silicone is common because they are difficult to fixate.

Recently, much controversy has surrounded silicone-gel breast implants as inducers of connective-tissue disease and autoimmune phenomena.[22-25] It should be noted that this association has not yet been conclusively proven statistically in a large cohort,[26] although some physicians believe that significant anecdotal evidence does exist. Furthermore, any perceived increase in connective-tissue disease is related to leakage of silicone gel. No such association has been attributed to solid-silicone implants. Despite this reassurance, many patients (and physicians) do not wish surgery with silicone implants. At present, the authors use porous polyethylene, microplates, or, in more severe deformities, calvarial bone grafts, for orbital reconstruction. Therefore, any concern by the patient and the referring physician about silicone implants is eliminated, while the patient is still provided with excellent reconstructive materials.

37-7-4 Microplates

One potential difficulty in late orbital reconstruction is the lack of stable platform or buttress points to support implants or soft tissue. This problem has been greatly alleviated with the introduction of rigid orbital plating systems (miniplates).[27]

Miniplates were first developed from stainless steel for fixation of long bones. Stainless steel, however, is too rigid for the contouring needed in orbital reconstruction. The recent development of both compression and noncompression microsystems made of cobalt (Vitallium) or titanium alloys has facilitated their use in the orbit.[28,29] These newer metals are less corrosive and more biocompatible than stainless steel and induce much less scatter on postoperative CT imaging. Because these metals are nonmagnetic, MRI can also be used postoperatively. It must be emphasized that the newer "micro" plating systems are ideal for use in and around the orbit. Although miniplates are suitable alternatives, the more conventional plates used in other anatomic sites are too large for facial skeletal reconstruction.

The disadvantages of miniplates and microplates include the expense of stocking a complete selection of plates and screws as well as the instruments to cut and secure the plates in place, all of which are specific to the manufacturer.[29] Each microplate set comes with a variety of plate shapes and self-tapping (threading) screws. The microplates have a variety of uses in and around the orbit, including orbital rim and wall reconstruction, as well as medial and lateral canthal angle re-formation. A great advantage of the miniplates and microplates over stainless-steel wires is twofold: the plates do not stretch with time, and they offer three-dimensional stability. The plates effectively resist deformation of the local bony anatomy by muscle or soft tissue pulling on healing bone;[29-31] interosseus wires are ineffective in this regard. Microplates are the one allograft that can be used in clean or contaminated wounds and need not necessarily be removed in the setting of postoperative infection. Indeed, the stability they offer to healing bone may be an aid in clearing infection.[29] Finally, most plating systems now include larger implants to replace the floor and walls of the orbit. Alloplastic implants or autogenous bone grafts can be placed on these stable platforms to augment orbital volume (see Figure 37-8C).

Once the surgical field is exposed, a plate of appropriate shape is chosen and cut with metal cutters to the necessary size. The shape of the plate is carefully tailored by bending to fit exactly over the bony defects. The shape and fit must be precise, because the bone will conform to the plate as the screws are tightened. A pneumatic drill is then used to drill pilot holes into bone while the assistant carefully protects the globe with malleable retractors and irrigates the drill tip. The plate is screwed into stable bone. Any unstable or comminuted fragments may then be secured to the stable plate, offering the necessary rigidity for osteosynthesis. The screws provide excellent purchase if they are threaded into both tables of the cortex. Additional implants or soft tissues may be sutured to the plate. Stainless-steel wires can be used on occasion to secure small, loose bone fragments or soft tissue to the plates.

The variety of shapes available, as well as the ability to provide specific contour to each individual case, makes the microplate system a useful tool for orbital reconstruction (Figure 37-9). At present, microplates represent the state-of-the-art method for orbital and facial skeletal reconstruction.

37-7-5 Hydroxyapatite

The use of "integrated" or "biocompatible" implants has grown significantly in recent years. These implants presumably have the advantages of both autogenous bone and alloplastic materials. Their ultrastructure allows for incorporation into adjacent bone by fibrovascular and bony ingrowth,[32,33] leading to more stability, less migration and extrusion, and possibly a lower incidence of infection. The lack of foreign-body reaction and inflammatory response to the implants may also allow for more long-term stability.[34] Integrated implants obviate the need for autogenous bone harvesting and eliminate any potential morbidity at the donor site. In addition, these implants spare potential bone-graft donor sites for future use in the event staged reconstruction is necessary.[35]

Hydroxyapatite, a material made from coral, has been used as an onlay bone-graft substitute in humans since 1984.

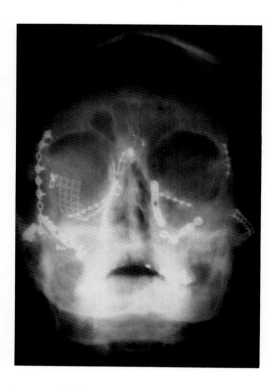

Figure 37-9 *Skull x-ray after extensive orbital reconstruction following a motor vehicle accident. Various microplates and miniplates were used to reapproximate normal orbital contours.*
Courtesy Peter A. D. Rubin, MD.

Two forms are presently available, porous and dense, and both have been used in facial reconstruction.[36] The porous type has the advantage of larger pore size, presently thought to be the definitive factor in the rate of bony ingrowth.[34] On the other hand, the dense form may have the advantage of a slower rate of resorption.[37] No conclusive data on either issue are available at present.

Several cautionary notes on hydroxyapatite are appropriate. The material is brittle, and sculpting with a pneumatic burr is experience-dependent. It also has the propensity to migrate in the early postoperative period, and may necessitate suturing to increase its stability in the orbit or orbital rim.[35] This is not the case with autogenous free bone grafts. Use of screws and wires is not advocated because of the material's inherent brittleness. Hydroxyapatite must also be covered with an adequate amount of soft tissue to prevent extrusion, as is true with other alloplastic materials. Although fibrovascular ingrowth occurs quickly, bony ingrowth will occur only in areas where hydroxyapatite is in direct contact with viable bone.[32,34] Despite these drawbacks, hydroxyapatite remains a promising material for use in orbital reconstruction and is in many ways superior to other alloplastic materials. Short-term data on fibrovascular and bony ingrowth and the lack of material resorption are very encouraging.[36]

37-7-6 Porous Polyethylene

Porous polyethylene, a material structurally similar to, but chemically different from, hydroxyapatite, has also been used in maxillofacial and orbital reconstruction.[38-40] The average pore size is slightly less than 200 μm,[38] the preferred minimum size thought to be necessary for osteon migration and bony ingrowth.[34] Thus, the rate of bony ingrowth may be slower than with hydroxyapatite.[41] (Recent studies have quoted a slightly larger average pore size for porous polyethylene of 240 μm.[42]) However, the rates of early fibrovascular ingrowth appear to be equivalent. Porous polyethylene is less brittle than hydroxyapatite and is therefore easier to mold into the necessary shape.[38] Despite its softer consistency, the material is structurally stable. The material can also be molded thermally, because it softens at temperatures of 110°C to 130°C.[38] Heating reportedly does not alter pore size.

37-7-7 Other Materials

A variety of other materials have been used for volume implantation in orbital reconstruction. Rib cartilage and bone have been used in the past. However, the complications of pleural penetration and pneumothorax or postoperative discomfort, when compared to the advantages of split-thickness calvarial bone grafts, make rib cartilage and bone grafts an outdated procedure. Glass-bead implantation, once quite popular for correcting enophthalmos in anophthalmic sockets, is no longer recommended because of the incidence of late migration of the beads, as well as an unacceptable incidence of inferior orbital nerve compression with subsequent hypesthesia and anesthesia of the cheek and maxilla. In unusual circumstances, the orbital and medial floors are absent and, in some cases of severe trauma, the orbital rim and even maxilla may be missing. Al-though facial slings with medial and lateral support via wires have been used to resuspend the globe, this technique has been replaced by the use of miniplates coupled with either calvarial bone grafts or porous polyethylene implants.

37-7-8 Implants and Antibiotics

The use of antibiotics prophylactically for repair of orbital fractures is controversial. Although orbital cellulitis has been reported after repair of orbital fractures,[43] presumably from paranasal sinus spread, others have pointed out that the sinuses are often sterile.[13] A survey of members of the American Society of Ophthalmic Plastic and Reconstructive Surgery showed that 85% favored the use of antibiotics if acute bony orbital trauma communicated with a paranasal sinus.[44] However, if bony trauma did not involve the sinuses, only half the respondents favored the use of antibiotics. For other bony orbital surgery, 57% did not use antibiotic prophylaxis. Conversely, if implants were to be used in orbital surgery, the percentage who did not use antibiotics dropped to 47%. Most of the respondents (68%) began intravenous antibiotic therapy either immediately before the operation or intraoperatively. Duration of antibiotic therapy is, again, controversial.

With respect to recommendations for antibiotic use in the late posttraumatic setting, it must first be recognized that no randomized prospective study is available. The recommendations are therefore based on other data and on clinical experience. In late posttraumatic orbital reconstruction, use of prophylactic antibiotics is suggested for three reasons. First, the presence of foreign bodies at a surgical site increases the risk of infection.[45] Second, studies have shown that porous (integrated) implants are difficult to sterilize once they are colonized by bacteria in the early postoperative period.[46] (Once vascularization has occurred, these implants have a lower rate of infection than other allografts.[47]) Finally, old traumatic wounds have a distinctly higher rate of infection (42%) than newly created traumatic wounds (18%).[48] In general, the authors advocate the use of intravenous antibiotics in the preoperative holding area immediately preceding surgery and 6 to 8 hours after surgery if the patient is admitted to the hospital.

37-8

SURGERY FOR TELECANTHUS

Transnasal wiring can be used to correct unilateral and bilateral telecanthus.[11,12,49] Since the surgical techniques for each are different, both will be described. As already mentioned, CT imaging is essential prior to attempted correction of orbital deformities. In addition, an assessment of preoperative lacrimal drainage function by probing and irrigation should be well documented.

37-8-1 Unilateral Transnasal Wiring

The superior recess of each nasal cavity is packed with neurosurgical cottonoids moistened with 4% cocaine, as for a dacryocystorhinostomy. After the induction of general endotracheal anesthesia, the medial canthal angle and medial orbital wall on the affected side are infiltrated with a mixture of lidocaine with 1:200,000 epinephrine and hyaluronidase. The skin and subcutaneous tissue just anterior to the medial canthus are also injected bilaterally. A crescent-shaped skin incision is made 2 to 3 mm anterior to the canthal angle on the affected side, with the apex centered over the canthal angle and pointing toward the dorsum of the nose. The incision may be tailored to incorporate any scar revision that may be necessary. This incision is dissected down to periosteum. Any abnormal subcutaneous tissue is excised before the periosteum is reflected temporally. Hypertrophic scar tissue is usually found following trauma to this area and must be trimmed to get a good result. Damage to the lacrimal canaliculi and sac must be avoided during the dissection, which is continued until the anterior and posterior lacrimal crests and superior portions of the lacrimal sac fossa are exposed. The periosteum may be quite adherent to bone in this area or incarcerated in a fracture following nasoethmoidal trauma. Although this makes the dissection difficult, the periosteum and adherent scar tissue must be dissected from the bone before proceeding. Access to the opposite side of the nose may be made in the thick skin anteriorly on the side of the nose for unilateral cases.

When adequate and proper exposure has been obtained, a cutting burr on a pneumatic drill is used to thin down the splayed bone in the region of the posterior lacrimal crest to the level of the ethmoidal air cells. This hyperostosis, formed during the healing of a nasoethmoidal fracture, must be removed to restore the normal bony configuration to the canthal angle prior to transnasal wiring. The hyperostotic bone often extends inferiorly into the lacrimal sac fossa and nasolacrimal canal. The location of the anterior ethmoidal artery and lamina cribrosa should always be considered during these manipulations, especially in a setting of traumatically disrupted normal anatomy.

It is important to understand the complex attachments of the medial canthal tendon and the direction of pull on the eyelids that is necessary to re-form the canthal angle properly. The force vector is not only directed medially, but also posteriorly (toward the posterior lacrimal crest) for proper configuration (Figure 37-10). Stable bone must therefore be present anterior to this position to prevent anterior

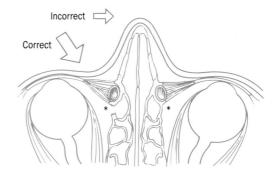

Figure 37-10 *Fracture of nasoethmoid complex (left) would result in avulsion of posterior limb of medial canthal tendon and telecanthus. Correct repair requires reapproximation of force vector of medial canthal tendon (large arrow) to posterior lacrimal crest (*). Anterior reapproximation (small arrow) will cause anterior migration of lid and poor lid-to-globe apposition.*

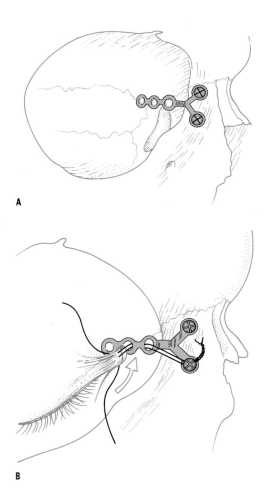

A

B

Figure 37-11 *Telecanthus repair with miniplates or microplates. (A) Y-shaped miniplate is secured anterior to anterior lacrimal crest with screws. Long arm of Y is cantilevered along disrupted posterior lacrimal crest and medial orbital wall. (B) Medial canthal tendon is anchored to appropriate hole of plate using either polypropylene suture or wire.*

migration of the wires postoperatively. Anterior fixation or migration will result in poor eyelid apposition to the globe. The bone anterior to the posterior lacrimal crest can be thinned a great deal to restore contour; however, it cannot be removed completely, as this will not allow for a posterior fixation of the wires. Occasionally, an intact nasal septum will stabilize the wires posteriorly. (Recently, in cases where poor bony support for the wires is encountered, the authors have used Y-shaped miniplates fixed to the nose to create a pseudoposterior lacrimal crest and have fixated the medial canthal tendon to the miniplate, as shown in Figure 37-11.[8])

The nasal packing is removed from each nostril, and a small hole is drilled in each lateral nasal wall where wires will subsequently be passed. A 16-gauge trocar is passed transnasally from the normal to the abnormal side through the previously drilled holes. The trocar will usually have to be tapped through the nasal septum with a small mallet. The globe must be carefully protected with malleable retractors during this procedure. When the trocar has been passed, the stylet is removed and a 32-gauge stainless-steel wire is bent on itself and the loop of the wire is passed through the lumen of the trocar transnasally so that the loop of the wire rests on the abnormal side. The trocar is then removed, leaving the loop in place. Because the wire is usually pinched at the apex of the loop as it passes through the trocar, thereby creating a weak point in the wire, the ends of the wire are adjusted so that this kink is brought to the unaffected side and cut off, leaving a smooth loop on the affected side ready for fixation to the eyelids.

The tissue in the area of the medial canthal tendon is secured to the loop of the wire using a 4-0 nonabsorbable suture. The wire itself should not be passed through the medial canthal tendon as it may "cheese-wire" through the soft tissue, leading to a recurrence of the telecanthus. The wire is now ready for tightening. To fixate it, a metal bolster pin is fashioned by cutting an 8-mm length from the central portion of the stylet of a 16-gauge angiocath (Figure 37-12). The pin is bent slightly in the middle and held against the lateral nasal bone on the unaffected side in a vertical orientation, resting between the ends of the wire, which are now twisted over the pin, anchoring the pin against the bone and providing excellent purchase for tightening the wire. The wire loop is further tightened by simultaneously pulling on the ends of the wires and twisting them over the pin until the telecanthus is slightly overcorrected. The ends of the wire are then cut, and the twisted wire is bent into the hole in the lateral nasal bone. The skin is closed with 6-0 nylon sutures.

Nose pads are usually not required in unilateral cases. A decision to use them, if necessary, must be made before the trocar is removed. If they are to be used, a second loop of 32-gauge wire is passed through the trocar and tagged. After the transnasal wiring has been completed, but before the skin is closed, the tags are removed and the loop of wire is cut, leaving two free "skin wires" exiting each skin incision. The skin is closed around the wires. The end of each wire is then passed through one of two silicone pads fashioned from trimmed silicone ocular conformers. The wires on each side are

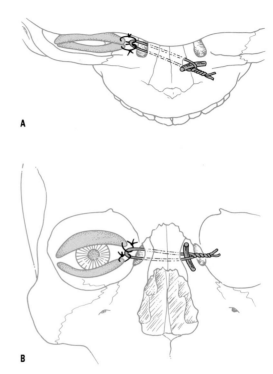

Figure 37-12 *Unilateral transnasal wiring. (A) Posterior fixation of transnasal wire is performed only on side with horizontal displacement of medial canthal angle. (B) Pin is fashioned from stylet of 16-gauge angiocath to hold transnasal wire on side opposite from medial canthal fixation loop.*

then twisted together over dental rolls to compress the skin in the canthal region, thus flattening out epicanthal folds and restoring normal consistency to the soft tissue in this area. The nose pads and skin sutures are left in place for 7 to 10 days, at which time the skin wires are clipped and the nose pads, skin wires, and skin sutures are removed. The deep, looped transnasal wire remains in place permanently.

Alternatively, as already mentioned, a Y-shaped miniplate or microplate can be attached to the nasal bone by two screws, with the long arm of the Y directed posteriorly.[8] The soft tissue of the medial canthus is engaged by either a wire on a free needle or a 4-0 nonabsorbable suture. The wire is then brought through the appropriate hole of the miniplate, mirroring the position of the posterior lacrimal crest. One of the previously placed screws is loosened, and the wire is wrapped around the head of the screw. As the assistant provides firm medial traction on the medial canthus, the wire is tightened by twisting the ends. Once the appropriate overcorrection of the telecanthus is obtained, the screw is retightened, the ends of the wire are cut, and the twisted wire is bent back into the miniplate.

This method is especially appropriate when there is little bony support in the area of the lacrimal sac fossa. The technique also obviates the need to correct the telecanthus transnasally, sparing a surgical incision on the opposite side.

37-8-2 Bilateral Transnasal Wiring

The surgical technique for bilateral transnasal wiring differs only slightly from that described for unilateral cases (Figure 37-13). The crescent-shaped skin incision is made bilaterally just anterior to the canthal angles. If an epicanthal fold exists, a small amount of skin may be excised; however, if no epicanthal fold is present, the skin excision is omitted. The subsequent dissection and removal of excess subcutaneous tissue and the thinning or hyperostosis are completed bilaterally. It is important to realize that abnormal bone is present even in congenital cases of telecanthus and that this bone must be properly trimmed to obtain the optimal postoperative result. Again, penetration of the bone must be at the level of the posterior lacrimal crest bilaterally, and intact bone must exist anterior to that position to avoid forward migration of the wires.

Once the trocar has been passed and its stylet removed, two looped 32-gauge stainless-steel wires are threaded through the trocar, which is then removed, leaving the two loops of wire in place. One loop and its two ends on the opposite side are tagged with hemostats; these will become the "skin wires." The other loop and its ends fixate the canthal tendons bilaterally. The kink in this loop of wire is removed, and the tissue of the medial canthal tendon is secured to the loop with 4-0 nonabsorbable suture. On the opposite side, a pin is not necessary (as in unilateral cases). Instead, the two ends of the wire

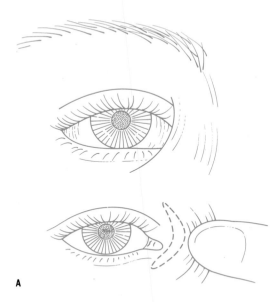

A

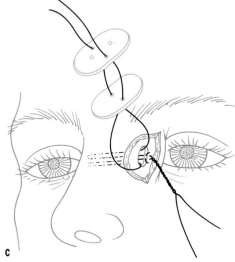

C

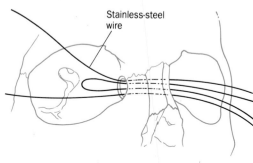

Stainless-steel wire

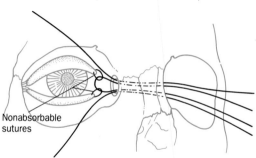

Nonabsorbable sutures

B

Figure 37-13 *Bilateral transnasal wiring. (A) Skin is excised only if prominent epicanthal fold is present. (B) Two looped wires have been passed through bony opening using 14-gauge trocar. One loop has been cut, creating external fixation wires. Remaining loop is fixed to medial canthal tendon with nonabsorbable suture and serves as internal fixation wire. (C) Nose pads are applied bilaterally (shown here prior to skin closure). Telfa pads are placed under silicone conformers to prevent maceration of skin. External wires will be tightened over dental rolls to provide pressure on medial canthal tissue.*

are twisted on themselves, forming a second loop, which is secured to the medial canthal tendon on that side with 4-0 nonabsorbable material. When the looped wire is tightened, each canthal angle is pulled toward the base of the nose, reforming the canthal angles bilaterally. The repositioning of the canthal angles to the base of the nose is accomplished by three manipulations taking place simultaneously. As the twisted wires are tightened, countertraction pulls the loop on the opposite side tight; at the same time, the nonabsorbable sutures on the twisted side are pushed inward, toward the base of the nose, with forceps. The sutures should slide very easily down the wire as the twisting takes place. After proper tightening is achieved, the twisted wire is cut short and the ends are inverted into deep tissue. The skin is closed with 6-0 nylon.

The "skin wires" that protrude through the skin will be tied over the nose pads to restore concavity to the soft tissues of the canthal angles. The tags are removed from the skin wires and the loop is cut, leaving two wires that will fixate the silicone nose pads and dental rolls as previously described. Postoperative management is identical to that after unilateral cases.

REFERENCES

1. Manson PN, Clifford CM, Su CT, et al: Mechanisms of global support and posttraumatic enophthalmos, I: the anatomy of the ligament sling and its relation to intramuscular cone orbital fat. *Plast Reconstr Surg* 1986;77: 193–202.

2. Manson PN, Grivas A, Rosenbaum A, et al: Studies on enophthalmos, II: the measurement of orbital injuries and their treatment by quantitative computed tomography. *Plast Reconstr Surg* 1986;77:203–214.

3. Bite U, Jackson IT, Forbes GS, Gehring DG: Orbital volume measurements in enophthalmos using three-dimensional CT imaging. *Plast Reconstr Surg* 1985;75:502–508.

4. Nelson LB, Catalano RA: *Atlas of Ocular Motility*. Philadelphia: WB Saunders Co; 1989: 118–119.

5. Markowitz BL, Manson PN, Sargent L, et al: Management of the medial canthal tendon in nasoethmoid orbital fractures: the importance of the central fragment in classification and treatment. *Plast Reconstr Surg* 1991;87: 843–853.

6. Yaremchuk MJ, Gruss JS, Manson PN, eds: *Rigid Fixation of the Craniomaxillofacial Skeleton.* Boston: Butterworth-Heinemann; 1992.

7. Lessell S: Indirect optic nerve trauma. *Arch Ophthalmol* 1989;107:382–386.

8. Shore JW, Rubin PA, Bilyk JR: Repair of telecanthus by anterior fixation of cantilevered miniplates. *Ophthalmology* 1992;99:1133–1138.

9. Nelson LB, Wagner RS, Calhoun JH: The adjustable suture technique in strabismus surgery. *Int Ophthalmol Clin* 1985;25:89–105.

10. Shore JW: Lateral canthal and inferior fornix approach in orbital trauma. *Ophthalmol Clin North Am* 1991;4:113–124.

11. McCord CD Jr, Shore JW, Moses JL: Orbital fractures and late reconstruction. In: McCord CD, Tanenbaum M, eds: *Oculoplastic Surgery*. 2nd ed. New York: Raven Press; 1987:155–168.

12. McCord CD Jr, Moses JL: Exposure of the inferior orbit with fornix incision and lateral canthotomy. *Ophthalmic Surg* 1979;10:53–63.

13. Westfall CT, Shore JW: Isolated fractures of the orbital floor: risk of infection and the role of antibiotic prophylaxis. *Ophthalmic Surg* 1991;22:409–411.

14. Putterman AM, Urist MJ: Treatment of anophthalmic narrow palpebral fissure after blowout fractures. *Ophthalmic Surg* 1977;6:45–49.

15. Craft PD, Sargent LA: Membranous bone healing and techniques in calvarial bone grafting. *Clin Plast Surg* 1989;16:11–19.

16. Hardesty RA, Marsh JL: Craniofacial onlay bone grafting: a prospective evaluation of graft morphology, orientation, and embryonic origin. *Plast Reconstr Surg* 1990;85:5–14.

17. Hunter D, Baker S, Sobol SM: Split calvarial grafts in maxillofacial reconstruction. *Otolaryngol Head Neck Surg* 1990;102:345–350.

18. Powell NB, Riley RW: Facial contouring with outer-table calvarial bone: a 4-year experience. *Arch Otolaryngol Head Neck Surg* 1989; 115:1454–1458.

19. Jackson IT, Pellett C, Smith JM: The skull as a bone graft donor site. *Ann Plast Surg* 1983; 11:527–532.

20. Young VL, Schuster RH, Harris LW: Intracerebral hematoma complicating split calvarial bone-graft harvesting. *Plast Reconstr Surg* 1990; 86:763–765.

21. Stuzin JM, Kawamoto HK: Saddle nasal deformity. *Clin Plast Surg* 1988;15:83–93.

22. Brozena SJ, Fenske NA, Cruse CW, et al: Human adjuvant disease following augmentation mammoplasty. *Arch Dermatol* 1988;124: 1383–1386.

23. Varga J, Schumacher HR, Jimenez SA: Systemic sclerosis after augmentation mammoplasty with silicone implants. *Ann Intern Med* 1989;111:377–383.

24. Sahn EE, Garen PD, Silver RM, Maize JC: Scleroderma following augmentation mammoplasty: report of a case and review of the literature. *Arch Dermatol* 1990;126:1198–1202.

25. Solomon G, Espinoza L, Silverman S: Breast implants and connective-tissue diseases. *N Engl J Med* 1994;331:1231–1232.

26. Gabriel SE, O'Fallon WM, Kurland LT, et al: Risk of connective-tissue diseases and other disorders after breast implantation. *N Engl J Med* 1994;330:1697–1702.

27. Rubin PA, Shore JW, Yaremchuk MJ: Complex orbital fracture repair using rigid fixation of the internal orbital skeleton. *Ophthalmology* 1992;99:553–559.

28. Munro IR: The Luhr fixation system for the craniofacial skeleton. *Clin Plast Surg* 1989; 16:41–48.

29. Marsh JL: The use of the Wurtzberg system to facilitate fixation in facial osteotomies. *Clin Plast Surg* 1989;16:49–60.

30. Davidson J, Nickerson D, Nickerson B: Zygomatic fractures: comparison of methods of internal fixation. *Plast Reconstr Surg* 1990;86: 25–32.

31. Rinehart GC, Marsh JL, Hemmer KM, Bresina S: Internal fixation of malar fractures: an experimental biophysical study. *Plast Reconstr Surg* 1989;84:21–28.

32. Rosen HM, McFarland MM: The biologic behavior of hydroxyapatite implanted into the maxillofacial skeleton. *Plast Reconstr Surg* 1990; 85:718–723.

33. Dutton JJ: Coralline hydroxyapatite as an ocular implant. *Ophthalmology* 1991;98:370–377.

34. Holmes RE, Wardrop RW, Wolford LM: Hydroxylapatite as a bone graft substitute in orthognathic surgery: histologic and histometric findings. *J Oral Maxillofac Surg* 1988;46: 661–671.

35. Salyer KE, Hall CD: Porous hydroxyapatite as an onlay bone-graft substitute for maxillofacial surgery. *Plast Reconstr Surg* 1989;84: 236–244.

36. Sutula FC, Rodgers IR: Hydroxyapatite in orbital reconstruction. *Ophthalmol Clin North Am* 1991;4:183–188.

37. Zide MF: Late posttraumatic enophthalmos corrected by dense hydroxylapatite blocks. *J Oral Maxillofac Surg* 1986;44:804–806.

38. Berghaus A: Porous polyethylene in reconstructive head and neck surgery. *Arch Otolaryngol* 1985;111:154–160.

39. Bilyk JR, Rubin PA, Shore JW: Correction of enophthalmos with porous polyethylene implants. *Int Ophthalmol Clin* 1992;32:151–156.

40. Rubin PA, Bilyk JR, Shore JW: Orbital reconstruction using porous polyethylene sheets. *Ophthalmology* 1994;101:1697–1708.

41. Maas CS, Merwin GE, Wilson J, et al: Comparison of biomaterials for facial bone augmentation. *Arch Otolaryngol Head Neck Surg* 1990;116:551–556.

42. Shanbhag A, Friedman HI, Augustine J, von Recum AF: Evaluation of porous polyethylene for external ear reconstruction. *Ann Plast Surg* 1990;24:32–39.

43. Goldfarb MS, Hoffman DS, Rosenberg S: Orbital cellulitis and orbital fractures. *Ann Ophthalmol* 1987;19:97–99.

44. Hurley LD, Westfall CT, Shore JW: Prophylactic use of antibiotics in oculoplastic surgery. *Int Ophthalmol Clin* 1992;32:165–178.

45. Elek SD, Conen PE: The virulence of *Staphylococcus pyogenes* for man: a study of the problems of wound infection. *Br J Exp Pathol* 1957;38:573–586.

46. Merritt K, Shafer JW, Brown SA: Implant site infection rates with porous and dense materials. *J Biomed Mater Res* 1979;13:101–108.

47. Rosen HM: The response of porous hydroxyapatite to contiguous tissue infection. *Plast Reconstr Surg* 1991;88:1076–1080.

48. Abramowiez M, ed: Antimicrobial prophylaxis in surgery. *Med Lett Drugs Ther* 1989; 31:105–108.

49. McCord CD Jr: The correction of telecanthus and epicanthal folds. *Ophthalmic Surg* 1980;11:446–454.

PART X

The Lacrimal System

CHAPTER 38

Evaluation of the Lacrimal System

Loan K. Nguyen, MD
John V. Linberg, MD

The common complaint of a watering eye may be caused by a variety of problems, including hyposecretion, hypersecretion, or blockage of the lacrimal drainage system. This system is a complex membranous channel whose function depends on the interaction of anatomy and physiology. Effective tear drainage depends on a variety of factors, including the volume of tear secretion, eyelid position, and anatomy of the lacrimal drainage passages. Epiphora is defined as an abnormal overflow of tears down the cheek. The patient with symptomatic tearing may have a normal lacrimal drainage system overwhelmed by primary or secondary (reflex) hypersecretion or a drainage system that is anatomically compromised and unable to handle normal tear production. On the other hand, a patient with partial drainage obstruction may have a concomitant reduction in tear production and therefore be completely asymptomatic or may even suffer from symptomatic dry eye syndrome.* Epiphora is determined by the balance between tear production and tear drainage, not by the absolute function or dysfunction of either one.

The causes of lacrimal drainage problems can be divided into two categories: anatomic and functional. Anatomic obstruction refers to a gross structural abnormality of the drainage system. The obstruction may be complete such as punctal occlusion, canalicular blockage, or nasolacrimal duct fibrosis, or partial caused by punctal stenosis, canalicular stenosis, or mechanical obstruction within the lacrimal sac (ie, dacryolith or tumor). In patients with functional obstruction, epiphora results not from anatomic blockage but from a failure of lacrimal drainage physiology. This failure may be caused by anatomic

---

*For more information about the dry eye syndrome, see Chapter 8, "Management of Ocular Surface Abnormalities," in Volume 1 of Ophthalmology Monograph 8, published in 1993.—ED.

deformity such as punctal eversion or other eyelid malpositions, but can also result from lacrimal pump inadequacy caused by weak orbicularis muscle action.

CLINICAL DIAGNOSTIC EVALUATION

It is helpful to determine whether the patient's complaint is true epiphora or a "wet eye." Detailed history-taking and careful examination will help direct the evaluation of a tearing eye. A host of clinical tests have been described, and the selection of appropriate tests will depend on the initial history and ophthalmic examination.

38-1-1 History-Taking

Any clinical evaluation should begin with a thorough history. A complaint of wet eye does not necessarily refer to a lacrimal drainage problem. Other possibilities including lacrimal secretory deficiency, ocular irritation, or allergy need to be considered. Sometimes, when basic lacrimal secretion is reduced moderately, the sensation of dryness will induce an intermittent increased reflex tear secretion. These patients complain of a foreign-body sensation with episodic tearing when, in fact, the basic problem is dry eye. In addition, some patients may describe a wet eye when, in fact, only a small amount of mucoid secretion is present in the conjunctival sac. Various sources of irritation including smoke, smog, wind, dry climate, and pollutants also may cause reflex hypersecretion.

Additional history may point to the cause of lacrimal drainage obstruction. Some topical medications, including such glaucoma medications as echothiophate iodide and chemotherapeutic agents (5-fluorouracil), are associated with lacrimal obstruction. A history of recurrent allergic or infectious conjunctivitis or ocular pemphigus should lead the physician to suspect canalicular occlusion or acquired punctal stenosis. A history of recurrent dacryocystitis strongly suggests distal nasolacrimal duct obstruction as well as potential stenosis of the proximal system.

A history of facial trauma, previous sinus surgery, or rhinostomy[1] should alert the physician to the possibility of nasolacrimal duct injury. Epiphora associated with bloody tears, nasal obstruction, or epistaxis should raise suspicion of a nasal, sinus, or lacrimal sac tumor. A review of systems may disclose a history of systemic disease that can involve the lacrimal system, such as sarcoidosis or Paget's disease, or a history of Bell's palsy as the cause of epiphora.

38-1-2 External and Slit-Lamp Examination

Together with a thorough history, a good external examination will guide the physician toward a diagnosis and specific diagnostic tests. As mentioned previously, complaint of a tearing eye should not divert attention from the possibility of a dry eye. Potential signs of dry eye syndrome include abnormalities in the quality or stability of the tear film, the size of the tear meniscus, and the condition of the corneal epithelium. There may be conjunctival hyperemia, loss of luster of the conjunctiva, limbal congestion, or tenacious conjunctival secretion. The corneal reflex is dull with superficial punctate corneal erosions, epithelial filaments, and sometimes corneal ulceration. Lacrimal hyposecretion may be present in all degrees, from the mildest to the most severe.

Numerous relatively minor abnormalities of the eyelids and conjunctiva may be responsible for reflex hypersecretion of tears. Conjunctival concretions, aberrant cilia, molluscum contagiosum, papillomata, and chalazia involving the eyelid margin may all cause excessive tearing.

Malformations and malpositions of the eyelid margins can be responsible for abnormal tearing. The most common of these are ectropion and entropion. Eversion of the lacrimal puncta may escape casual inspection but can be observed by having the patient rotate the eye maximally upward. If the punctum can be seen without manual eversion of the eyelid, its position is not normal and may be responsible for the epiphora. Because the orbicularis oculi muscle is the source of the tear pump mechanism, deficiency in orbicularis function will result in epiphora. A patient with a seventh cranial nerve (facial) paralysis, or lower eyelid laxity, may exhibit epiphora.

A careful biomicroscopic evaluation may disclose punctal stenosis. Mucoid reflux with lacrimal sac massage is pathognomonic for a lower system obstruction. Mass lesions in the medial canthal region, such as a sac mucocele, may cause mechanical obstruction of the tear drainage. Mass lesions extrinsic to the lacrimal drainage system, such as an ethmoid mucocele, may also compress the sac and cause obstruction.

Chronic canaliculitis is characterized by epiphora, fullness in the region of the canaliculus, and the appearance of creamy pus when pressure is applied over the canaliculus. Canaliculitis tends to affect only one eyelid and for some reason generally does not involve the adjacent lacrimal sac. Canaliculitis may be caused by infection with bacterial, viral, chlamydial, or mycotic organisms. However, the most common cause is the filamentous gram-positive rod *Actinomyces israelii*. The diagnosis can sometimes be confirmed by instilling a drop of topical anesthesia into the conjunctival sac and then gently massaging the canaliculus between two cotton applicators to express the concretions. The diagnosis can also be made by microscopic examination of the purulent secretion without stain, after adding a drop of potassium hydroxide. Mycelia may be found in such fresh wet preparations.

30-1-3 Tear Production Measurement

Approximate measurement of tear production is provided by the Schirmer test without topical anesthetic. The Schirmer I test is used to assess stimulated tear production. The test should be performed in subdued lighting, and both eyes may be tested simultaneously. One end of the filter paper strip is folded and hooked over the lateral third of the inferior eyelid margin. Wetting of the strip is measured at 5 minutes; the average normal measurement is between 10 and 30 mm. Unfortunately, the stimulus to the eye from the filter paper strip is great, and the reflex tearing measured by this test may not reflect normal physiology. The amount of ocular stimulation can be reduced, but not eliminated, by anesthetizing the conjunctiva with topical agents. When the Schirmer test is performed with topical anesthetic, the term *basic secretion* is often used, suggesting that basal secretion is not related to reflex stimuli. A broad range of recent research indicates that all tears are produced in response to neurologic ("reflex") stimuli, so that the simplistic distinction between reflex and basal secretion may be inaccurate. A Schirmer test result of less than 5 mm of wetting, using topical anesthesia, is abnormal. All Schirmer testing is highly variable, and the test should be repeated in an effort to verify the results of an initial test.

Rose bengal is a chloride-substituted iodinated fluorescein dye that stains devitalized epithelial cells. Increased staining of the conjunctival and corneal epithelium is a sensitive indicator of inadequate tear function regardless of the Schirmer test results.

The tear breakup time (BUT) is a simple test for evaluation of the tear film stability that depends on the basal mucous layer. One drop of fluorescein is placed in the eye, and the patient is asked to blink once. The tear film on the cornea is observed with cobalt-blue light until the film breaks up, exposing dry spots on the cornea. Normal breakup time is 15 to 30 seconds. A tear breakup time of less than 10 seconds is abnormal. The presence or absence of the tear meniscus or its height is a useful finding in ascertaining dry or wet eye. Enhancing the tear meniscus with fluorescein allows better visualization of the strip and its contents.

38-2

LACRIMAL DRAINAGE EVALUATION

After examination of tear secretion and the ocular surface, the lacrimal drainage system may be evaluated with the following tests in recommended order:

1. Fluorescein dye disappearance test
2. Lacrimal irrigation
3. Probing of canaliculi
4. Dacryocystography
5. Nasal endoscopy

38-2-1 Fluorescein Dye Disappearance Test

The fluorescein dye disappearance (FDD) test is a quick, simple, and physiologic method for assessing the lacrimal drainage system.[2] The FDD test is an extremely valuable and practical clinical tool, since it is entirely safe, painless, and requires no special instrumentation. The test is most meaningful when both eyes are compared simultaneously. One drop of 2% fluorescein is instilled into the lower fornix of each eye. The patient is instructed not to touch or dab the eye and to blink normally. Both the intensity of the color and the volume of tears are assessed after 5 minutes. As originally described by Zappia and Milder,[2] a residual of 0 or +1 dye is designated as a positive test, indicating probable normal drainage outflow; whereas a residual of +2 to +4 represents a negative test, indicating partial or complete obstruction or pump failure. Other authors have found it more practical to grade the residual dye in only three grades, and use the more common medical convention that defines an abnormal test result as positive.[3] In this version, trace or no residual dye is considered a negative test (normal); minimal residual dye (+1) is considered a low positive; and marked residual dye (+2) is considered a high positive test suggestive of a delay or impairment in tear drainage.

Although the FDD test is simple to perform and effective as an initial screening test, it is nonspecific and may give false-positive results in the elderly and in dry-eyed patients secondary to excessive conjunctival staining. If the FDD test results are normal, significant lacrimal drainage dysfunction is very unlikely. However, intermittent obstruction from allergy, dacryolith, or nasal polyps may still be a possibility. If the fluorescein dye disappearance is delayed, the test cannot distinguish between physiologic and anatomic causes of drainage dysfunction, nor can it determine whether the abnormality is in the upper or lower outflow system. Thus, a delayed fluorescein dye disappearance is an indication for further testing; and the authors' next step is lacrimal irrigation.

38-2-2 Lacrimal Irrigation

Gentle irrigation should be performed to evaluate the anatomic patency of the lacrimal drainage system. A drop of topical anesthetic is instilled into the conjunctival sac.* The punctum is dilated with a punctal dilator (Figure 38-1A), and a 23-gauge cannula is inserted about 5 to 6 mm into one canaliculus to irrigate saline. The irrigation is initially performed without occlusion of the opposite punctum. It is important to hold the irrigation cannula gently in the anatomic position of the canaliculus (Figure 38-1B), because kinking or pressure against the wall of the canaliculus will produce a false sensation of obstruction.

In a normal drainage system, the fluid will easily flow into the nasopharynx, with little or no reflux from the opposite punctum. Reflux in the opposite punctum documents patent canaliculi, but suggests distal obstruction. Irrigation with occlusion of the opposite punctum documents mechanical patency at nonphysiologic pressures if fluid passes into the nasopharynx. However, these elevated pressures may force fluid through a partially or physiologically obstructed drainage system.

---

*Some examiners anesthetize the medial conjunctival cul-de-sac, using 4% lidocaine on a cotton pledget or applicator prior to probing and/or irrigation.—ED.

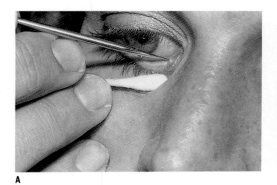

A

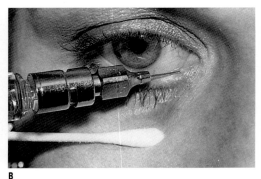

B

38-2-3 Probing of Canaliculi

When the irrigation test indicates obstruction, gentle probing using a No. 0000 probe should be performed to palpate the site of the obstruction. If a small probe is used, it is rarely necessary to dilate. The probe is gently advanced through the canaliculus until an obstruction is encountered; force is not appropriate. The probe can be grasped with forceps at the punctum, and then withdrawn to measure the distance from the punctum to the obstruction (Figure 38-2). The nasolacrimal duct in adults should never be probed because the probing is not therapeutic and causes significant pain. Thus, gentle probing is used to localize a site of obstruction within the canaliculi, but not in the lacrimal sac or nasolacrimal duct. The degree of stenosis can sometimes be estimated by using progressively larger probes, but a large probe should never be forced through an obstruction. Probing is diagnostic, not therapeutic, in the evaluation of epiphora. Occasionally, the examiner will detect a gritty sensation during probing, which suggests concretions associated with canaliculitis.

Figure 38-1 *Lacrimal irrigation. (A) Punctum is dilated with punctal dilator. (B) Cannula is held in anatomic position in canaliculus.*

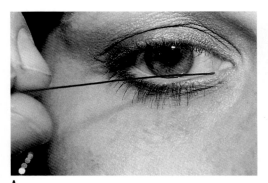

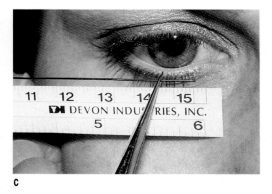

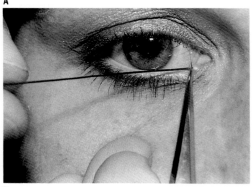

Figure 38-2 *Canalicular probing is performed when irrigation test indicates obstruction. (A) No. 0000 probe is passed into canalicular system without force until it comes to obstruction. (B) Forceps are used to mark how far probe is advanced from punctum. (C) Probe is withdrawn and distance of stenosis or blockage is measured.*

38-2-4 Jones Dye Test

In any discussion of the evaluation of the lacrimal drainage system, the Jones dye test should be included. The interpretation of the results of the protocol needs to be understood by ophthalmologists. In 1961, Jones described the use of fluorescein to test lacrimal outflow function.[4] In the primary dye test (Jones I), one drop of 2% fluorescein is instilled into the conjunctival sac. After the nose has been sprayed with 4% cocaine for comfort, a fine cotton-tipped applicator is inserted beneath the inferior turbinate at 2 minutes and again at 5 minutes. If fluorescein is recovered, the test is positive and indicates a patent system.

If no fluorescein is recovered in the primary test, the secondary dye test (Jones II) is performed. A topical anesthetic is instilled in the conjunctival cul-de-sac and residual fluorescein is flushed from the conjunctival sac. The patient's head is tilted over an emesis basin, and the canaliculus is irrigated with clear saline. If the irrigant is fluorescein-stained, the test is positive, indicating a patent proximal system. If the irrigant is clear, the test is negative, suggesting stenosis of the punctum or canaliculus. If fluid does not reach the nose at all, then complete obstruction of the system exists.

A positive dye test (Jones I) indicates a normal drainage system. Unfortunately, it is possible for fluorescein dye to pass through a normal drainage system and into the nasal cavity without being detected by the examiner. Even in expert hands, the primary dye test has a high incidence of false-negative results.[5] In addition, the secondary dye test is not physiologic. It does not establish the functional condition of the lacrimal sac, because the irrigating solution is forced into the nose under nonphysiologic pressures (Table 38-1). Although the Jones fluorescein dye tests have been widely used since they were first described in 1961, the present authors have not found them to be useful or practical. Since we have found it difficult to obtain consistent results with these tests, we use alternate tests including the fluorescein dye disappearance test, irrigation, probing, dacryocystography, and nasal endoscopy.

38-2-5 Dacryocystography

Dacryocystography (DCG) provides visualization of anatomic details that are not available by any other nonoperative technique. The authors do not routinely employ special imaging techniques in the everyday evaluation of patients with lacrimal problems. However, dacryocystography is indicated for patients with suspected lacrimal sac tumors or those who may have abnormal anatomy (whether due to trauma, reoperations, or congenital

TABLE 38-1

Results of Primary and Secondary Jones Tests

Jones I		
+		Patent system, probable normal physiologic function
−		False-negative: physiologic dysfunction, anatomic obstruction
Jones II		
+	Dye in nose	Partial block at lower sac or duct
−	Saline in nose	Punctal or canalicular stenosis
−	Regurgitation at opposite punctum with dye	Complete nasolacrimal duct obstruction
−	Regurgitation at opposite punctum without dye	Complete common canaliculus obstruction
−	Regurgitation at same punctum with dye	Complete common canaliculus obstruction

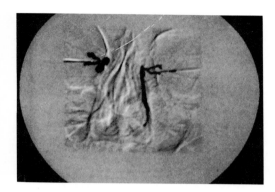

Figure 38-3 *Computerized digital subtraction dacryocystogram in patient with unilateral epiphora after facial trauma. Right lacrimal sac is dilated and obstruction is noted at sac–duct junction. Left side shows normal-caliber lacrimal system.*

anomalies). In addition, DCG may be indicated in selected patients with partial or functional obstruction of the nasolacrimal duct. We recommend the use of computerized digital subtraction dacryocystography over standard DCG to obtain better imaging of the lacrimal system (Figure 38-3).

This study can be performed in the angiography suite of the radiology department. The patient is placed supine on the angiography table. Topical anesthetic drops are placed over the puncta of both eyes. The lower puncta are dilated with a punctal dilator. A sialography catheter is inserted into the lower canaliculus of each eye and taped in place on the patient's cheek and forehead for later injection of contrast material. Then, the patient is positioned underneath the x-ray beam to allow simultaneous imaging of both lacrimal systems. Each catheter is connected to a 3-cc syringe filled with a warmed contrast agent (iophendylate). The imaging starts as the lacrimal system in both eyes is injected simultaneously with 2 to 3 cc of contrast material. The lacrimal system is visualized on the monitor screen as the contrast agent flows down the pathway. Selected prints can be made to illustrate the flow through the system. Films can be obtained 10 minutes later to evaluate dye retention. Visualization of the site of the obstruction or stenosis by DCG helps determine the surgical plan.

If a functional or partial obstruction of the nasolacrimal duct is suspected with a normal irrigation to the nose, a simplified dacryocystogram can be ordered. Only the late film is of interest in these cases, because retention of contrast material in the sac after 10 minutes is clear evidence of distal functional obstruction. The contrast agent can be injected in the clinic, and the patient sent to radiology for a single posteroanterior Waters view film. This approach avoids the need for a separate appointment with radiology and the expense of a full dacryocystogram.

38-2-6 Dacryoscintigraphy

Dacryoscintigraphy uses radionuclei tracer [^{99m}Tc] pertechnetate in saline or technetium sulfur colloid to image the lacrimal system. The drop of the tracer is instilled in the conjunctival cul-de-sac and the lacrimal system is imaged with a gammagram. The advantages of using the isotope study are its sensitivity, ease of performance, and noninvasiveness. Dacryoscintigraphy and contrast dacryocystography provide different types of information. Scintigraphy is more sensitive for the diagnosis of incomplete blocks, especially in the upper system.[6] In addition, the amount of radiation exposure to the lens is less than 2% of that for a complete dacryocystogram. However, dacryoscintigraphy does not provide the detailed anatomic visualization available with contrast DCG.

38-2-7 Computed Tomography

Computed tomography (CT) of the lacrimal system is generally not utilized in the evaluation of a tearing patient. However, when epiphora follows trauma and other studies have demonstrated nasolacrimal duct obstruction, CT may reveal orbital rim or maxillary fractures compressing the sac or duct. In the evaluation of an infant with a congenital cystic mass in the medial canthus, a CT scan may be necessary to differentiate an amniocele from a meningocele. In cases of suspected malignancy, a CT scan will demonstrate a soft-tissue mass of the sac or adjacent paranasal sinuses and guide the approach to surgical excision.

38-2-8 Nasal Endoscopy

Nasal endoscopy has revolutionized the visualization of nasal anatomy and has become an important tool for the otolaryngologist in sinus surgery. In the past, the results of lacrimal surgery have generally been evaluated in terms of functional success rather than actual visual inspection of an anatomic result. For the ophthalmologist, the endoscope provides excellent visualization of the intranasal aspect of lacrimal surgery and takes the guesswork out of postoperative evaluations.

Two areas of principal interest in lacrimal surgery are (1) the opening of the nasolacrimal duct under the inferior turbinate and (2) the site of a dacryocystorhinostomy ostium anterior to the middle turbinate (Figure 38-4). These areas are accessible to rigid endoscopes with conventional solid optical elements. The authors are experienced with the Hopkins telescopic endoscope, which is used in a variety of other fields such as urology, la-

A

B

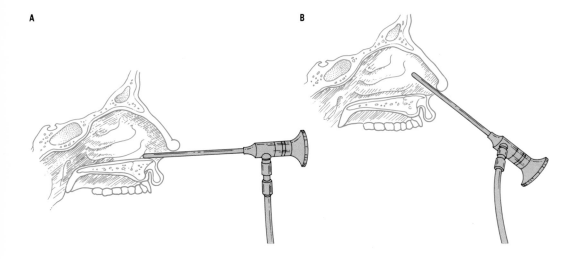

Figure 38-4 *Correct position of endoscope for visualization of (A) nasolacrimal duct ostium under inferior turbinate (B) area of intranasal DCR ostium or Jones tube anterior to middle turbinate.*

paroscopy, arthroscopy, and otorhinolaryngoscopy.[7] This instrument is widely available in most general hospitals so that the lacrimal surgeon can utilize endoscopy without having to purchase one. For the initial attempt with endoscopy, the ophthalmologist may want to ask for assistance from an otolaryngologist.

The technique is simple and easily performed in an outpatient setting using topical anesthesia and no sedation: 4% lidocaine hydrochloride applied with a nasal atomizer works well. Nasal decongestion with a 0.25% or 0.5% phenylephrine hydrochloride or Afrin nose spray will shrink the nasal mucosa and facilitate manipulation of the endoscope. A good view of the dacryocystorhinostomy ostium is obtained using the 5.5-mm-diameter Hopkins telescopic endoscope with a 30° view angle or the 0° wide-angle instrument. The examiner introduces the rod through the nares with its axis parallel to the septum and at an angle of about 45° in relation to the frontal plane of the face. The viewing port is directed laterally away from the midline.

The opening of the nasolacrimal duct under the inferior turbinate is more difficult to visualize because of limited space. A smaller-diameter (2.4-mm) endoscope is introduced through the nares along the floor of the nose, with the viewing port directed upward. Packing the area briefly with a cocaine-moistened pledget of cotton will shrink the mucosa to increase the available space and comfort.

Endoscopy can be very useful in the evaluation of dacryocystorhinostomy failures. The distinction between closure of the nasal ostium and common canalicular stenosis is sometimes difficult to establish by probing or irrigation. Endoscopy is especially helpful in the postoperative care of Jones tubes, because visualization assists in the diagnosis and management of problem cases. In addition, skill in using an endoscope is essential for laser-assisted dacryocystorhinostomy.

38-3

PEDIATRIC LACRIMAL PROBLEMS

Congenital obstruction of lacrimal drainage systems is present in 6% of newborns. The most common cause is a membranous obstruction of the nasolacrimal duct at the valve of Hasner. Less common congenital anomalies include punctal atresia, canalicular absence, lacrimal sac fistula, and supernumerary puncta and canaliculi. Amniocele is another cause of tearing in newborns. Nonlacrimal causes of tearing are congenital glaucoma, epiblepharon with lashes rubbing against the eye, and distichiasis. Acquired conditions include conjunctivitis, foreign body, or other ocular inflammations. An evaluation of a tearing infant should be made to rule out the more serious ocular conditions that require urgent therapy.

38-3-1 Diagnosis in Children and Infants

The symptoms of children with congenital nasolacrimal duct obstruction usually include epiphora and chronic or recurrent conjunctivitis, but dacryocystitis is rare. An infant with nasolacrimal duct obstruction usually has mucus accumulation in the eye or on the lashes. Tearing is present, but no redness unless there is a superimposed conjunctivitis or dacryocystitis. Pressure over the lacrimal sac may produce regurgitation of mucus and tears from the puncta.

Amniocele (congenital lacrimal sac mucocele) is a rare condition of newborns, appearing as a soft bluish mass in the medial canthus, usually not associated with infection. The dilated lacrimal sac is filled with mucus and possibly amniotic fluid. This condition must be differentiated from meningocele and orbital hemangioma, which may have a similar appearance. A CT scan may be necessary to make the differential diagnosis.

A child with punctal atresia has tearing without reflux of mucus from the punctum, because the obstruction is proximal. Examination will show a punctal dimple with a membrane occluding the orifice. Frequently, both the upper and the lower puncta are involved.

A congenital lacrimal sac fistula is unusual and might be better described as an extra aberrant canaliculus. The patient demonstrates a small dimple and opening below the medial canthal tendon that communicates with the lacrimal sac. The complaint is tearing; more specifically, the tears roll down the cheek. The remainder of the ocular examination is usually normal.

Tearing may be caused by corneal or ocular surface defects. Careful examination of the position of the eyelid and lashline is important to identify abnormal lashes, an extra row of lashes, or epiblepharon, which forces lashes against the cornea. Epiblepharon is more apparent when the child looks downward. Fluorescein staining should be used to detect epithelial surface defects.

Irrigation or probing of the lacrimal system in infants and children is usually impossible, unless they are sedated. However, a fluorescein dye disappearance test can be performed. In most cases, the diagnosis is based on history, symptoms, signs, and physical examination. A dacryocystogram may be helpful for infants with multiple congenital anomalies, because they often have abnormal anatomy.

38-3-2 Treatment of Children and Infants

Treatment of a patient with congenital nasolacrimal duct obstruction depends on the child's age and symptoms, and some aspects remain controversial. When there is a history of epiphora but no evidence of infection, the patient may be treated conservatively, with the expectation of spontaneous resolution. Approximately 90% of all congenital nasolacrimal duct obstructions resolve spontaneously in the first year of life. The parents are instructed to massage the sac, stroking it firmly in a downward direction several times daily. The hydrostatic pressure generated by massage may force an opening in the distal end. Also, massage minimizes the accumulation of mucopurulent material within the sac and thus decreases the risk of dacryocystitis. If there is mucopurulent discharge associated with epiphora, a drop of antibiotic solution can be instilled in the eye before each massage treatment.

Amniocele can often be cured with massage. Topical antibiotics should also be given, because the incidence of infection is quite high. If massage is not successful within 5 to 7 days, probing should be done before the sac becomes infected. Congenital amniocele is one of the few indications for early probing, and immediate probing may be necessary in cases of dacryocystitis.

In some patients with punctal atresia, the canaliculus may be normal. A sharp dilator or a sterile safety pin can be used to break through the membrane covering the punctum; then the patency of the rest of the drainage system should be evaluated.

If a congenital lacrimal sac fistula causes significant symptoms, the tract can be excised. These tracts are often contiguous with the normal canaliculi or common canaliculus, and care must be taken to avoid scarring of these normal structures.

38-3-3 Probing in Children and Infants

In infants under the age of 3 to 6 months, some authorities suggest that irrigation and probing can be accomplished without inhalation anesthesia. The authors almost always recommend sedation by a trained anesthesiologist, so that probing may be accomplished in a painless and controlled manner.

The goal of probing is to open the membrane at the distal end of the naso-lacrimal duct. The puncta are gently dilated, and fluorescein solution is irrigated through the canaliculus to determine the patency of the system and to clear the sac of any mucous material. A fine suction catheter is inserted into the corresponding nostril. If fluorescein-stained fluid is recovered from the nose, then the system is patent. If dye refluxes from the opposite punctum, then there is probably a naso-lacrimal duct obstruction, especially if there is mucus mixed with the fluid.

When probing infants, the examiner must remember that the distance between the punctum and the floor of the nose is usually no more than 20 mm. Therefore, it is helpful to place a mark on the probe at 20 mm as a guide. A pledget may be moistened with cocaine solution (dose < 3 mg/kg) and inserted along the floor of the nose adjacent to the inferior turbinate. A No. 0 or 00 lacrimal probe is passed through the lower or upper canaliculus into the lacrimal sac. Once the probe touches the lacrimal bone, it is rotated into a vertical position and passed down through the nasolacrimal canal without excessive force. The probe should be advanced toward the floor of the nose until a "pop" is felt, when the obstruction is penetrated. Using a nasal speculum, the surgeon may visualize the probe in the nose. To confirm the success of the probing, fluorescein solution is irrigated through the lacrimal drainage system and recovered from the nasopharynx.

Because one lacrimal probing is 90% successful in opening a congenital obstruction, it is not necessary to keep infants with recurrent infections "under observation" until the age of 6 to 8 months. If probing is necessary, best results are obtained within the first 13 months of life. The success rate drops to about 50% after 18 months of age.[8]

Although lacrimal probing usually solves the problem of congenital nasolacrimal duct obstruction, 5% to 10% of these procedures are less successful. If the first probing is performed in a careful manner and the probe clearly passes into the nose, the authors would not repeat the probing. If the initial probing was technically difficult, it may be helpful to repeat the procedure after infracture of the inferior turbinate.

38-3-4 Treatment When Probing Fails

If a careful probing combined with infracturing the inferior turbinate has not resulted in a cure, then silicone intubation is indicated. Silicone intubation is at least 85% successful for infants with congenital nasolacrimal duct obstruction.[9-13] Although successful intubation of the nasolacrimal system has been reported in children as old as 16 years of age, the best results are obtained in children less than 5 years.

Dacryocystorhinostomy is an appropriate treatment when probing and silicone intubation fail. However, the authors would recommend dacryocystorhinostomy, instead of silicone intubation, for children older than 5 years of age with a history of dacryocystitis and failed probing. For a younger child who failed silicone intubation, surgery is usually delayed until the child is 18 months old. However, dacryocystorhinostomy can be performed at any age if the infant has problems with recurrent infections. The authors have had the occasion to perform this operation on infants ranging in age from 2 weeks to 1 year, with no unusual complications or failures. Although the anatomy of infants is small in size, the surgery is not exceptionally difficult, and dacryocystorhinostomy is performed in the same manner as for adults.

REFERENCES

1. Flanagan JC: Epiphora following rhinoplasty. *Ann Ophthalmol* 1978;10:1239–1242.

2. Zappia RJ, Milder B: Lacrimal drainage function, 2: the fluorescein dye disappearance test. *Am J Ophthalmol* 1972;74:160–162.

3. Meyer DR, Antonello A, Linberg JV: Assessment of tear drainage after canalicular obstruction using fluorescein dye disappearance. *Ophthalmology* 1990;97:1370–1374.

4. Jones LT: An anatomical approach to problems of the eyelids and lacrimal apparatus. *Arch Ophthalmol* 1961;66:111–150.

5. Zappia RJ, Milder B: Lacrimal drainage function, 1: the Jones fluorescein test. *Am J Ophthalmol* 1972;74:154–159.

6. Rose JD, Clayton CB: Scintigraphy and contrast radiography for epiphora. *Br J Radiol* 1985;58:1183–1186.

7. Linberg JV: Endoscopy. In: Linberg JV, ed: *Lacrimal Surgery.* New York: Churchill Livingstone; 1988:297–314.

8. Katowitz JA, Welsh MG: Timing of initial probing and irrigation in congenital nasolacrimal duct obstruction. *Ophthalmology* 1987;94:698–705.

9. Leone CR Jr, Van Gemert JV: The success rate of silicone intubation in congenital lacrimal obstruction. *Ophthalmic Surg* 1990;21:90–92.

10. Crawford JS: Intubation of obstructions in the lacrimal system. *Can J Ophthalmol* 1977;12:289–292.

11. Durso F, Hand SI Jr, Ellis FD, Helveston EM: Silicone intubation in children with nasolacrimal obstruction. *J Pediatr Ophthalmol Strab* 1980;17:389–393.

12. Dortzbach RK, France TD, Kushner BJ, Gonnering RS: Silicone intubation for obstruction of the nasolacrimal duct in children. *Am J Ophthalmol* 1982;94:585–590.

13. Pashby RC, Rathbun JE: Silicone tube intubation of the lacrimal drainage system. *Arch Ophthalmol* 1979;97:1318–1322.

SUGGESTED READINGS

Dutton JJ: Diagnostic tests and imaging techniques. In: Linberg JV, ed: *Lacrimal Surgery.* New York: Churchill Livingstone; 1988:19–47.

Leone CR Jr: The management of pediatric lacrimal problems. *Ophthalmic Plast Reconstr Surg* 1989;5:34–39.

Milder B: Diagnostic tests of lacrimal function. In: Milder B, Weil BA, eds: *The Lacrimal System.* Norwalk, CT: Appleton; 1983:71.

Millman AL, Liebeskind A, Putterman AM: Dacryocystography: the technique and its role in the practice of ophthalmology. *Radiol Clin North Am* 1987;25:781–786.

CHAPTER 39

Surgery of the Lacrimal System

John L. Wobig, MD
Roger A. Dailey, MD

Obstruction of the tear outflow system can occur anywhere along its course from the tear lake to the inferior meatus of the nose. Surgical techniques designed to relieve this functional or complete obstruction have been available for a long time. Toti of Italy described the dacryocystorhinostomy (DCR) procedure in 1908 as a treatment modality for obstruction of the nasolacrimal duct. His technique did not make use of mucosal flaps. Dupuy-Dutemps of France, on the other hand, encouraged use of flaps. He recommended suturing together the nasal mucosal and lacrimal sac flaps. The success rate of the operation improved dramatically. Today the external dacryocystorhinostomy procedure makes use of modifications of both of these historically described procedures.

In recent years, intranasal DCR has enjoyed renewed popularity. This procedure had been performed by Lester Jones and others for years, but was dropped because the success rate was 80% at best. Although the use of endoscopic techniques and laser technology has been advocated by some authorities, the success rate (approximately 70%) with relatively short-term followup has limited its acceptance. More recently, Javate and associates reported a series of patients undergoing endoscopic DCR with the radiofrequency Ellman unit. Their reported success rate of 90% compared favorably with a 94% success rate in 50 age-matched patients undergoing external DCR with a followup of 9 months. This rate also compares favorably to the present authors' success rate of approximately 95% in uncomplicated cases undergoing external DCR. Therefore, the laser does not appear to offer any significant advantage over more traditional intranasal approaches, and the cost may actually be a financial disincentive to its use. The addition of mitomycin to the internal fistula at the time of surgery is currently being investigated and may prove to be a beneficial adjunct.

While the DCR works well for lacrimal sac or nasolacrimal duct obstruction, it does not address obstructions of the puncta and canaliculi. Multiple procedures are available to the lacrimal surgeon for obstructions in the upper system and are discussed in this chapter. The definitive procedure for significant canalicular obstruction is the conjunctivodacryocystorhinostomy (CDCR), which was initially described by Lester Jones. The DCR was performed to the point of mucosal flaps and then a polyethylene tube was placed from the medial canthus into the nasal cavity posterior to the anterior lacrimal sac mucosal flap and the nasal mucosal flap. Because of the improved capillary attraction of glass, these were later changed to Pyrex tubes, which demonstrated improved effectiveness, and they remain the standard today despite efforts to find substitute autogenous and synthetic materials.

39-1

DACRYOCYSTORHINOSTOMY

Dacryocystorhinostomy, as performed today, has proved to be beneficial for the treatment of acute or chronic nasolacrimal duct obstruction, as well as functional obstruction of the lacrimal outflow system. Functional obstruction is diagnosed using the Jones dye tests. The Jones I in this case would be negative (no dye), and the Jones II would be positive, indicating that the dye was unable to pass from the eye to the nose in approximately 10 minutes without assistance; however, fluid can be forced through the duct by the examiner using a syringe and cannula. This procedure, performed through an external incision, facilitates the identification and removal of dacryoliths and benign or malignant lacrimal sac tumors.

39-1-1 Anesthesia

Cooperative adult patients are urged to have the procedure performed with local infiltrative anesthetic combined with intravenous sedation or monitored anesthesia care (MAC). Recovery is generally shorter and easier for the patient and there is less intraoperative hemorrhage than with general anesthesia.

The eye is topically anesthetized with proparacaine hydrochloride. Subcutaneous infiltration of 2% lidocaine with epinephrine (1:100,000) in the operative area below the medial canthus and in the region of the infratrochlear nerve above the medial canthal tendon is performed. Half-inch packing gauze or cottonoids saturated with cocaine hydrochloride 4% to 5% and phenylephrine hydrochloride 2% are packed into the nose in the region of the anterior tip of the middle turbinate. When general anesthetic is used, the same infiltration and nasal packing are employed.

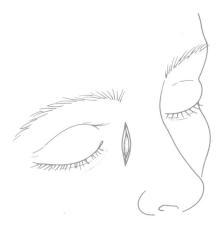

Figure 39-1 *Skin incision for dacryocysto-rhinostomy.*

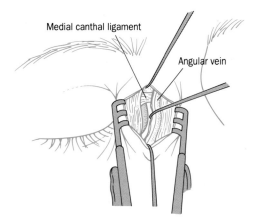

Medial canthal ligament

Angular vein

Figure 39-2 *Deeper dissection revealing medial canthal tendon and angular vein.*

39-1-2 Technique

The skin incision is made 11 mm nasal to the medial commissure, starting just superior to the insertion of the medial canthal tendon and extending inferiorly and slightly laterally for about 20 mm (Figure 39-1). The knife should not cut deeper than the subcutaneous fascia. After cutting through the remaining subcutaneous tissue with sharp Stevens scissors, the surgeon should insert a self-retaining, spring-type retractor such as the Agrikola. Hemostasis is obtained with a battery cautery unit, which facilitates initial orbicularis fiber separation as well.

With two Freer elevators, the angular artery and vein are located as they cross the medial canthal tendon (Figure 39-2). The vessels are retracted to the medial or lateral side with one elevator, while the other elevator begins the separation of the muscle and periosteum exactly beneath the point where the medial canthal tendon attaches to the bone. With pressure against the bone, the tip of the elevator is directed inferiorly and outwardly until the region below the spine of the anterior lacrimal crest is reached. The periosteal division will be about 3 to 5 mm medial and will extend inferiorly to the margin of the anterior lacrimal crest. The periosteum is elevated on both sides of this incision and reflected over the anterior lacrimal crest; then the sac is elevated posteriorly beneath the tendon to the posterior lacrimal crest. Next, the nasolacrimal duct is freed from the bone inferiorly as far as possible in the nasolacrimal canal.

The lacrimal sac is infiltrated with local anesthetic, and a 0.5-inch square cottonoid is inserted between the soft tissue of the lacrimal sac and the bony lacrimal fossa. The cottonoid serves three purposes: hemostasis, anesthesia, and protection of the sac during bone removal.

At this time, the spring retractor is exchanged for one with longer teeth, such as a Goldstein, which will reach the periosteum and give better deep exposure.* The nasal packing is removed in preparation for bone removal. Using the Hall drill or a similar drill with a 4- to 5-mm dental burr, the surgeon removes an oblong area of bone anterior to the lacrimal crest, taking care not to injure the nasal mucoperiosteum (Figure 39-3). Irrigation is done to prevent excessive heat buildup and to facilitate visualization. The nasal mucoperiosteum is separated from the underside of the bone with a dental burnisher or Clev-dent No. 1. The cottonoid is extracted and the nasal mucoperiosteum is injected with the local anesthetic.

A 45° Kerrison punch is then used to enlarge the vertical dimensions of the bony opening (Figure 39-4). The most important area to remove is just in front of the posterior lacrimal crest and under the medial canthal tendon. The tendon can be elevated but typically is not, as it is a most important guide to adequate removal of the bone beneath its insertion.

The bony bridge of anterior lacrimal crest that remains is then removed with a rongeur. This step occasionally leads the surgeon into the anterior ethmoid air cells, typically posing no problem. The authors

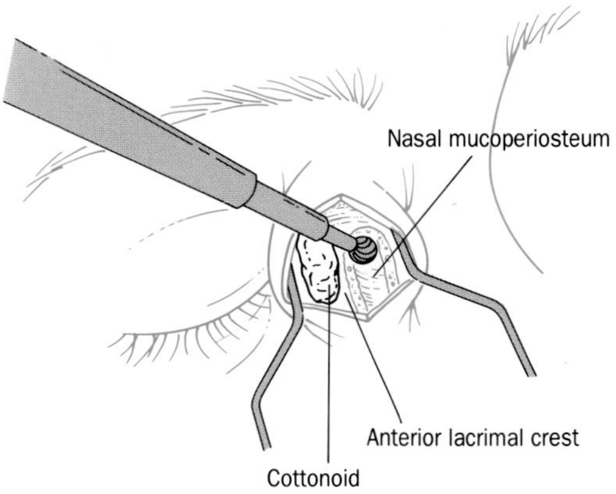

Figure 39-3 *Dental burr used to create bony ostium.*

Nasal mucoperiosteum

Anterior lacrimal crest

Cottonoid

---

*Some surgeons prefer the use of traction sutures to self-retaining retractors.—ED.

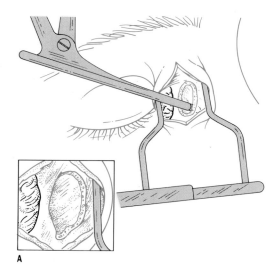

A

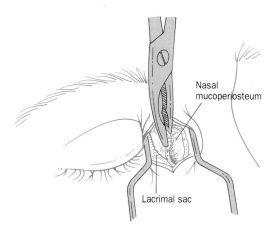

Nasal mucoperiosteum

Lacrimal sac

B

Figure 39-4 *Enlarging bony ostium. (A) Using Kerrison punch to enlarge vertical dimensions of bony opening. (B) Further enlargement of bony ostium with removal of medial wall of naso-lacrimal duct.*

suggest a conservative "deskeletonization" of these cells. The last portion of bone to be removed is the medial half of the naso-lacrimal canal. First the nasal mucoperiosteum is separated from the canal down to the inferior turbinate. A rongeur can then be used to remove this bone, thereby avoiding the postoperative "sump" syndrome described by Richard Welham, MD. The Kerrison rongeur is helpful to smooth the rough edges of the bone where the anterior and posterior lacrimal crests meet inferiorly. A good rule in all tear sac surgery is never to have a bony margin closer than 5 mm to the common canaliculus.

Attention is now focused on the tear sac. The Goldstein retractor is loosened and a No. 0 probe inserted through either canaliculus "tents" the medial wall toward the nasal mucoperiosteum (Figure 39-5). A No. 11 Bard-Parker blade is used to cut through both the periosteal and the mucosal layers of the medial wall of the sac slightly lateral to the tip of the probe. When the wall has been perforated, the scalpel is removed and one blade of a sharp curved Stevens or iris scissors is inserted into the sac. The incision is extended to the top of the fundus and to the bottom of the exposed nasolacrimal duct. A similar incision is made in the nasal mucoperiosteum adjacent to and parallel with the one in the tear sac. The posterior flap of the tear sac and nasal mucoperiosteum is removed with forceps and scissors. There is no need to sew these flaps together.*

Both canaliculi are now intubated by malleable silver probes with silicone tubing. The silicone is brought out through the nose, and at the end of surgery is tied with a square knot, cut, and allowed to retract into the nose. The surgeon should ensure that there is no tension on the puncta, which could lead to punctal erosion. If bleeding is a problem, 0.5-inch gauze with petroleum jelly can be placed up the nose as an anterior pack, or an adequate amount of Instat, a collagen absorbable hemostat, can be placed beneath the flaps anterior to the tip of the middle turbinate (Figure 39-6).

Silicone tubing is not always necessary; it is suggested for pediatric patients, canalicular stenosis, and reoperations. The alternative is to place a Metamyd ointment–soaked strip of 0.25-inch packing gauze behind the anterior nasal and sac flaps.

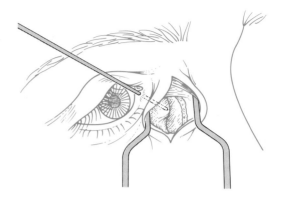

Figure 39-5 *Tenting of lacrimal sac to allow for fenestration.*

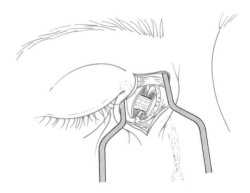

Figure 39-6 *Instat in place deep to silicone tubing.*

---

*Some surgeons preserve both anterior and posterior nasal and lacrimal sac mucosal flaps and prefer anterior and posterior mucosal flap anastomoses.—ED.

The packing is removed through the nose in approximately 2 weeks. This can be impossible to do in infants or children and in adult patients who are uncooperative unless a general anesthetic is used.

The anterior flap of the tear sac is now approximated with the anterior-based flap of the nasal mucosa using two interrupted 5-0 polyglactin 910 sutures on a P-2 needle. The retractor is removed. The periosteum and orbicularis muscle are now closed as a single layer using running or interrupted 6-0 polyglactin 910 sutures. An absorbable subcuticular suture is used to close skin, and can be reinforced with a 6-0 plain fast-absorbing gut running horizontal mattress suture.

An antibiotic–corticosteroid ointment is then placed on the wound, and the eye is mildly pressure-patched for 1 day. If petroleum-jelly gauze was used for hemostasis, it is removed through the nose the following day. If Instat was used, it can remain. The sutures are removed within 7 days, and the silicone tubing is usually retained for 6 weeks. The tubing can be removed through the nose after being cut in the medial canthus, or it is cut and then pulled through the upper canaliculus.

39-2

CANALICULAR ABNORMALITIES

The lacrimal drainage system may be divided into the upper system (eyelid margins, punctum, and canaliculi) and the lower system (lacrimal sac and nasolacrimal duct). This section deals primarily with diseases and surgery of the upper system. Disorders of the upper lacrimal system may result from congenital disorders, such as agenesis, atresia, or supernumerary channels or diverticula, or may be acquired after trauma, inflammation, neoplastic disease, or medications (idoxuridine or echothiophate iodide).

39-2-1 Punctal Disorders

Stenosis of the punctum is treated conservatively by dilating first with a Jones punctum dilator and then the Ziegler dilator. If inspection reveals a closed punctum, it can frequently be opened using a No. 75 Beaver blade or a No. 11 Bard-Parker scalpel blade. Once the punctum has been opened, weekly dilation is advisable until it remains open. Loupes, a biomicroscope, or an operating microscope can be helpful.

Chronic spastic closure of the punctum and conditions leading to phimosis of the punctum are repaired by a one-snip technique. This simple office procedure preserves the pumping action of the ampulla. Proparacaine is instilled in the conjunctival cul-de-sac, and cocaine solution on a cotton-tipped applicator is applied to the punctum for several minutes. One blade of an iris scissors is inserted vertically into the ampulla, while the other blade re-

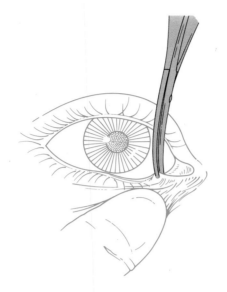

A

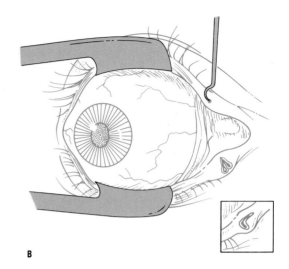

B

mains on the conjunctival side of the eyelid. To avoid pain, the scissors are closed quickly, snipping the canal vertically (Figure 39-7). If the one-snip procedure fails, then a second snip is made at the inferior margin of the vertical incision, progressing medially for 3 mm.

Eversion of the punctum due to mild medial eyelid ectropion is repaired by a diamond-shaped wedge resection (Figure 39-8). A diamond-shaped section of the conjunctival and subconjunctival tissue is removed just inferior to the punctum. The conjunctiva and submucosa are grasped with forceps inferior to the punctum. When the forceps are elevated, small curved iris scissors are placed horizontally beneath the forceps, pushed toward the eyelid, and brought together. This procedure removes an ellipse or diamond-shaped piece of tissue. The wound is then closed with an interrupted 7-0 polygly-

Figure 39-7 *One-snip technique for chronic spastic closure of punctum. (A) Iris scissors in punctum of right lower lid. (B) Scissors snip canal vertically. Inset shows two-snip procedure done after failure of one-snip.*

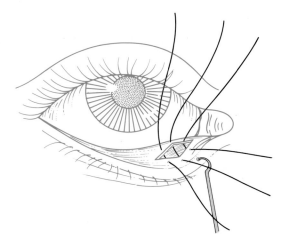

Figure 39-8 *Closure of diamond-shaped wedge excision for punctal eversion.*

colic acid suture. An alternative is the "window-shade procedure," in which a rectangular flap of conjunctiva–tarsus is dissected toward the punctum. The flap is resected, and its edges are sutured to the cut in the cul-de-sac with a 7-0 polyglycolic acid suture.*

For patients who suffer secondary reflex hypersecretion in association with keratitis sicca, closing the punctum may provide a great deal of relief. If all tests confirm that the patient's epiphora is the result of reflex tearing due to sicca problems such as foreign-body sensation, contact-lens intolerance, or corneal damage, collagen plugs may be placed in the ampulla to temporarily retard or completely block lacrimal outflow. Gentle thermal cautery or electrocautery directed into the punctum may be performed to produce the same temporary effect. If the patient notes definite improvement in symptoms without troublesome epiphora, more vigorous cautery to the entire ampulla epithelial surface can be used to close the ducts permanently. The canaliculus may also be surgically interrupted by dissecting out the canaliculus, while it is defined by a probe, and excising a portion.

39-2-2 Canalicular Disease

Scarring of the canaliculi may follow severe conjunctival infections, inflammations, allergies, burns, and reactions to drugs, such as glaucoma medications. Idiopathic canalicular obliteration is present in a small percentage of patients, who may

---

*See also Chapter 15, "Classification and Correction of Ectropion," in Volume 2 of Ophthalmology Monograph 8, published in 1994.—ED.

develop closure at any point in the canalicular system. Sealing frequently commences at the common canaliculus and progresses to complete obliteration over time, without evidence of trauma or infection. Canaliculitis is rarely bacterial. However, cultures should be obtained and any potentially causative organisms treated with appropriate antibiotic therapy. Concretions in the canaliculi are usually caused by infection with *Actinomyces israelii*. Some fungi can also be causative. One or both canaliculi may become so dilated that the concretions may be removed with a small ear curette or "milked out" with a glass rod. When all granules appear to have been removed, the canaliculi should be irrigated with normal saline or antifungal solutions. The treatment may be repeated at weekly intervals. Occasionally, a *Streptothrix* granule forms a plug, which must be dislodged.

If the foreign material is not removed, the canaliculus should be opened by an incision into the horizontal limb along the posterior aspect of the eyelid. The vertical limb of the canaliculus and the punctum must be left undisturbed while the canaliculus and ampulla are curetted. Usually, horizontal incisions do not need to be sutured, but if a vertical tear develops in the eyelid margin, it should be closed to prevent gaping and fistulization.

39-2-3 Punctal and Canalicular Lacerations

Atraumatic technique is essential in handling tissues that have been lacerated. No sharp instrument should be used until all parts of the lacerated lacrimal system have been identified. It is important that all skin and muscle tissues be preserved.

Although repair of lacrimal lacerations should be done as early as safety permits, it is usually wise to delay surgery 12 to 24 hours if local swelling or hemorrhage is present. Surgery is best undertaken with an operating microscope and an experienced surgical team. An interim treatment consists of compresses and local antibiotics. Lacerations of the punctum on the conjunctival side may be left alone if they are vertical and minimal or if they create a large punctal opening but do not affect the lacrimal pump mechanism.

For skin lacerations and lacerations extending into one or both canaliculi, the Jones dye test will quickly determine if at least one canaliculus is still functioning. An undamaged canaliculus alone may handle the lacrimal drainage. Surgical intervention may not be needed, other than for anatomic repair of the involved canaliculus in the event of a future injury.

When the lateral 2 to 3 mm of the canaliculus has been destroyed by burns or lacerations and is irreparable but the medial canaliculus can be identified, marsupializing the open end of the medial canaliculus may cure the obstruction. It may be necessary to slit the canaliculus to enlarge the ostium or to perform a canaliculo-conjunctival anastomosis. The proximal end of the lacerated canaliculus can often be identified more easily with the operating microscope. Saline may be helpful in identifying the lacerated end of the canaliculus by retrograde flow when instilled through the intact part of the system, or the wound can be filled with saline and then air injected through the intact portion of the system. The air bubbles emanate from the end of the lacerated canaliculus, allowing its identification. A flap of skin and muscle may be turned down for better exposure. The medial palpebral tendon may be elevated so that the area of injury is exposed.

The canaliculus is identified and a fine lacrimal probe is passed through the punctum and the lateral canaliculus, across the laceration, and into the medial end of the canaliculus. The probe is replaced by a stent before repair begins. The most popular stent consists of silicone tubing. As popularized by Quickert and Dryden, silicone tubing is attached to a probe that is passed through the lacrimal system. The probe is guided out the nose with the help of a groove director or under direct visualization (Figure 39-9). The canaliculus is approximated with 9-0 or 10-0 nylon, after which the pretarsal orbicularis muscle, conjunctiva, and skin are closed to complete the repair.

39-2-4 Strictures at the Common Canaliculus

Strictures at the common canaliculus may require slitting or excising, often under direct visualization after the lacrimal sac is opened. The stricture, pushed into view in the open sac with a lacrimal probe, may then be incised or excised around the probe. Various methods have been suggested to stent the stricture and prevent its recurrence. This stenting of the opened stricture or obstruction is as essential to the success of the surgical procedure as the actual lysis of the tissues.

A 3-0 nylon suture may be passed into the sac, past the stricture site, and out the canaliculus. To this may be attached several additional sutures, which can then be pulled into the stricture; eventually, material as thick as umbilical tape may be added. The external ends of the suture are fixed to the face with adhesive tape. After several weeks, the tape or suture can be pulled through the nose.

An alternative stent has been suggested by Werb and modified by Quickert and others. This procedure consists of exposing and excising the stricture and passing silicone tubing through both the upper and the lower canalicular systems and out the nose, where the two ends of the silicone are attached to each other by a sleeve or suture, or tied in a square knot. The Quickert probes can be used to guide the silicone tubing. The continuous loop of silicone tubing may be directed from the opened internal punctum through the anastomosis of sac and nasal mucosa membrane in the middle meatus during dacryocystorhinostomy. In some cases, the Quickert probes may be inserted through

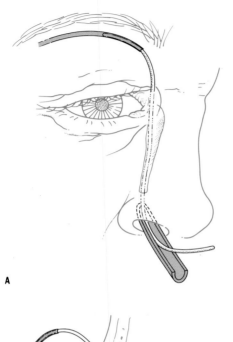

A

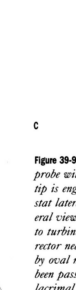

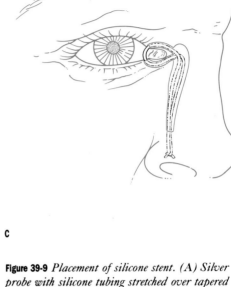

C

B

Figure 39-9 *Placement of silicone stent. (A) Silver probe with silicone tubing stretched over tapered tip is engaged in grooved director or with hemostat laterally in inferior meatus. (B) Right lateral view shows relationship of lacrimal passages to turbinates. Probe initially engages grooved director near valve of Hasner, which is represented by oval marking. (C) Both ends of tubing have been passed, and tubing lies freely movable in lacrimal drainage system with knot in inferior meatus.*

the occluded common canaliculus and directed down the nasolacrimal duct under the inferior turbinate without the necessity of the accompanying dacryocystorhinostomy.

39-3

CANALICULODACRYOCYSTOSTOMY

Canaliculodacryocystostomy is done when both canaliculi are obstructed near their juncture with the sac and at least 8 mm of the lower canaliculus is in good condition. Because of the high failure rate, the authors often place a Pyrex tube at the same time. After the silicone has been removed, the Pyrex tube is temporarily obstructed. If the anastomosis stays open, the Pyrex tube can be removed.

The skin incision, beginning at the level of the medial palpebral tendon 11 mm nasal to the medial commissure of the eye, is carried downward and slightly outward for about 20 mm. The lacrimal sac is exposed and the fundus dissected free. A probe is passed into the canaliculus and pressed into the wound beneath and posterior to the orbicularis muscle and tendon. The sac is carefully dissected free at its medial 3 or 4 mm, and a cut is made obliquely into the blind end of the sac so that the resulting beveled opening will be

present downward. The dissection is carried around the common canaliculus, and the stricture is resected (Figure 39-10). Silicone tubing or malleable probes are passed as a stent through the canaliculus and sac and out the nares. The canaliculus is sutured to the sac with 7-0 polyglycolic acid suture so that its mucosa will extend into the sac about 1 to 2 mm. The wound is closed in the usual manner, and the silicone is tied, cut, and allowed to retract into the nose.

39-4

CONJUNCTIVODACRYOCYSTORHINOSTOMY

Conjunctivodacryocystorhinostomy is done when a flaccid canaliculus or complete paralysis of the lacrimal pump is present or when both canaliculi are absent or obliterated. The dacryocystorhinostomy is performed to the point of anastomosis of the anterior lacrimal flap, without detaching the medial palpebral tendon. If prominent, the caruncle is excised, with care being taken to remove as little conjunctiva as possible. A sharp, slightly curved 22-gauge hypodermic needle, 20 mm long, is inserted into the lacrimal lake 2.5 mm posterior to the cutaneous margin at the medial canthal angle. The needle is pushed in a direction that will permit the point to emerge just posterior to the anterior lacrimal sac flap, midway between its fundus and isthmus (Figure 39-11A). Several attempts may be necessary to get the point to emerge in exactly the right place. It must be anterior to the body of the middle turbinate, the anterior end of which should be resected if it interferes

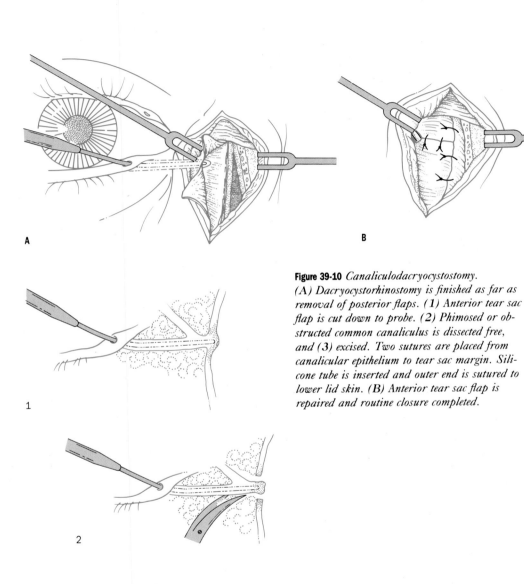

A

B

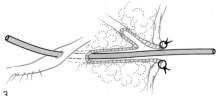

1

2

3

Figure 39-10 *Canaliculodacryocystostomy.*
(A) Dacryocystorhinostomy is finished as far as
removal of posterior flaps. (1) Anterior tear sac
flap is cut down to probe. (2) Phimosed or ob-
structed common canaliculus is dissected free,
and (3) excised. Two sutures are placed from
canalicular epithelium to tear sac margin. Sili-
cone tube is inserted and outer end is sutured to
lower lid skin. (B) Anterior tear sac flap is
repaired and routine closure completed.

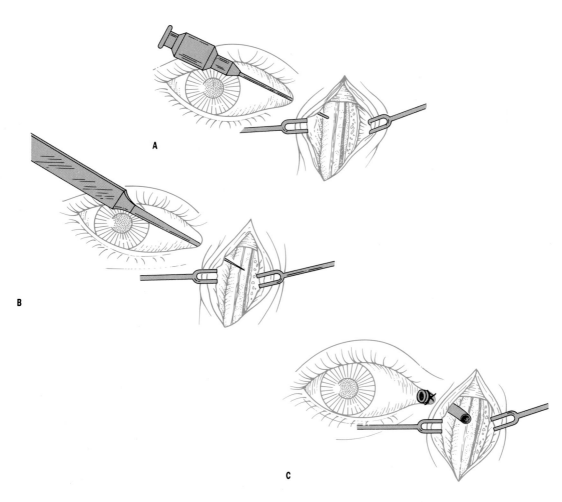

Figure 39-11 *Conjunctivodacryocystorhinostomy. (A) Hypodermic needle has been placed in position between conjunctival sac and dacryocystorhinostomy. (B) Needle replaced by cataract knife. (C) Cataract knife replaced by Pyrex tube.*

with the needle. A cataract knife is advanced from the lacrimal lake into the sac, following the guide needle (Figure 39-11B). The needle is then removed, and the knife enlarges the passage superiorly and inferiorly, sufficiently to allow insertion of a 17-mm Pyrex tube (Jones tube) with a 4-mm collar (Figure 39-11C). The length should be matched to the length of the passage. The Pyrex tube is

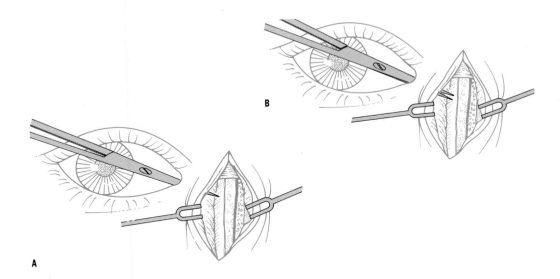

threaded over a No. 1 Bowman probe, which is slipped through the new opening into the nose. The tube is passed down the probe and secured in place with a 5-0 polyglycolic acid suture passed around the collar of the tube. The tube is tied in place, and the suture is passed through the skin of the canthus and tied to prevent dislodging of the tube.

An alternative to the cataract knife is curved iris scissors to make the same opening (Figure 39-12). A 2-mm trephine can be used to make the passage between the caruncle and the lacrimal sac. The remainder of the closure is the same as for dacryocystorhinostomy.

Postoperatively, patients are seen at 1 day, 1 week, and 6 weeks. At the time of surgery, the authors typically place longer tubes than will ultimately be necessary, to prevent mucosal overgrowth from the nasal sidewall. Because of this length, the tube will occasionally be obstructed by

Figure 39-12 *Conjunctivodacryocystorhinostomy performed with iris scissors instead of with hypodermic needle and cataract knife.*

the mucosa of the nasal septum. At the 6-week visit, the tube can be exchanged for a shorter one and the collar size reduced to 3.5 mm to minimize the tube's visibility in the medial canthus.

Patients are warned to hold the tubes or squeeze their eyes closed tightly when blowing the nose, sneezing, or coughing. If the tube becomes dislodged, it must be replaced as soon as possible, because the fistula will close down completely within hours. Patients are instructed to snuff in artificial tears through the tubes, while pinching the nostrils closed, twice a day to help maintain patency. The tubes are removed in the office and cleaned with alcohol every year.

39-5

CONGENITAL NASOLACRIMAL DUCT OBSTRUCTION

Management of epiphora in the neonate or infant depends heavily on the diagnosis. In general, neonates presenting with an amniocele or a dacryocele are probed, using topical anesthesia, in the neonatal intensive care unit within hours to days of birth. The situation becomes urgent if the condition is bilateral and associated with intranasal airway obstruction due to the amniocele, because neonates are obligate "nose breathers." The authors have not found neuroimaging to be necessary in these cases, and general anesthesia with intranasal manipulation is only rarely required.

Often, infants develop epiphora with mucopurulent discharge several weeks after birth as the initial manifestation of congenital nasolacrimal duct obstruction. These patients are typically managed with antibiotic eyedrops and nasolacrimal sac massage under the direction of the family pediatrician. The authors' experience suggests that the most effective and cost-efficient method of managing these problems is in-office probing with topical anesthesia for infants between 3 and 10 months of age. The morbidity is minimal and the procedure no more traumatic to the patient than an immunization injection.

Patients who fail initial probing are usually given a general anesthetic and probed in the operating room. In addition, the inferior turbinate is infractured with either a Freer elevator or a hemostat. The lacrimal drainage system is then intubated with silicone tubing. The tube is tied in a square knot, cut, and allowed to retract into the nose without fixation. The puncta should be checked to relieve any excessive tension and thus avoid "cheese-wiring." After 6 weeks, the tube is removed in the office by cutting the loop and briskly pulling the small knot through the upper canaliculus.

Occasionally, patients present with epiphora and on examination the tearing is shown to emanate from a small opening in the medial canthal or lower eyelid area. This condition represents a lacrimal anlage. The authors recommend resecting this epithelium-lined tract of tissue, usually with a probe in place to aid in the dissection, followed by 6 weeks of silicone stenting.

In children with punctal agenesis, epiphora is a problem but there is no mucopurulent discharge. These patients require placement of a Jones Pyrex tube, but often this procedure can and should be delayed for several years because of the potential difficulties of postoperative tube management, requiring multiple administrations of general anesthesia for tube cleaning and changing.

SUGGESTED READINGS

Dailey RA, Wobig JL: Use of collagen absorbable hemostat in dacryocystorhinostomy. *Am J Ophthalmol* 1988;106:109–110.

Javate RM, Campomanes BSA Jr, Co ND, et al: The endoscope and the radiofrequency unit in DCR surgery. *Ophthalmic Plast Reconstr Surg* 1995;11:54–58.

Jones LT, Linn ML: The diagnosis of the causes of epiphora. *Am J Ophthalmol* 1969;67: 751–754.

Jones LT, Marquis MM, Vincent NJ: Lacrimal function. *Am J Ophthalmol* 1972;73:658–659.

Luff HJ, Wobig JL, Dailey RA: The bubble test: an atraumatic method for canalicular laceration repair. *Ophthalmic Plast Reconstr Surg.* In press.

Mustarde JC, Jones LT, Callahan A: *Ophthalmic Plastic Surgery: Up-to-Date*. Birmingham, AL: Aesculapius Publishing Co; 1970:100.

Reifler DM: Results of endoscopic KTP laser–assisted dacryocystorhinostomy. *Ophthalmic Plast Reconstr Surg* 1993;9:231–236.

Wobig JL, Dailey RA: Surgery of the lacrimal apparatus. In: Lindquist TD, Lindstrom RL, eds: *Ophthalmic Surgery: Looseleaf and Update Service*. St Louis: Year Book Medical Publishers; 1990:VE1–VE17.

CME Accreditation

The American Academy of Ophthalmology is accredited by the Accreditation Council for Continuing Medical Education to sponsor continuing medical education for physicians.

CME credit hours in Category 1 of the Physician's Recognition Award of the American Medical Association may be earned for completing the study of any monograph in the Ophthalmology Monographs series. The Academy designates the number of credit hours for each monograph based on the scope and complexity of the material covered.

CME Credit Report Form

The Academy designates Ophthalmology Monograph 8, *Surgery of the Eyelid, Orbit, and Lacrimal System*, Volume 3, for up to 25 credit hours. To claim credit, complete the answer sheet for the self-study examination and sign the statement below.

I hereby certify that I have spent _____ (up to 25) hours of study on this monograph and that I have completed the self-study examination.

_____

Signature   Date

Send the completed answer sheet and signed statement to:

American Academy of Ophthalmology
P.O. Box 7424
San Francisco, CA 94120-7424
ATTN: Clinical Education Division

The Academy upon request will send you a transcript of the credit claimed on this form. Check the box below if you wish credit verification now.

☐ Please send credit verification now.

PLEASE PRINT

_____

Last Name   First Name   MI

_____

Mailing Address

_____

City

_____

State   ZIP Code

_____

Telephone   ID Number*

*Your ID Number is located following your name on most Academy mailing labels, in your membership directory, and on your monthly statement of account.

OPHTHALMOLOGY MONOGRAPH 8, Volume 3
Surgery of the Eyelid, Orbit, and Lacrimal System

Circle the letter of the response option that you regard as the "best" answer to the question.

Question	Answer					Question	Answer				
1	a	b	c	d	e	21	a	b	c	d	e
2	a	b	c	d	e	22	a	b	c	d	e
3	a	b	c	d	e	23	a	b	c	d	e
4	a	b	c	d	e	24	a	b	c	d	e
5	a	b	c	d	e	25	a	b	c	d	e
6	a	b	c	d	e	26	a	b	c	d	e
7	a	b	c	d	e	27	a	b	c	d	e
8	a	b	c	d	e	28	a	b	c	d	e
9	a	b	c	d	e	29	a	b	c	d	e
10	a	b	c	d	e	30	a	b	c	d	e
11	a	b	c	d	e	31	a	b	c	d	e
12	a	b	c	d	e	32	a	b	c	d	e
13	a	b	c	d	e	33	a	b	c	d	e
14	a	b	c	d	e	34	a	b	c	d	e
15	a	b	c	d	e	35	a	b	c	d	e
16	a	b	c	d	e	36	a	b	c	d	e
17	a	b	c	d	e	37	a	b	c	d	e
18	a	b	c	d	e	38	a	b	c	d	e
19	a	b	c	d	e	39	a	b	c	d	e
20	a	b	c	d	e	40	a	b	c	d	e

SELF-STUDY EXAMINATION

The self-study examination provided for each book in the Ophthalmology Monographs series is intended for use after completion of the monograph. The examination for *Surgery of the Eyelid, Orbit, and Lacrimal System*, Volume 3, consists of 40 multiple-choice questions followed by the answers to the questions and a discussion of each answer. The Academy recommends that you not consult the answers until you have completed the entire examination.

Questions

The questions are constructed so that there is one "best" answer. Despite the attempt to avoid ambiguous selections, disagreement may occur about which selection constitutes the optimal answer. After reading a question, record your initial impression on the answer sheet (facing page).

Answers and Discussions

The "best" answer to each question is provided after the examination. The discussion that accompanies the answer is intended to help you confirm that the reasoning you used in determining the most appropriate answer was correct. If you missed a question, the discussion may help you decide whether your "error" was due to poor wording of the question or to your misinterpretation. If, instead, you missed the question because of miscalculation or failure to recall relevant information, the discussion may help fix the principle in your memory.

QUESTIONS

Chapter 25

1. All of the following clinical signs are characteristic of the congestive stage of thyroid-related orbitopathy *except*
   a. eyelid erythema
   b. chemosis and conjunctival injection
   c. compressive optic neuropathy
   d. eyelid edema
   e. strabismus

2. Idiopathic sclerosing inflammation of the orbit is a type of orbital inflammation that
   a. represents a burned-out chronic sequela of acute idiopathic orbital inflammation
   b. typically resolves with corticosteroid therapy
   c. may present with infiltration of tissues and destruction of function
   d. may be observed for some time before treatment is undertaken
   e. all of the above

Chapter 26

3. A large discrete intraconal mass, inferior to the optic nerve and posterior to the globe, is best removed through
   a. a medial conjunctival orbitotomy
   b. an extraperiosteal orbitotomy
   c. an anterior orbitotomy
   d. a combined medial and lateral orbitotomy
   e. a lateral bony orbitotomy

4. When an anterosuperior nasal extraperiosteal orbitotomy is performed, care must be taken to avoid damage to the
   a. ethmoidal arteries
   b. supraorbital nerve and trochlea
   c. infraorbital nerve and artery
   d. zygomaticofacial nerve
   e. palpebral lobe of the lacrimal gland

5. All of the following complications may occur after an extensive lateral bony orbitotomy *except*
   a. diplopia
   b. ptosis
   c. visual loss
   d. pupillary changes
   e. infraorbital nerve hypesthesia

Chapter 27

6. All of the following are indications for orbital decompression surgery in thyroid-related orbitopathy *except*
   a. severe exophthalmos
   b. severe eyelid retraction

c. compressive optic neuropathy

d. recurrent subluxation of the globe anterior to the eyelids

e. severe proptosis with exposure keratopathy

7. If optic neuropathy persists after orbital decompression surgery, the first step should be

a. orbital radiation

b. plasmapheresis

c. high-dose intravenous corticosteroids

d. a second orbital CT scan to assess the extent of decompression

e. reoperation to remove residual bone

8. All of the following complications may occur after a transconjuntival orbital decompression *except*

a. maxillary sinusitis

b. diplopia

c. oroantral fistula

d. hypoglobus

e. preseptal cellulitis

9. When orbital decompression surgery is planned, the *least* important consideration is

a. size of the maxillary sinus

b. severity of proptosis

c. presence of optic neuropathy

d. preoperative diplopia

e. eyelid retraction

Chapter 28

10. The prime indication for optic nerve sheath decompression (ONSD) is

a. visual loss due to nonarteritic anterior ischemic optic neuropathy (NAION)

b. visual loss due to central retinal vein occlusion (CRVO)

c. visual loss due to chronic papilledema

d. headache

e. none of the above

11. Optic nerve sheath decompression may be performed with

a. general anesthesia

b. peribulbar anesthesia

c. retrobulbar anesthesia

d. infiltrative anesthesia

e. all of the above

Chapter 29

12. All of the following are craniosynostosis syndromes *except*

a. Goldenhar's

b. Apert's

c. Crouzon's

d. Pfeiffer's

e. plagiocephaly

13. All of the following benefits are achieved by rigid fixation of bone grafts *except*

    a. early revascularization

    b. elimination of shearing motion

    c. three-dimensional alignment

    d. normal expansion of growth centers

    e. reduced resorption of bone

14. Removing additional bone posterior to a standard lateral orbitotomy may expose the

    a. middle cranial fossa

    b. anterior cranial fossa

    c. posterior cranial fossa

    d. auditory fossa

    e. trochlear fossa

15. The most dense and rigid bone graft available for orbital reconstruction is

    a. iliac crest

    b. split calvaria

    c. rib

    d. femur

    e. tibia

Chapter 30

16. During evisceration surgery, if the scleral pouch is found to be too small to hold an adequate implant, the surgeon may

    a. convert to an enucleation

    b. make an incision in the posterior sclera and place a 12-mm sphere in the muscle cone; then close the posterior sclera and place an 8-mm sphere in the scleral pouch

    c. perform expansion radial sclerotomies

    d. close the scleral pouch without an implant, and at a later date place a subperiosteal Medpor secondary implant

    e. do all of the above

17. The biggest disadvantage of a dermis–fat graft is

    a. unpredictable rate of absorption

    b. conjunctival cysts and granulomas

    c. socket keratinization

    d. retention of cilia

    e. all of the above

Chapter 31

18. Orbital exenteration involves removal of the

    a. eye, orbital soft tissues, and periorbita

    b. eye only

    c. contents of the globe, leaving the scleral shell intact

d. tumor within the orbit, leaving the eye undisturbed

e. bone adjacent to the orbit, such as the paranasal sinuses

19. Frozen-section evaluation should not be relied on for

    a. making a determination at the time of initial biopsy on whether to proceed with exenteration

    b. monitoring cutaneous margins for resection of skin cancer that has spread to the orbit

    c. monitoring the orbital apex for adequacy of apical resection

    d. determining the adequacy of a biopsy specimen

    e. differentiating a basal cell carcinoma from a sebaceous cell carcinoma

Chapter 32

20. All of the following are frequently encountered deformities of the anophthalmic socket *except*

    a. enophthalmos

    b. tissue atrophy

    c. ptosis

    d. ectropion

    e. proptosis

21. All of the following are usually helpful in treating contracted sockets *except*

    a. mucous membrane grafting

    b. eyelid shortening

    c. conjunctivoplasty

    d. lateral canthotomy

    e. tarsomüllerectomy

Chapter 33

22. All of the following statements concerning the advantages of plastic over glass for fabricating ocular prostheses are true *except*

    a. Plastic is not easily damaged.

    b. Plastic allows for a precise fit.

    c. Plastic does not etch, because of the alkalinity of tears.

    d. Plastic can be repaired or polished if scratched.

    e. Plastic can be fabricated into many designs and shapes.

23. The *most* important consideration in placing a conformer is

    a. A silicone conformer can be sterilized easily without damage by autoclave, chemical agents, and gas. It can also be trimmed to any size by cutting.

    b. An acrylic conformer is more comfortable than a silicone conformer because acrylic is smoother.

c. A conformer should not be too large, as an oversized conformer can place pressure on the suture line and create a pressure necrosis or stretch the socket.

d. The patient should be informed that a conformer will be inserted at the time of surgery.

e. A conformer prevents particulate matter from entering the socket and causing irritation.

24. In the treatment of congenital anophthalmos or microphthalmos, the objective of encouraging the development of orbital tissue and the bony orbit is best obtained by

    a. placing increasingly larger conformers soon after birth

    b. oversizing the conformers to help stimulate growth and reduce contraction

    c. placing conformers of increasing size in rapid succession to expand the socket

    d. opening the lateral commissure to allow for a larger conformer

    e. placing an ocular implant to enhance orbital volume so that a small conformer can be used

Chapter 34

25. Once an infectious process has been ruled out, the most common cause of excessive mucus discharge and conjunctival irritation associated with a properly fitting prosthesis is usually

    a. conjunctival shrinkage

    b. poor motility

    c. implant migration

    d. ptosis

    e. poor surface condition

26. To evaluate an ocular prosthesis properly, it is essential to

    a. obtain a patient history

    b. use magnification

    c. perform a Schirmer test

    d. remove the prosthesis from the socket

    e. evaluate the motility of the prosthesis

Chapter 35

27. Which of the following statements about the use of corticosteroids following head trauma is true?

    a. Prolonged use of corticosteroids is indicated to reduce edema.

    b. Corticosteroids should be tapered after a 2-week trial.

    c. Corticosteroids should be given only intermittently.

    d. Prolonged use of corticosteroids is contraindicated.

e. Prolonged use of corticosteroids is indicated to prevent late scar-tissue formation.

28. Which of the following statements about orbital emphysema is true?

  a. It is always associated with diplopia.

  b. It occurs with nasal bone fractures.

  c. It is indicative of incarceration of an extraocular muscle.

  d. It is indicative of an orbital fracture communicating with a sinus cavity.

  e. It cannot be detected by palpation.

29. Numbness of the upper molar and bicuspid teeth in a patient with an orbital floor fracture is suggestive of a

  a. fracture of the anterior portion of the orbital floor

  b. rim fracture

  c. medial wall fracture

  d. fracture of the posterior one third of the orbital floor

  e. palate fracture

30. Which of the following statements about vertical diplopia following orbital trauma is true?

  a. It is pathognomonic of an orbital fracture.

  b. It can be related to an intraorbital hemorrhage.

  c. It is always associated with injury to the infraorbital nerve.

  d. It does not occur with small orbital floor fractures.

  e. It never resolves spontaneously.

Chapter 36

31. All of the following are mechanisms for the development of enophthalmos following an orbital floor blowout fracture *except*

  a. orbital fat atrophy

  b. an increase in orbital volume

  c. tethering of the globe by an entrapped inferior rectus muscle

  d. prolapse of inferior orbital tissues into the maxillary antrum

  e. trapping of orbital septa into a small fracture

32. All of the following are current indications for repair of an orbital floor blowout fracture *except*

  a. fracture size greater than 50% of the orbital floor

  b. cosmetically unacceptable enophthalmos

  c. orbital emphysema

  d. an entrapped inferior rectus muscle as revealed by orbital scanning

  e. diplopia in primary gaze or reading position and associated with positive forced ductions

33. All of the following are usually associated with an acute orbital floor blowout fracture *except*

   a. infraorbital nerve hypesthesia

   b. trauma caused by an object smaller than the diameter of the orbital opening

   c. enophthalmos

   d. diplopia secondary to inferior rectus muscle entrapment

   e. ecchymosis and eyelid edema

Chapter 37

34. All of the following mechanisms are involved in the development of posttraumatic enophthalmos *except*

   a. enlargement of the bony orbit

   b. cicatricial contracture of the maxillary sinus

   c. soft-tissue cicatrix formation in the posterior orbit

   d. resorption of orbital soft tissues

   e. displacement of orbital soft tissues

35. All of the following statements are true *except*

   a. Traumatic telecanthus usually presents with rounding of the medial canthal angle.

   b. Clinical manifestations of a tripod (trimalar) fracture may include lateral canthal dystopia, malar flattening, and orbital rim stepoff deformity.

   c. In hypo-ophthalmos or hypoglobus, a translatory displacement of the globe always results in severe vertical diplopia.

   d. In nasoethmoidal-complex fractures, the patient may complain of tearing.

   e. Le Fort I fractures do not involve the orbit.

36. All of the following statements regarding orbital implants are true *except*

   a. Hydroxyapatite and porous polyethylene are considered "integrated" implants.

   b. One advantage of miniplates over stainless-steel wire in facial and orbital reconstruction is that miniplates offer three-dimensional stability.

   c. Most orbital surgeons favor the use of perioperative and postoperative antibiotics during orbital reconstruction for acute injury if communication with a paranasal sinus exists.

   d. One disadvantage of split-thickness calvarial bone grafts is that, with time, they resorb more than iliac crest bone grafts.

   e. Alloplastic materials should be avoided if an anatomic communication (such as with an exposed sinus cavity) is present.

Chapter 38

37. All of the following statements regarding lacrimal drainage system evaluation are true *except*

    a. The Jones dye tests are most useful in evaluating the lacrimal drainage system.

    b. Computed tomography (CT) of the lacrimal system may be very useful in evaluating certain cases of epiphora.

    c. Dacryocystography provides better anatomic visualization than does dacryoscintigraphy.

    d. The fluorescein dye disappearance (FDD) test is most meaningful when both eyes are compared simultaneously.

    e. If, during the irrigation of a lacrimal canaliculus, the cannula is held improperly, pressure against the canalicular wall will produce a false sensation of obstruction.

38. The treatment of children under 13 months of age with nasolacrimal duct obstruction includes

    a. observation and massage if no complications develop

    b. probing and irrigation

    c. probing and infracture of the inferior turbinate

    d. dacryocystorhinostomy

    e. all of the above

Chapter 39

39. Dacryocystorhinostomy (DCR) is indicated for the relief of epiphora due to

    a. dry eye

    b. punctal agenesis

    c. nasolacrimal duct obstruction

    d. medial lower eyelid ectropion

    e. canalicular obstruction

40. Acceptable treatment of congenital nasolacrimal duct obstruction includes

    a. topical antibiotics and massage

    b. office probing

    c. silicone intubation

    d. infracture of the ipsilateral inferior turbinate

    e. all of the above

ANSWERS AND DISCUSSIONS

Chapter 25

1. Answer—a. The congestive phase of thyroid-related orbitopathy is characterized by venous congestion caused by apical compression of venous outflow from large extraocular muscles. Active inflammation has died down by this stage, and therefore eyelid erythema is not typical. Chemosis and swelling, however, can be present based on venous congestion. Conjunctival injection can be present based on irritation from exposure keratopathy as well as venous congestion. Strabismus and compressive optic neuropathy can occur because of the enlarged and tight extraocular muscles.

2. Answer—c. Nonspecific sclerosing orbital inflammation represent a distinct clinical pathologic entity, not "burned-out" acute inflammation. It often does not respond to corticosteroid therapy; however, cytotoxic therapy and radiotherapy may be beneficial. The condition sometimes follows a clinically aggressive course, with destruction of function and even extension beyond the boundaries of the orbit.

Chapter 26

3. Answer—e. The lateral orbitotomy offers the best exposure to the intraconal space and is the safest way to remove most intraconal masses. Medial anterior tumors can be removed via a conjunctival approach, and medial posterior tumors may need a combined medial/lateral orbitotomy. The extraperiosteal approach is not useful for intraconal lesions and is reserved for lesions adjacent to the periosteum or involving bone. An anterior orbitotomy can be performed to remove anterior masses or to biopsy certain more posterior masses; however, total removal of an intraconal posterior mass is difficult without the exposure provided by a lateral orbitotomy.

4. Answer—b. When the superior extraperiosteal space is explored, the periosteum near the trochlea should be kept intact, reflected, and replaced. The supraorbital nerve should not be transected if it can be moved out of the way. The ethmoidal arteries exit via more posterior foramina in the medial wall and are not encountered in an anterior dissection. The infraorbital nerve and artery are encountered along the orbital floor. The zygomaticofacial nerve exits via a small foramen in the zygoma.

5. Answer—e. Diplopia, ptosis, pupillary changes, and visual loss may occur after a lateral orbitotomy. Infraorbital nerve hypesthesia occurs after blowout floor fractures and their repair. It also occurs after orbital decompressions of the floor for thyroid-related orbitopathy.

Chapter 27

6. Answer—b. Indications for orbital decompression surgery in thyroid-related orbitopathy include compressive optic neuropathy, severe exophthalmos (which either is a threat to vision from exposure keratopathy or is cosmetically objectionable), and recurrent subluxation of the globe anterior to the eyelids. Orbital decompression surgery does not correct eyelid retraction.

7. Answer—d. Ordering a second orbital CT scan should be the first step in evaluating persistent optic neuropathy after orbital decompression surgery. The purpose is to rule out residual optic nerve compression from incomplete bone removal at the orbital apex. If no residual bone is found, oral corticosteroids should be maintained and the patient should be referred for orbital radiation therapy. Patients are often maintained on oral corticosteroids perioperatively, but rarely continued on intravenous corticosteroids for more than a few days. The role of plasmapheresis in the treatment of thyroid optic neuropathy is unknown.

8. Answer—c. Possible complications of the transconjunctival approach to orbital decompression include maxillary sinusitis, preseptal cellulitis, diplopia, and hypoglobus. The development of oroantral fistulas is seen only with the transantral approach through the mouth.

9. Answer—a. The degree of proptosis, the presence of optic neuropathy, and preoperative diplopia and eyelid retraction should all be considered when planning the approach and extent of orbital decompression surgery. Barring any major anatomic deformity, the size of the maxillary sinus is the the least important of these considerations.

Chapter 28

10. Answer—c. Visual loss due to chronic papilledema may be arrested and even reversed with a timely and carefully performed ONSD. It is important to intervene before extensive loss of optic nerve fibers and ensuing optic atrophy occur. A recent controlled clinical trial confirmed the ineffectiveness of ONSD in treating visual loss due to NAION, so this condition is no longer an indication except in special circumstances. The use of ONSD in treating visual loss due to CRVO has its advocates, but its benefits are as yet unproven. About 50% to 60% of patients with chronic papilledema report relief from the intracranial pressure after ONSD. This is an interesting secondary benefit, but not a prime indication for ONSD. Headaches in these patients are best treated medically or with neurosurgical shunting procedures.

11. Answer—e. It is important to realize that ONSD can be performed using a variety of anesthesia techniques. Experienced surgeons are switching to infiltrative intraoperative anesthesia, thereby avoiding the risks inherent in general anesthesia, especially in the elderly, sick, and markedly obese individuals. Peribulbar anesthesia and retrobulbar anesthesia risk elevating the intraorbital pressure, which may further compromise an already compromised optic nerve. Infiltrative intraoperative anesthesia avoids the risk of general anesthesia and other regional anesthetics. There is no elevation of intraorbital pressure and no risk of globe perforation. It is becoming the anesthetic procedure of choice for ONSD.

Chapter 29

12. Answer—a. Goldenhar's syndrome is a lateral facial hypoplasia that is classified as a clefting syndrome. Apert's, Crouzon's, Pfeiffer's, and plagiocephaly are due to premature closure of a cranial suture (craniosynostosis).

13. Answer—d. Rigid fixation of bone grafts seems to minimize resorption of the graft by eliminating any shearing motion that may limit early revascularization. In addition, rigid fixation allows precise three-dimensional alignment of bone segments and grafts. Rigid fixation in children may be associated with retardation of facial development.

14. Answer—a. The posterior half of the lateral orbital wall comprises the greater wing of the sphenoid bone and is not typically removed during a standard lateral orbitotomy. If this bone is burred away or resected, the middle cranial fossa (containing the temporal lobe of the brain) will be exposed.

15. Answer—b. Split calvaria is the only bone graft listed that is membranous bone. The others are endochondral (cancellous) and do not have the density and rigidity of calvaria. Conversely, because the iliac crest, rib, and femur are less dense, they can be more easily bent or contoured without breaking.

Chapter 30

16. Answer—c. Expansion radial sclerotomies are an excellent way of enlarging a scleral pouch to hold an adequate implant. Converting to an enucleation is a complicated way of solving the problem. A doubly-placed implant in the muscle cone and scleral pouch will maintain orbital volume, but may not enhance prosthetic motility. A secondary implant does not meet the criteria of the anophthalmic socket.

17. Answer—e. The biggest disadvantage of dermis–fat grafts is unpredictable fat atrophy combined with volume loss. This problem can be avoided by using a wide piece of dermis and handling the adjacent fat carefully. Conjunctival cysts and granulomas, socket keratinization, and retention of cilia are other disadvantages.

Chapter 31

18. Answer—a. Orbital exenteration is removal of the eye, orbital soft tissues, and periorbita. Enucleation is removal of the eye. Evisceration is removal of intraocular contents, leaving the sclera (and sometimes the cornea) undisturbed. Orbital tumors are removed by orbitotomy procedures without disturbing the eye. Removal of orbital bones can be used in decompression surgery and in providing surgical exposure to the posterior orbit. "Extended" exenteration may include removal of periorbital bones in some circumstances.

19. Answer—a. Permanent histopathologic sections allow for greater cellular detail, the ability to share slides with other observers, and the chance to process additional tissue for special testing. Exenteration should proceed based on an interpretation of permanent histopathologic sections showing malignancy. Frozen-section control is excellent for monitoring the margins of the surgical field in cases of skin cancer. To a lesser degree, it is adequate for monitoring the apical margin of surgical resection. Frozen-section evaluation of a biopsy specimen can result in a report that the tissue is "adequate" for diagnostic studies on permanent section.

Chapter 32

20. Answer—e. Ectropion due to stretching of the lower eyelid and its tendons by the weight of the ocular prosthesis is common, but entropion of the lower eyelid is not. Ptosis of the upper eyelid, often found, may include lash ptosis, but rarely does the upper eyelid invert. Anophthalmic enophthalmos, rather than proptosis, is the rule. Proptosis should spur investigation for orbital disease, either localized (orbital cysts or tumors, adjacent sinus masses) or part of systemic disease (eg, thyroid ophthalmopathy).

21. Answer—e. Contracted sockets are helped by addition of tissue to the socket (mucous membrane grafting), eyelid reconstruction to support a prosthesis (eyelid shortening), lateral canthotomy to enlarge the surface area of the socket, and conjunctivoplasty to recess conjunctiva into the inferior fornix. Tarsomüllerectomy robs the socket surface of palpebral conjunctiva, making the surface area of the socket smaller.

Chapter 33

22. **Answer—c.** Plastic materials (eg, polymethylmethacrylate) are the current standard of care in fabricating ocular prostheses because of their durability, precision in fitting, and ability to be repaired or polished if scratched and to be incorporated into refitting. Glass ocular prostheses are concave on the posterior surface and rest largely on the peripheral edges. This leaves a space where tears and mucus can collect, stagnate, and become a fertile environment for bacterial growth. Because of the working properties of glass, not all shapes can be obtained. Obtaining a close coaptation between socket and prosthesis is nearly impossible.

23. **Answer—c.** All of the choices are correct, but the *most* important consideration is proper sizing. Placing a conformer that does not damage the socket or create an environment requiring further surgery is paramount.

24. **Answer—a.** Because most of the growth of the orbit and surrounding tissue takes place in the early years (birth to age 4), the greatest effect of encouraging volume expansion of the orbit occurs during this time. Oversizing a conformer can create entropion, and placing conformers in rapid succession will not allow time for growth of the orbit.

Chapter 34

25. **Answer—e.** Poor surface condition of the ocular prosthesis is often the source of excessive mucous discharge and conjunctival irritation due to either protein buildup or abrasiveness. With continual wear of the prosthesis, the protein deposits thicken, becoming a rough surface and indicating the need to remove the prosthesis and clean it. Surface defects on the plastic surface include scratches, cracks, chips, tool marks, sharp edges, and tooth marks. The defects often result from improper handling by the patient or inadequate polishing by the ocularist. The corrective measure involves proper polishing by an ocularist and patient education on the proper, nonabrasive care of the prosthesis.

26. **Answer—d.** Removal of the prosthesis is essential to determine the proper fit, to evaluate the condition of the anophthalmic socket and its contents, and to rule out any medical conditions such as infection, conjunctival cysts, implant exposure, or neoplastic processes. Only by comparison of the posterior aspect of the prosthesis and the socket configuration can the fit be properly evaluated. Implant position and function can be determined to help evaluate motility. Close examination of the surface with magnification can help identify sources of irritation and excessive discharge.

Chapter 35

27. Answer—d. Prolonged use of corticosteroids in a person with severe head injuries is contraindicated because death rates from infection are significantly higher in patients with multiple injuries when corticosteroids are continued. An aseptic necrosis of bone can occur even after only a few weeks of corticosteroid use.

28. Answer—d. Air from a contiguous sinus cavity enters the orbit through the fracture site. Orbital emphysema is aggravated by sneezing or blowing the nose.

29. Answer—d. Fractures in the posterior one third of the orbital floor cause numbness of the upper molar and bicuspid teeth because of trauma to the posterior portion of the superior alveolar nerve.

30. Answer—b. An intraorbital hemorrhage can cause vertical diplopia secondary to extraocular muscle compression or mechanical limitation of globe movement.

Chapter 36

31. Answer—e. The orbital septa constitute a complex system of support, interconnection, and linkage of orbital soft tissues. Trapped orbital septa within a small orbital floor fracture site would most likely lead to restriction in upgaze, not enophthalmos.

32. Answer—c. Orbital emphysema usually occurs after medial wall fractures and can be exacerbated by nose blowing or sneezing. It usually resolves spontaneously and does not require treatment unless severe proptosis with elevated intraocular pressure and compromise of ocular blood supply occurs.

33. Answer—b. Orbital blowout fractures typically occur from an object larger than the orbital diameter. This leads to posterior displacement of the globe and an increase in intraorbital pressure, causing the weakest area in the orbital floor to break.

Chapter 37

34. Answer—b. Cicatricial contracture of the maxillary sinus, usually due to chronic sinusitis, is a cause of *spontaneous* enophthalmos and is not associated with trauma in the majority of cases; it is known as the *silent sinus syndrome*. All of the other possibilities may cause posttraumatic enophthalmos either by themselves or in combination. Of the four mechanisms, enlargement of the bony orbit has been shown by imaging studies to play the greatest role.

35. Answer—c. Translatory displacement of the globe is often well tolerated by the patient. Conversely, even a small degree of angular displacement usually results in symptomatic diplopia (see Figure 37-2). Choices **a** and **b** are the classic clinical signs of traumatic telecanthus and tripod fractures, respectively. In addition to causing telecanthus, nasoethmoidal-complex fractures may involve the lacrimal drainage system, resulting in epiphora. Le Fort I fractures involve the lower maxilla, and patients complain of malocclusion; the orbit is spared.

36. **Answer—d.** The membranous bone of the calvaria resorbs far less (15% to 30%) than the endochondral bone of the iliac crest (60% to 80%); this is one of the chief advantages of split-thickness calvarial bone grafting. Because both hydroxyapatite and porous polyethylene are porous and allow for fibrovascular ingrowth, they are considered "integrated" implants. Unlike miniplates, stainless-steel wire provides only two-dimensional stability, making it less desirable than miniplates in facial reconstruction. During the healing phase, the face cannot be splinted and imobilized like other anatomic sites, and the overlying facial musculature induces distortional forces on the fractured facial bones. In a survey of members of the American Society of Ophthalmic Plastic and Reconstructive Surgery, the majority favored the use of antibiotics prophylactically during repair of acute orbital trauma with paranasal sinus communication, based on anecdotal evidence.

Chapter 38

37. **Answer—a.** Although the Jones dye tests have been widely used, it is difficult to obtain consistent results. Recommended alternate procedures include the FDD test, irrigation, probing, dacryocystography, and nasal endoscopy. A CT scan may reveal orbital rim or maxillary fractures compressing the lacrimal sac or nasolacrimal duct after trauma. In the evaluation of an infant with a congenital cystic mass in the medial canthus, a CT scan may be necessary to differentiate an amniocele from a meningocele. If malignancy is suspected, a CT scan will show a soft-tissue mass of the sac or adjacent paranasal sinuses.

38. **Answer—e.** Dacryocystorhinostomy (DCR) is appropriate when probing and silicone intubation fail. DCR can be performed at any age if the infant has problems with recurrent infections.

Chapter 39

39. **Answer—c.** Punctal and canalicular abnormalities generally require placement of a Pyrex tube. Surgical treatment of dry eye is most often punctal occlusion with plugs, heat cautery, or epithelial excision and primary closure. Medial lower eyelid ectropion with resultant loss of punctal apposition to the globe is best treated with eyelid surgery.

40. **Answer—e.** All of the choices listed are acceptable in managing congenital nasolacrimal duct obstruction. Infracture of the inferior turbinate alone has been shown by Ralph E. Wesley, MD, to have a high success rate.

INDEX

NOTE: An *f* following a page number indicates a figure, and a *t* following a page number indicates a table. Drugs are listed under their generic names; when a drug trade name is listed, the reader is referred to the generic name.

A

Acrylic conformers, 135
Acuity (visual), assessment of, in orbital/periorbital fractures, 175
Acute retinal necrosis syndrome, optic nerve sheath decompression for, 51
Afferent pupillary defect, in supraorbital fractures, 193–194
Allen orbital implant, 86, 149, 153
Alveolar nerves, in orbital/periorbital fractures, 173–174
Amniocele, 265
  treatment of, 266
Anesthesia
  for dermis–fat grafting, 105
  for optic nerve sheath decompression, 51, 52–53
  for orbital fracture repair, 180
  for orbital surgery, 34
Angiography
  carotid, for craniofacial preoperative evaluation, 62
  magnetic resonance (MRA), in orbital disease, 11
    guidelines for ordering, 9*t*
Anophthalmic socket. *See also specific aspect*
  deformities of, 119–132
    contracture, 129–132
    enophthalmos, 119–128
    prosthesis modification and, 141–147
  enucleation and, 85–99
  evisceration and, 99–104
  exenteration of orbit and, 112–118
  ideal characteristics of, 84
  ocular prostheses and
    management and care of, 159–166
    overview of, 133–158
    scleral shell prostheses compared with, 160

Anophthalmos, ocular prostheses for, 135, 136*f*
Anterior orbital translocation, 76–77
Anterior orbitotomy, 21–24
  extraperiosteal, 23–24
  medial conjunctival, 22
  transconjunctival, 21–23
  transseptal, 23
Antibiotics
  after Berke-Reese lateral orbitotomy, 25
  for prophylaxis, with late repair of posttraumatic deformities, 243–244
Antral clouding, in inferior orbital rim fractures, 195
Apert's syndrome, 72*f*, 72*t*
  bipartitioning for, 75–76
Arruga orbital implant, 149
Arteriography, in orbital disease, 11
  guidelines for ordering, 9*t*
Auriculotemporal nerve, in zygomatic fractures, 186–187

B

Ball orbital implant, 149
Basal cell carcinoma, exenteration for, 113*t*
Base-down prism, for improved appearance of prosthetic eye, 156, 166
Berke-Reese lateral orbitotomy, 25–29
Biomatrix orbital implant. *See* Hydroxyapatite orbital implants
Biomicroscopy, slit-lamp, in epiphora evaluation, 255–256
Bipartitioning, for craniofacial deformities, 75–76

Cumulative Index

A